WBI LEARNING RESOURCES SERIES

Analyzing Health Equity Using Household Survey Data

A Guide to Techniques and Their Implementation

Owen O'Donnell

Eddy van Doorslaer

Adam Wagstaff

Magnus Lindelow

The World Bank
Washington, D.C.

ISBN: 978-0-8213-6933-3

eISBN: 978-0-8213-6934-0

DOI: 10.1596/978-0-8213-6933-3

Library of Congress Cataloging-in-Publication Data

Analyzing health equity using household survey data : a guide to techniques and
their implementation / Owen O'Donnell ... [et al.].
   p. ; cm.
 Includes bibliographical references and index.
 ISBN-13: 978-0-8213-6933-3
 ISBN-10: 0-8213-6933-4
 1. Health surveys--Methodology. 2. Health services
accessibility--Resarch--Statistical methods. 3. Equality--Health
aspects--Research--Stastistical methods. 4. World health--Research--Statistical
methods. 5. Household surveys. I. O'Donnell, Owen (Owen A.) II. World Bank.
 [DNLM: 1. Quality Indicators, Health Care. 2. Data Interpretation,
Statistical. 3. Health Services Accessibility. 4. Health Surveys. 5. World
Health. W 84.1 A532 2007]
 RA408.5.A53 2007
 614.4'2072--dc22

                                    2007007972

Contents

Boxes

Figures

Tables

Foreword

Health outcomes are invariably worse among the poor—often markedly so. The chance of a newborn baby in Bolivia dying before his or her fifth birthday is more than three times higher if the parents are in the poorest fifth of the population than if they are in the richest fifth (120‰ compared with 37‰). Reducing inequalities such as these is widely perceived as intrinsically important as a development goal. But as the World Bank's 2006 World Development Report, *Equity and Development*, argued, inequalities in health reflect and reinforce inequalities in other domains, and these inequalities together act as a brake on economic growth and development.

One challenge is to move from general statements such as that above to monitoring progress over time and evaluating development programs with regard to their effects on specific inequalities. Another is to identify countries or provinces in countries in which these inequalities are relatively small and discover the secrets of their success in relation to the policies and institutions that make for small inequalities. This book sets out to help analysts in these tasks. It shows how to implement a variety of analytic tools that allow health equity—along different dimensions and in different spheres—to be quantified. Questions that the techniques can help provide answers for include the following: Have gaps in health outcomes between the poor and the better-off grown in specific countries or in the developing world as a whole? Are they larger in one country than in another? Are health sector subsidies more equally distributed in some countries than in others? Is health care utilization equitably distributed in the sense that people in equal need receive similar amounts of health care irrespective of their income? Are health care payments more progressive in one health care financing system than in another? What are catastrophic payments? How can they be measured? How far do health care payments impoverish households?

Typically, each chapter is oriented toward one specific method previously outlined in a journal article, usually by one or more of the book's authors. For example, one chapter shows how to decompose inequalities in a health variable (be it a health outcome or utilization) into contributions from different sources—the contribution from education inequalities, the contribution from insurance coverage inequalities, and so on. The chapter shows the reader how to apply the method through worked examples complete with Stata code.

Most chapters were originally written as technical notes downloadable from the World Bank's Poverty and Health Web site (www.worldbank.org/povertyand health). They have proved popular with government officials, academic researchers, graduate students, nongovernmental organizations, and international organization staff, including operations staff in the World Bank. They have also been used in training exercises run by the World Bank and universities. These technical notes were all extensively revised for the book in light of this "market testing." By collecting these revised notes in the form of a book, we hope to increase their use and usefulness and thereby to encourage further empirical work on health equity that ultimately will help shape policies to reduce the stark gaps in health outcomes seen in the developing world today.

François J. Bourguignon
Senior Vice President
and Chief Economist
The World Bank

Preface

This volume has a simple aim: to provide researchers and analysts with a step-by-step practical guide to the measurement of a variety of aspects of health equity. Each chapter includes worked examples and computer code. We hope that these guides, and the easy-to-implement computer routines contained in them, will stimulate yet more analysis in the field of health equity, especially in developing countries. We hope this, in turn, will lead to more comprehensive monitoring of trends in health equity, a better understanding of the causes of these inequities, more extensive evaluation of the impacts of development programs on health equity, and more effective policies and programs to reduce inequities in the health sector.

Owen O'Donnell
Eddy van Doorslaer
Adam Wagstaff
Magnus Lindelow

1

Introduction

Equity has long been considered an important goal in the health sector. Yet inequalities between the poor and the better-off persist. The poor tend to suffer higher rates of mortality and morbidity than do the better-off. They often use health services less, despite having higher levels of need. And, notwithstanding their lower levels of utilization, the poor often spend more on health care as a share of income than the better-off. Indeed, some nonpoor households may be made poor precisely because of health shocks that necessitate out-of-pocket spending on health.

Most commentators accept that these inequalities reflect mainly differences in constraints between the poor and the better-off—lower incomes, higher time costs, less access to health insurance, living conditions that are more likely to encourage the spread of disease, and so on—rather than differences in preferences (cf. e.g., Alleyne et al. 2000; Braveman et al. 2001; Evans et al. 2001a; Le Grand 1987; Wagstaff 2001; Whitehead 1992). Such inequalities tend therefore to be seen not simply as inequalities but as *inequities* (Wagstaff and van Doorslaer 2000).

Some commentators, including Nobel prize winners James Tobin (1970) and Amartya Sen (2002), argue that inequalities in health are especially worrisome—more worrisome than inequalities in most other spheres. Health and health care are integral to people's capability to function—their ability to flourish as human beings. As Sen puts it, "Health is among the most important conditions of human life and a critically significant constituent of human capabilities which we have reason to value" (Sen 2002). Society is not especially concerned that, say, ownership of sports utility vehicles is low among the poor. But it *is* concerned that poor children are systematically more likely to die before they reach their fifth birthday and that the poor are systematically more likely to develop chronic illnesses. Inequalities in out-of-pocket spending matter too, because if the poor—through no fault of their own—are forced into spending large amounts of their limited incomes on health care, they may well end up with insufficient resources to feed and shelter themselves.

The rise of health equity research

Health equity has, in fact, become an increasingly popular research topic during the course of the past 25 years. During the January–December 1980 period, only 33 articles with "equity" in the abstract were published in journals indexed in Medline. In the 12 months of 2005, there were 294 articles published. Of course, the *total* number of articles in Medline has also grown during this period. But even as a share of the total, articles on equity have shown an increase: during the 12 months

Figure 1.1 *Equity Articles in Medline, 1980–2005*[1]

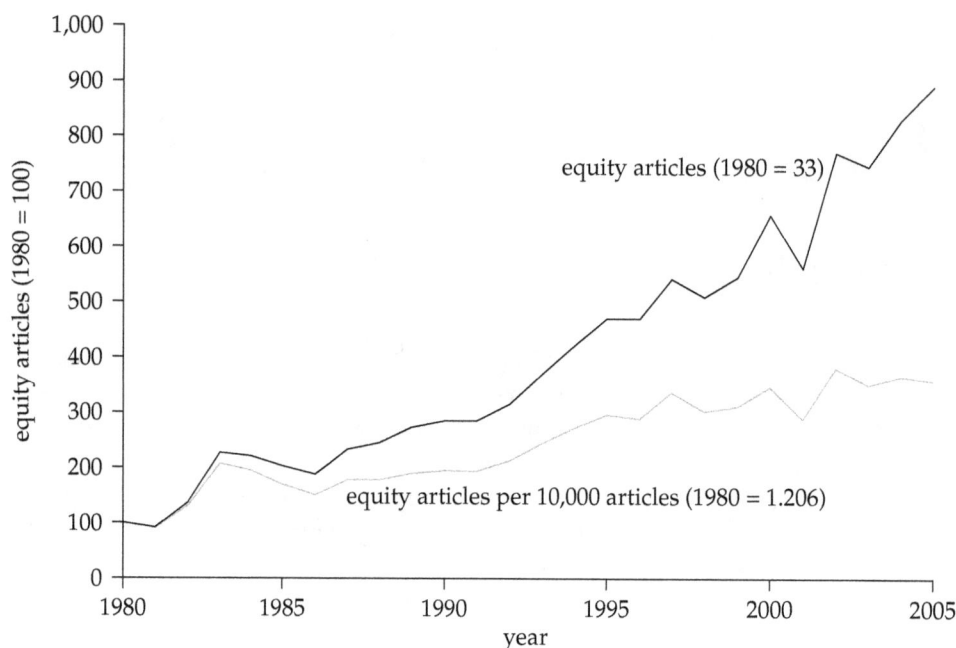

Source: Authors.

of 1980, there were just 1.206 articles on equity published per 10,000 articles in Medline. In 2005, the figure was 4.313, a 260 percent increase (Figure 1.1).

The increased popularity of equity as a research topic in the health field most likely reflects a number of factors. Increased demand is one. A growth of interest in health equity on the part of policy makers, donors, nongovernmental organizations, and others has been evident for some time. Governments in the 1980s typically were more interested in cost containment and efficiency than in promoting equity. Many were ideologically hostile to equity; one government even went so far as to require that its research program on health inequalities be called "health variations" because the term "inequalities" was deemed ideologically unacceptable (Wilkinson 1995). The 1990s were kinder to health equity. Researchers in the field began to receive a sympathetic hearing in many countries, and by the end of the decade many governments, bilateral donors, international organizations, and charitable foundations were putting equity close to—if not right at—the top of their health agendas.[2] This emphasis continued into the new millennium, as equity research became increasingly applied, and began to focus more and more on policies and programs to reduce inequities (see, e.g., Evans et al. 2001b; Gwatkin et al. 2005).

---

[1] The chart refers to articles published in the year in question, *not* cumulative numbers up to the year in question. The numbers are index numbers, the baseline value of each series being indicated in the legend to the chart.

[2] Several international organizations in the health field—including the World Bank (World Bank 1997) and the World Health Organization (World Health Organization 1999)—now have the improvement of the health outcomes of the world's poor as their primary objective, as have several bilateral donors, including, for example, the British government's Department for International Development (Department for International Development 1999).

Supply-side factors have also played a part in contributing to the growth of health equity research:

- Household data sets are more plentiful than ever before. The European Union launched its European Community Household Panel in the 1990s. The Demographic and Health Survey (DHS) has been fielded in more and more developing countries, and the scope of the exercise has increased too. The World Bank's Living Standards Measurement Study (LSMS) has also grown in coverage and scope. At the same time, national governments, in both the developing and industrialized world, appear to have committed ever more resources to household surveys, in the process increasing the availability of data for health equity research.
- Another factor on the supply side is computer power. Since their introduction in the early 1980s, personal computers have become increasingly more powerful and increasingly cheaper in real terms, allowing large household data sets to be analyzed more and more quickly, and at an ever lower cost.
- But there is a third supply-side factor that is likely to be part of the explanation of the rise in health equity research, namely, the continuous flow (since the mid-1980s) of analytic techniques to quantify health inequities, to understand them, and to examine the influence of policies on health equity. This flow of techniques owes much to the so-called ECuity project,[3] now nearly 20 years old (cf., e.g., van Doorslaer et al. 2004; Wagstaff and van Doorslaer 2000; Wagstaff et al. 1989).

The aim of the volume and the audience

It is those techniques that are the subject of this book. The aim is to make the techniques as accessible as possible—in effect, to lower the cost of computer programming in health equity research. The volume sets out to provide researchers and analysts with a step-by-step practical guide to the measurement of a variety of aspects of health equity, with worked examples and computer code, mostly for the computer program Stata. It is hoped that these step-by-step guides, and the easy-to-implement computer routines contained in them, will complement the other favorable demand- and supply-side developments in health equity research and help stimulate yet more research in the field, especially policy-oriented health equity research that enables researchers to help policy makers develop and evaluate programs to reduce health inequities.

Each chapter presents the relevant concepts and methods, with the help of charts and equations, as well as a worked example using real data. Chapters also present and interpret the necessary computer code for Stata (version 9).[4] Each chapter contains a bibliography listing the key articles in the field. Many suggest

---

[3] The project's Web site is at http://www2.eur.nl/bmg/ecuity/.

[4] Because of the narrow page width, some of the Stata code breaks across lines. The user will need to ensure breaks do not occur in the Stata do-files. Although Stata 9 introduces many innovations relative to earlier versions of Stata, most of the code presented in the book will work with earlier versions. There are however some instances in which the code would have to be adjusted. That is the case, for example, with the survey estimation commands used in chapters 2, 9, 10, and 18. Version 9 also introduces new syntax for Stata graphs. For further discussion of key differences, see http://www.stata.com/stata9/.

further reading and provide Internet links to useful Web sites. The chapters have improved over time, having been used as the basis for a variety of training events and research exercises, from which useful feedback has been obtained.

The target audience comprises researchers and analysts. The volume will be especially useful to those working on health equity issues. But because many chapters (notably chapters 2–6 and chapters 10 and 11) cover more general issues in the analysis of health data from household surveys, the volume may prove valuable to others too.

Some chapters are more complex than others, and some sections more complex than others. Nonetheless, the volume ought to be of value even to those who are new to the field or who have only limited training in quantitative techniques and their application to household data. After working through chapters 2–8 (ignoring the sections on dominance checking in chapter 7 and on statistical inference in chapter 8), such a reader ought to be able to produce descriptive statistics and charts showing inequalities in the more commonly used health status indicators. Chapters 16, 18, and 19 also provide accessible guides to the measurement of progressivity of health spending and the incidence of catastrophic and impoverishing health spending. Chapter 14 provides an accessible guide to benefit incidence analysis. The bulk of the empirical literature to date is based on methods in these chapters. The remaining chapters and the sections on dominance checking and inference in chapters 7 and 8 are more advanced, and the reader would benefit from some previous study of microeconometrics and income distribution analysis. The econometrics texts of Greene (1997) and Wooldridge (2002) and Lambert's (2001) text on income distribution and redistribution cover the relevant material.

Focal variables, research questions, and tools

Typically, health equity research is concerned with one or more of four (sets of) focal variables.[5]

- Health outcomes
- Health care utilization
- Subsidies received through the use of services
- Payments people make for health care (directly through out-of-pocket payments as well as indirectly through insurance premiums, social insurance contributions, and taxes)

In the case of health, utilization, and subsidies, the concern is typically with inequality, or more precisely inequalities between the poor and the better-off. In the case of out-of-pocket and other health care payments, the analysis tends to focus on progressivity (how much larger payments are as a share of income for the poor than for the better-off), the incidence of catastrophic payments (those that exceed a prespecified threshold), or the incidence of impoverishing payments (those that cause a household to cross the poverty line).

---

[5]For a review of the literature by economists on health equity up to 2000, see Wagstaff and van Doorslaer (2000).

In each case, different questions can be asked. These include the following:

1. *Snapshots.* Do inequalities between the poor and better-off exist? How large are they? For example, how much more likely is it that a child from the poorest fifth of the population will die before his or her fifth birthday than a child from the richest fifth? Are subsidies to the health sector targeted on the poor as intended? Wagstaff and Waters (2005) call this the snapshot approach: the analyst takes a snapshot of inequalities as they are at a point in time.

2. *Movies.* Are inequalities larger now than they were before? For example, were child mortality inequalities larger in the 1990s than they had been in the 1980s? Wagstaff and Waters (2005) call this the movie approach: the analyst lets the movie roll for a few periods and measures inequalities in each "frame."

3. *Cross-country comparisons.* Are inequalities in country X larger than they are in country Y? For example, are child survival inequalities larger in Brazil than they are in Cuba? Examples of cross-country comparisons along these lines include van Doorslaer et al. (1997) and Wagstaff (2000).

4. *Decompositions.* What are the inequalities that generate the inequalities in the variable being studied? For example, child survival inequalities are likely to reflect inequalities in education (the better educated are likely to know how to feed a child), inequalities in health insurance coverage (the poor may be less likely to be covered and hence more likely to pay the bulk of the cost out-of-pocket), inequalities in accessibility (the poor are likely to have to travel farther and for longer), and so on. One might want to know how far each of these inequalities is responsible for the observed child mortality inequalities. This is known as the decomposition approach (O'Donnell et al. 2006). This requires linking information on inequalities in each of the determinants of the outcome in question with information on the effects of each of these determinants on the outcome. The effects are usually estimated through a regression analysis; the closer analysts come to successfully estimating causal effects in their regression analysis, the closer they come to producing a genuine explanation of inequalities. Decompositions are also helpful for isolating inequalities that are of normative interest. Some health inequalities, for example, might be due to differences in preferences, and hence not inequitable. In principle at least, one could try to capture preferences empirically and use the decomposition method to isolate the inequalities that are *not* due to inequalities in preferences. Likewise, some utilization inequalities might reflect differences in medical needs, and therefore are not inequitable. The decomposition approach allows one to isolate utilization inequalities that do not reflect need inequalities.

5. *Cross-country detective exercises.* How far do differences in inequalities across countries reflect differences in health care systems between the countries, and how far do they reflect other differences, such as income inequality? For example, the large child survival inequalities in Brazil may have been even larger, given Brazil's unequal income distribution, had it not been for Brazil's universal health care system. The paper on benefit incidence by O'Donnell et al. (2007), which tries to explain why subsidies are better targeted on the poor in some Asian countries than in others, is an example of a cross-country detective exercise.

6. *Program impacts on inequalities.* Did a particular program narrow or widen health inequalities? This requires comparing inequalities as they are with inequalities as they would have been without the program. This latter counterfactual distribution is, of course, never observed. One approach, used in some of the studies in Gwatkin et al. (2005), is to compare inequalities (or changes in inequalities over time) in areas where the program has been implemented with inequalities in areas where the program has not been implemented. Or inequalities can be compared between the population enrolled in the program and the population not enrolled in it. This approach is most compelling in instances in which the program has been placed at random in different areas or in instances in which eligibility has been randomly assigned. Where this is not the case, biases may result. Methods such as propensity score matching can be used to try to reduce these biases. Studies in this genre are still relatively rare; examples include Jalan and Ravallion, who look at the differential impacts at different points in the income distribution of piped water investments on diarrhea disease incidence, and Wagstaff and Yu (2007), who look inter alia at the impacts of a World Bank-funded health sector reform project on the incidence of catastrophic out-of-pocket spending.

Answering all these questions requires quantitative analysis. This in turn requires at least three if not four ingredients.

- First, a suitable data set is required. Because the analysis involves comparing individuals or households in different socioeconomic circumstances, the data for health equity analysis often come from a household survey.
- Second, there needs to be clarity on the measurement of key variables in the analysis—health outcomes, health care utilization, need, subsidies, health care payments, and of course living standards.
- Third, the analyst requires a set of quantitative methods for measuring inequality, or the progressivity of health care payments, the incidence and intensity of catastrophic payments, and the incidence of impoverishing payments.
- Fourth, if analysts want to move on from simple measurement to decomposition, cross-country detective work, or program evaluation, they require additional quantitative techniques, including regression analysis for decomposition analysis and impact evaluation methods for program evaluation in which programs have been nonrandomly assigned.

This volume will help researchers in all of these areas, except the last—impact evaluation—which has only recently begun to be used extensively in the health sector and has been used even less in health equity analysis.

Organization of the volume

Part I addresses data issues and the measurement of the key variables in health equity analysis. It is also likely to be valuable to health analysts interested in health issues more generally.

- *Data issues.* Chapter 2 discusses the data requirements for different types of health equity analysis. It compares the advantages and disadvantages of different types of data (e.g., household survey data and exit poll data) and summarizes the key characteristics of some of the most widely used household surveys, such as the DHS and LSMS. The chapter also offers a brief discussion and illustration of the importance of sample design issues in the analysis of survey data.

- *Measurement of health outcomes.* Chapters 3–5 discuss the issues involved in the measurement of some widely used health outcome variables. Chapter 3 covers child mortality. It describes how to compute infant and under-five mortality rates from household survey data using the direct method of mortality estimation using Stata and the indirect method using QFIVE. It also explains how survey data can be used to undertake disaggregated mortality estimation, for example, across socioeconomic groups. Chapter 4 discusses the construction, interpretation, and use of anthropometric indicators, with an emphasis on infants and children. The chapter provides an overview of anthropometric indicators, discusses practical and conceptual issues in constructing anthropometric indicators from physical measurements, and highlights some key issues and approaches to analyzing anthropometric data. The chapter presents worked examples using both Stata and EpiInfo. Chapter 5 is devoted to the measurement of self-reported adult health in the context of general population health inequalities. It illustrates the use of different types of adult health indicators—medical, functional, and subjective—to describe the distribution of health in relation to socioeconomic status (SES). It shows how to standardize health distributions for differences in the demographic composition of SES groups and so provide a more refined description of socioeconomic inequality in health. The chapter also discusses the extent to which measurement of health inequality is biased by socioeconomic differences in the reporting of health.
- *Measurement of living standards.* A key theme throughout this volume and throughout the bulk of the literature on health equity measurement is the variation in health (and other health sector variables) across the distribution of some measure of living standards. Chapter 6 outlines different approaches to living standards measurement, discusses the relationship between and the merits of different measures, shows how different measures can be constructed from survey data, and provides guidance on where further information on living standards measurement can be obtained.

Part II outlines quantitative techniques for interpreting and presenting health equity data.

- *Inequality measurement.* Chapters 7 and 8 present two key concepts—the concentration curve and the concentration index—that are used throughout health equity research to measure inequalities in a variable of interest across the income distribution (or more generally across the distribution of some measure of living standards). The chapters show how the concentration curve can be graphed in Stata and how the concentration index—and its standard error—can be computed straightforwardly.
- *Extensions to the concentration index.* Chapter 9 shows how the concentration index can be extended in two directions: to allow analysts to explore the sensitivity of their results to imposing a different attitude to inequality (i.e., degree of inequality aversion) to that implicit in the concentration index and

to allow a summary measure of "achievement" to be computed that captures both the mean of the distribution as well as the degree of inequality between rich and poor.

- *Decompositions.* What are the underlying inequalities that explain the inequalities in the health variable of interest? For example, child survival inequalities are likely to reflect inequalities in education (the better educated are more likely to know how to feed a child efficiently), in health insurance coverage, in accessibility to health facilities (the poor are likely to have to travel farther), and so on. One might want to know the extent to which each of these inequalities can explain the observed child mortality inequality. This can be addressed using decomposition methods (O'Donnell et al. 2006), which are based on regression analysis of the relationships between the health variable of interest and its correlates. Such analyses are usually purely descriptive, revealing the associations that characterize the health inequality, but if data are sufficient to allow the estimation of causal effects, then it is possible to identify the factors that generate inequality in the variable of interest. In cases in which causal effects have not been obtained, the decomposition provides an explanation in the statistical sense, and the results will not necessarily be a good guide to policy making. For example, the results will not help us predict how inequalities in Y would change if policy makers were to reduce inequalities in X, or reduce the effect of X and Y (e.g., by expanding facilities serving remote populations if X were distance to provider). By contrast, if causal effects *have* been obtained, the decomposition results ought to shed light on such issues. Decompositions are also helpful for isolating inequalities that are of normative interest. Some health inequalities, for example, might be due to differences in preferences and hence are not inequitable. In principle at least, one could try to capture preferences empirically and use the decomposition method to isolate the inequalities that are *not* due to inequalities in preferences. Likewise, some utilization inequalities might reflect differences in medical needs and therefore are not inequitable. The decomposition approach allows one to isolate utilization inequalities that do not reflect need inequalities.

Part III presents the application of these techniques in the analysis of equity in health care utilization and health care spending.

- *Benefit incidence analysis.* Chapter 14 shows how benefit incidence analysis (BIA) is undertaken. In its simplest form, BIA is an accounting procedure that seeks to establish to whom the benefits of government spending accrue, with recipients being ranked by their relative economic position. The chapter confines its attention to the distribution of average spending and does not consider the benefit incidence of marginal dollars spent on health care (Lanjouw and Ravallion 1999; Younger 2003). Once a measure of living standards has been decided on, there are three principal steps in a BIA of government health spending. First, the utilization of public health services in relation to the measure of living standards must be identified. Second, each individual's utilization of a service must be weighted by the unit value of the public subsidy to that service. Finally, the distribution of the subsidy must be evaluated against some target distribution. Chapter 14 discusses each of these three steps in turn.

- *Equity in health service delivery.* Chapter 15 discusses measurement and explanation of inequity in the delivery of health care. In health care, most attention—both in policy and research—has been given to the horizontal equity principle, defined as "equal treatment for equal medical need, irrespective of other characteristics such as income, race, place of residence, etc." The analysis proceeds in much the same way as the standardization methods covered in chapter 5: one seeks to establish whether there is differential utilization of health care by income after standardizing for differences in the need for health care in relation to income. In empirical work, need is usually proxied by expected utilization given characteristics such as age, gender, and measures of health status. Complications to the regression method of standardization arise because typically measures of health care utilization are nonnegative integer counts (e.g., numbers of visits, hospital days, etc.) with highly skewed distributions. As discussed in chapter 11, nonlinear methods of estimation are then appropriate. But the standardization methods presented in chapter 5 do not immediately carry over to nonlinear models—they can be rescued only if relationships can be represented linearly. Chapter 15 therefore devotes most of its attention to standardization in nonlinear settings. Once health care use has been standardized for need, inequity can be measured by the concentration index. Inequity can then be explained by decomposing the concentration index, as explained in chapter 13. In fact, with the decomposition approach, standardization for need and explanation of inequity can be done in one step. This procedure is described in the final section of chapter 15.
- *Progressivity and redistributive effect of health care finance.* Chapter 16 shows how one can assess the extent to which payments for health care are related to ability to pay (ATP). Is the relationship proportional? Or is it progressive—do health care payments account for an increasing proportion of ATP as the latter rises? Or, is there a regressive relationship, in the sense that payments comprise a decreasing share of ATP? The chapter provides practical advice on methods for the assessment and measurement of progressivity in health care finance. Progressivity is measured in regard to departure from proportionality in the relationship between payments toward the provision of health care and ATP. Chapter 17 considers the relationship between progressivity and the redistributive impact of health care payments. Redistribution can be vertical and horizontal. The former occurs when payments are disproportionately related to ATP. The chapter shows that the extent of vertical redistribution can be inferred from measures of progressivity presented in chapter 16. Horizontal redistribution occurs when persons with equal ability to pay contribute unequally to health care payments. Chapter 17 shows how the total redistributive effect of health payments can be measured and how this redistribution can be decomposed into its vertical and horizontal components.
- *Catastrophe and impoverishment in health spending.* One conception of fairness in health finance is that households should be protected against catastrophic medical expenses (World Health Organization 2000). A popular approach has been to define medical spending as "catastrophic" if it exceeds some fraction of household income or total expenditure within a given period, usually one year. The idea is that spending a large fraction of the household

budget on health care must be at the expense of consumption of other goods and services. Chapter 18 develops measures of catastrophic health spending, including the incidence and intensity of catastrophic spending, as well as a measure that captures not just the incidence or intensity but also the extent to which catastrophic spending is concentrated among the poor. Chapter 19 looks at the measurement of impoverishing health expenditures—expenditures that result in a household falling below the poverty line, in the sense that had it not had to make the expenditures on health care, the household could have enjoyed a standard of living above the poverty line.

References

Alleyne, G. A. O., J. Casas, and C. Castillo-Salgado. 2000. "Equality, Equity: Why Bother?" *Bulletin of the World Health Organization* 78(1): 76–77.

Braveman, P., B. Starfield, and H. Geiger. 2001. "World Health Report 2000: How It Removes Equity from the Agenda for Public Health Monitoring and Policy." *British Medical Journal* 323: 678–80.

Department for International Development. 1999. *Better Health for Poor People.* London: Department for International Development.

Evans, T., M. Whitehead, F. Diderichsen, A. Bhuiya, and M. Wirth. 2001a. "Introduction." In *Challenging Inequities in Health: From Ethics to Action,* ed. T. Evans, M. Whitehead, F. Diderichsen, A. Bhuiya, and M. Wirth. Oxford: Oxford University Press.

Evans, T., M. Whitehead, F. Diderichsen, A. Bhuiya, and M. Wirth. 2001b. *Challenging Inequities in Health: From Ethics to Action.* Oxford: Oxford University Press.

Greene, W. 1997. *Econometric Analysis.* Upper Saddle River, NJ: Prentice-Hall Inc.

Gwatkin, D. R., A. Wagstaff, and A. Yazbeck. 2005. *Reaching the Poor with Health, Nutrition, and Population Services: What Works, What Doesn't, and Why.* Washington, DC: World Bank.

Lambert, P. 2001. *The Distribution and Redistribution of Income: A Mathematical Analysis.* Manchester, United Kingdom: Manchester University Press.

Lanjouw, P., and M. Ravallion. 1999. "Benefit Incidence, Public Spending Reforms and the Timing of Program Capture." *World Bank Economic Review* 13(2).

Le Grand, J. 1987. "Equity, Health and Health Care." *Social Justice Research* 1: 257–74.

O'Donnell, O., E. van Doorslaer, and A. Wagstaff. 2006. "Decomposition of Inequalities in Health and Health Care." In *The Elgar Companion to Health Economics,* ed. A. M. Jones. Cheltenham, United Kingdom: Edward Elgar.

O'Donnell, O., E. van Doorslaer, R. P. Rannan-Eliya, A. Somanathan, S. R. Adhikari, D. Harbianto, C. G. Garg, P. Hanvoravongchai, M. N. Huq, A. Karan, G. M. Leung, C.-w. Ng, B. R. Pande, K. Tin, L. Trisnantoro, C. Vasavid, Y. Zhang, and Y. Zhao. 2007. "The Incidence of Public Spending on Health Care: Comparative Evidence from Asia." *World Bank Economic Review,* in press.

Sen, A. 2002. "Why Health Equity?" *Health Economics* 11(8): 659–66.

Tobin, J. 1970. "On Limiting the Domain of Inequality." *Journal of Law and Economics* 13: 263–78.

van Doorslaer, E., A. Wagstaff, H. Bleichrodt, S. Calonge, U. G. Gerdtham, M. Gerfin, J. Geurts, L. Gross, U. Hakkinen, R. E. Leu, O. O'Donnell, C. Propper, F. Puffer, M. Rodriguez, G. Sundberg, and O. Winkelhake. 1997. "Income-Related Inequalities in Health: Some International Comparisons." *Journal of Health Economics* 16: 93–112.

van Doorslaer, E., X. Koolman, and A. M. Jones. 2004. "Explaining Income-Related Inequalities in Doctor Utilisation in Europe." *Health Econ* 13(7): 629–47.

Wagstaff, A. 2000. "Socioeconomic Inequalities in Child Mortality: Comparisons across Nine Developing Countries." *Bulletin of the World Health Organization* 78(1): 19–29.

Wagstaff, A. 2001. "Economics, Health and Development: Some Ethical Dilemmas Facing the World Bank and the International Community." *Journal of Medical Ethics* 27(4): 262–67.

Wagstaff, A., and E. van Doorslaer. 2000. "Equity in Health Care Finance and Delivery." In *North Holland Handbook in Health Economics,* ed. A. Culyer and J. Newhouse, 1804–1862. Amsterdam, Netherlands: North Holland.

Wagstaff, A., and H. Waters. 2005. "How Were the Reaching the Poor Studies Done?" In *Reaching the Poor with Health, Nutrition and Population Services: What Works, What Doesn't, and Why,* ed. D. Gwatkin, A. Wagstaff, and A. Yazbeck. Washington, DC: World Bank.

Wagstaff, A., and S. Yu. 2007. "Do Health Sector Reforms Have Their Intended Impacts? The World Bank's Health VIII Project in Gansu Province, China." *Journal of Health Economics,* 26(3): 505–535.

Wagstaff, A., E. van Doorslaer, and P. Paci. 1989. "Equity in the Finance and Delivery of Health Care: Some Tentative Cross-Country Comparisons." *Oxford Review of Economic Policy* 5: 89–112.

Whitehead, M. 1992. "The Concepts and Principles of Equity and Health." *International Journal of Health Services* 22(3): 429–45.

Wilkinson, R. G. 1995. "'Variations' in Health." *British Medical Journal* 311: 1177–78.

Wooldridge, J. M. 2002. *Econometric Analysis of Cross Section and Panel Data.* Cambridge, MA.: MIT Press.

World Bank. 1997. *Health, Nutrition and Population Sector Strategy.* Washington, DC: World Bank.

World Health Organization. 1999. *The World Health Report 1999: Making a Difference.* Geneva, Switzerland: World Health Organization.

World Health Organization. 2000. *World Health Report 2000.* Geneva, Switzerland: World Health Organization.

Younger, S. D. 2003. "Benefits on the Margin: Observations on Marginal Benefit Incidence Analysis." *World Bank Economic Review* 17(1): 89–106.

2

Data for Health Equity Analysis: Requirements, Sources, and Sample Design

The first step in health equity analysis is to identify appropriate data and to understand their potential and their limitations. This chapter provides an overview of the data needs for health equity analysis, considering how data requirements may vary depending on the analytical issues at hand. The chapter also provides a brief guide to different sources of data and their respective limitations. Although there is some scope for using routine data, such as administrative records or census data, survey data tend to have the greatest potential for assessing and analyzing different aspects of health equity. With this in mind, the chapter also provides examples of different types of survey data that analysts may be able to access. Finally, it offers a brief discussion and illustration of the importance of sample design issues in the analysis of survey data.

Data requirements for health equity analysis

Health outcomes and health-related behavior

Data on health outcomes are a basic building block for health equity analysis. But how can health be measured? Murray and Chen (1992) have proposed a classification of morbidity measures that distinguishes between self-perceived and observed measures (see table 2.1).

For most of these measures, data are not collected routinely and can be obtained only through surveys. However, as is discussed further below, surveys differ substantially, both in the range of measures covered and in the approach to measurement. For example, some surveys include only short questions about illness episodes. Other surveys, such as the Indonesia Family Life Survey, use trained health workers in enumerator teams and collect detailed "observed" morbidity data, including measured height, weight, hemoglobin status, lung capacity, blood pressure, and the speed with which the respondent was able to stand up five times from a sitting position.

Health equity analysis can also be concerned with health-related behavior. The most obvious question in this respect concerns the utilization of and payment for health services. Questions on these issues have been included in many surveys, although the level of detail has varied considerably. But health-related behavior extends beyond the utilization of health services. Other variables relevant to health equity analyses include (i) behavior with an effect on health status (smoking,

Table 2.1 *A Classification of Morbidity Measures*

	Self-Perceived
Symptoms and impairments	Occurrence of illness or specific symptoms during a defined time period
Functional disability	Assessment of ability to carry out specific functions and tasks, or restrictions on normal activities (activities of daily living, e.g., dressing, preparing meals, or performing physical movement)
Handicap	Self-perceived functional disability within a specifically defined context
	Observed
Physical and vital signs	Aspects of disease or pathology that can be detected by physical examination (e.g., blood pressure and lung capacity)
Physiological and pathophysiological indicators	Measures based on laboratory examinations (e.g., blood, urine, feces, and other bodily fluids), body measurements (anthropometry)
Physical tests	Demonstrated ability to perform specific functions, both physical and mental (e.g., running, squatting, blowing up a balloon, or performing an intellectual task)
Clinical diagnosis	Assessment of health status by a trained health professional based on an examination and possibly specific tests

Source: Authors.

drinking, and diet), (ii) sexual practices, and (iii) household-level behavior (cooking practices, waste disposal, sanitation, sources of water). Some data on health service use are collected through routine information systems and population censuses (e.g., immunizations), but more detailed data are likely to be available only through surveys.

In the case of both health outcomes and health-related behaviors, it is important to keep in mind that variation in the variable of interest may arise for many reasons. Some of these relate to health system characteristics—for example, features of health financing or service delivery arrangements. But there is also likely to be variation due to biological, environmental, social, and other factors. Although it is often difficult to identify the contribution of different factors in practice, this is clearly an important issue to address in thinking about the policy implications of health equity analysis.

Living standards or socioeconomic status

Concerns for health equity arise in the relationships between health, or health-related behavior, and a variety of individual characteristics, such as social class, ethnic group, sex, age, and location. This book is concerned primarily with health equity defined in relation to socioeconomic status or living standards. The goal is to assess and to understand how health outcome or health-related behaviors vary with some measure of socioeconomic status or living standards. This is not to say that other types of comparisons are not of interest or relevant to policy—they clearly are. However, comparisons across, say sex, ethnic group, or geographic location, typically are not amenable to the techniques described in this book and hence receive less attention in what follows.

For the purposes of analyzing socioeconomic health inequalities, health-related information must be complemented by data on living standards or socioeconomic status. As is discussed in detail in chapter 6, there are many approaches to living standards measurement, including direct approaches (e.g., income, expenditure, or consumption) and proxy measures (e.g., asset index). In practice, the choice of living standards measure is often driven by data availability. Nonetheless, the choice of measure may influence the conclusions, so it is important for analysts to be aware of both the assumptions that underpin the chosen measure and the potential sensitivity of findings.

It is also important to distinguish between cardinal and ordinal measures of living standards. In the case of cardinal measures—for example, income or consumption in dollars or units of another currency—numbers convey comparable information about magnitude. Ordinal measures only rank individuals or households and do not permit comparisons of magnitudes across units. Some forms of health equity analysis require a cardinal measure of living standards. This is the case, for example, with financing progressivity and the poverty impact of health payments or health events. But in some cases, a ranking of households by some measure of living standards suffices. For example, measures of inequality in health and health care.

Other complementary data

For some forms of health equity analysis, data on the relevant health variables and a measure of living standards suffice. Often, however, other complementary data are required. For example, if multivariate analysis of health-related variables is to be used to better understand why observed inequalities arise, then data on community, household, and individual characteristics are required. This could include, for example, availability and characteristics of health care providers, environmental and climatic characteristics of the community, housing characteristics, education, sex, ethnicity, and so on.

Complementary data are also required to identify the distribution of public health expenditure in relation to living standards, so-called benefit-incidence analysis. The primary requirement is data on unit subsidies to health services. This information tends to be based on public expenditure data, but in some cases, more detailed cost information is available. Taking account of regional variation in unit costs requires data on the geographic location of the individual. Extending the analysis to examine variation in utilization with, for example, sex and ethnicity, requires data on the relevant demographics. Analysis of health financing fairness and progressivity depends on detailed data on user payments for health care.

The data requirements of different types of health equity analysis are summarized in table 2.2. As discussed in the rest of this chapter, the richest data for health equity analysis are likely to be from household surveys, but routine administrative data can also prove useful.

Table 2.2 *Data Requirements for Health Equity Analysis*

	Health variables	Utilization variables	Living standards measure (ordinal)	Living standards measure (cardinal)	Unit subsidies	User payments	Background variables
Health inequality	✓		✓				
Equity in utilization		✓	✓				
Multivariate analysis	✓ or	✓		✓			✓
Benefit-incidence analysis		✓	✓		✓		(✓)
Health financing							
– Progressivity				✓		✓	
– Catastrophic payments				✓		✓	
– Poverty impact				✓		✓	

Source: Authors.

Data sources and their limitations

Household surveys and other nonroutine data

Household surveys are implemented on a regular basis in many countries and are probably the most important source of data for health equity analysis. Some household surveys are designed as multipurpose surveys, with a focus on a broad set of demographic and socioeconomic issues, whereas other surveys focus explicitly on health. Surveys sample from the population and are representative, or can be made representative, of the population as a whole (or whatever target population is defined for the survey). They have the advantage of permitting more detailed data collection than is feasible in a comprehensive census. Although many surveys are conducted on an ad hoc basis, there are an increasing number of multiround integrated survey programs. These include the Living Standards Measurement Study (World Bank), the Demographic and Health Surveys (ORC Macro), the Multiple Indicator Cluster Surveys (UNICEF), and the World Health Surveys (WHO).[1] The Living Standards Measurement Surveys are different from the other surveys in that they collect detailed expenditure data, income data, or both. In that sense, the Living Standards Measurement Surveys are a type of household budget survey.[2] Many countries implement household budget surveys in some form or other on a semiregular basis. A core objective of these surveys is to capture the essential elements of the household income and expenditure pattern. In some countries, the surveys focus exclusively on this objective and are hence of limited use for health equity analysis. However, it is also common for household budget surveys to include additional modules—for example, on health and nutrition—making them

---

[1]Some surveys, in particular the *Demographic and Health Surveys* and some budget surveys, are repeated on a regular basis and can in that sense be considered "semiroutine" data.
[2]These surveys are sometimes called "family expenditure surveys," "expenditure and consumption surveys," or "income and expenditure surveys."

ideal for detailed analysis of the relationship between economic status and health variables.

Aside from large-scale household surveys, there are often a wealth of other non-routine data that can be used for health equity analysis. This may include small-scale, ad hoc household surveys and special studies. It may also be possible to analyze data from facility-based surveys of users (exit polls) from an equity perspective. Relative to household surveys, exit polls are cheap to implement (in particular if they are carried out as a component of a health facility survey) and are an efficient means of collecting data on health service use and perceptions. With exit polls it is also easier to associate outcomes of health-seeking behavior (e.g., client perceptions of quality, payments, receipt of drugs) with a particular provider and care-seeking episode. This is often difficult in general household surveys, in which typically specific providers are not identified and in which recall periods of up to 4 weeks can result in considerable measurement error. However, unlike a household survey, an exit poll provides information only about users of health services.

Although survey data can be of considerable value for health equity analysis, it is important to be aware of their limitations. For one thing, large-scale surveys are expensive to conduct and, as a result, they tend to be implemented only periodically. Moreover, the scope, focus, and measurement approaches can vary across surveys and over time, limiting the scope for comparisons. Another challenge concerns the way the survey sample is selected and what this implies for making inferences from the data. It is important for analysts to be aware of the "representativeness" of the survey data and to take this into account when drawing conclusions about the wider population. It is also important to be aware of how to adjust the analysis for departures from simple random sampling, arising from, for example, stratification or multistage sampling. These issues are discussed in more detail below. Finally, survey data can be misleading, or "biased," because of problems in both the sample design and the way the survey is implemented (see box 2.1). Both of these problems can lead analysts to draw inappropriate inferences from survey data.

Box 2.1 *Sampling and Nonsampling Bias in Survey Data*

When analyzing survey data, analysts must be aware of potential sources of sampling and nonsampling bias. Sampling bias refers to a situation in which the sample is not representative of the target population of interest. For example, it is inappropriate to draw inferences about the general population on the basis of a sample drawn from users of health facilities. The reason is that different groups in the population use health facilities to different degrees—for example, due to differences in access or need. Sampling bias can also arise from the practice of "convenience sampling" aimed at avoiding remote or inaccessible areas or from the use of an inaccurate or inappropriate sampling frame. These potential problems point to the need for analysts to be well aware of the sampling procedure.

There are also many potential forms of nonsampling bias that can arise in the process of survey implementation. For example, nonresponse or measurement errors may be systematically related with variables of interest—for example, nonresponse about utilization of health services may be higher among the poor. If this were the case, analysts should be cautious in interpreting results and drawing inferences about the general population. In some cases, it may be possible to correct for this bias by modeling nonresponse. Other potential sources of nonsampling bias include errors in recording or data entry.

Source: Authors.

Routine data: health information systems and censuses

Some forms of routine data may be suitable for health equity analysis. Health information systems (HIS) collect a combination of health data through ongoing data collection systems. These data include administrative health service statistics (e.g., from hospital records or patient registration), epidemiological and surveillance data, and vital events data (registering births, deaths, marriages, etc.). HIS data are used primarily for management purposes, for example, for planning, needs assessments, resource allocation, and quality assessments. However, in some contexts, HIS data include demographic or socioeconomic variables that permit equity analysis. This is the case, for example, in Britain, where mortality data based on death certificates have been used for tabulations of mortality rates by occupational group since the 19th century. Similar analysis has been undertaken in other countries by ethnic group or educational level. Although many HIS do not routinely record socioeconomic or demographic characteristics, this may change in the future as the importance of monitoring health system equity becomes more recognized.

Periodic population and housing censuses are another form of routine data. Censuses are an important source of data for planning and monitoring of population issues and socioeconomic and environmental trends, in both developed and developing countries. National population and housing censuses also provide valuable statistics and indicators for assessing the situation of various special population groups, such as those affected by gender issues, children, youth, the elderly, persons with a disability, and the migrant population. Population censuses have been conducted in most countries in recent years.[3] Census data often contain only limited information on health and living standards, but have sometimes been used to study health inequalities by linking the information to HIS data. For example, socioeconomic differences in disease incidence and hospitalization have been studied by linking cause-of-death or hospital discharge records with census data. In the United States, there have also been efforts to link public health surveillance data with area-based socioeconomic measures based on geocoding. Although poor data quality and availability may currently preclude such linking in low-income countries, census data may be used to study equity issues by constructing need indicators for geographic areas based on demographic and socioeconomic profiles of the population.

Notwithstanding the potential for using routine data for health equity analysis, it is important to be aware of the common weaknesses of such data. In particular, coverage is often incomplete and data quality may be poor. For example, as a result of spatial differences in the coverage of health facility infrastructure, routine data are likely to be more complete and representative in urban than in rural areas. Similarly, better-off individuals are more likely to seek and obtain medical care and, hence, to be recorded in the HIS. Moreover, in cases in which routine data are used for management purposes, there may exist incentives for staff to record information inaccurately.

Data sources and their limitations are summarized in table 2.3.

---

[3]Information about dates of censuses in different countries can be found on http://unstats. un.org/unsd/demographic/census/cendate/index.htm.

Table 2.3 *Data Sources and Their Limitations*

Type of data	Examples	Advantages	Disadvantages
Survey data (household)	Living Standards Measurement Study (LSMS), Demographic and Health Surveys (DHS), Multiple Indicator Cluster Surveys (MICS), World Health Surveys (WHS)	Data are representative for a specific population (often nationally), as well as for subpopulations Many surveys have rich data on health, living standards, and other complementary variables Surveys are often conducted on a regular basis, sometimes following households over time	Sampling and nonsampling errors can be important Survey may not be representative to of small subpopulations of interest
Survey data (exit poll)	Ad hoc surveys, often linked to facility surveys	Cost of implementation is relatively low Detailed information that can be related to provider characteristics is provided about users of health services Data on payments and other characteristics of visit are more likely to be accurate	Exit polls provide no information about nonusers Data often contain limited information about household and socioeconomic characteristics Survey responses may be biased from "courtesy" to providers or fear of repercussions
Administrative data	HIS, vital registration, national surveillance system, sentinel site surveillance	Data are readily available	Data may be of poor quality Data may not be representative for the population as a whole Data contain limited complementary information, e.g., about living standards
Census data	Implemented on a national scale in many countries	Data cover the entire target population (or nearly so)	Data contain only limited data on health Data collection is irregular Data contain limited complementary information, e.g., about living standards

Source: Authors.

Examples of survey data

Demographic and Health Surveys (DHS and DHS+)

The Demographic and Health Surveys (DHS) have been an important source of individual and household-level health data since 1984[4] The design of the DHS drew on the experiences of the World Fertility Surveys[5] (WFS) and the Contraceptive Prevalence Surveys, but included an expanded set of indicators in the areas of population, health, and nutrition. DHS are nationally representative, with sample sizes typically ranging from 5,000 to 30,000 households.

The standard Demographic and Health Surveys consist of a household questionnaire and a women's questionnaire (ages 15–49). The core questionnaire concentrates on basic indicators and is standardized across countries. The household questionnaire covers basic demographic data for all household members, household and dwelling characteristics, and nutritional status of young children and women ages 15 through 49. The women's questionnaire contains information on general background characteristics, reproductive behavior and intentions, contraception, maternity care, breastfeeding and nutrition, children's health, status of women, AIDS and other sexually transmitted diseases, husband's background, and other topics. Some surveys also include special modules tailored to meet particular needs.

Aside from the standard DHS, interim surveys are sometimes implemented to collect information on a reduced set of performance-monitoring indicators. These surveys have a smaller sample size and are often conducted between rounds of DHS. In addition, many of the DHS have included tools to collect community-level data (Service Availability Modules). More recently, detailed facility surveys—Service Provision Assessments—have been implemented alongside household surveys with a view to providing information about the characteristics of health services, including their quality, infrastructure, utilization, and availability.

Further information, including a list of past and ongoing surveys, survey reports, questionnaires, and information on how to access the data, can be found on http://www.measuredhs.com.

The Living Standards Measurement Study

The Living Standards Measurement Study (LSMS) was established by the World Bank in 1980 to explore ways of improving the type and quality of household data collected by government statistical offices in developing countries. LSMS surveys are multitopic surveys, designed to permit four types of analysis: (i) simple descriptive statistics on living standards, (ii) monitoring of poverty and living standards

---

[4]For further information about the history of DHS, see http://www.measuredhs.com/about-dhs/history.cfm. In 1997 DHS changed its name to DHS+ to reflect the integration of DHS activities under the MEASURE program. Under that mandate, DHS+ is charged with collecting and analyzing demographic and health data for regional and national family planning and health programs.

[5]The WFSs were a collection of internationally comparable surveys of human fertility conducted in 41 developing countries in the late 1970s and early 1980s. The project was conducted by the International Statistical Institute (ISI), with funding from USAID and UNFPA.

over time, (iii) description of the incidence and coverage of government programs, and (iv) measurement of the impact of policies and programs on household behavior and welfare (Grosh et al. 2000). The first surveys were implemented in Côte d'Ivoire and Peru. Other early surveys followed a similar format, although considerable variation has been introduced over time.

The household questionnaire forms the heart of the LSMS survey. Typically, it includes a health module that provides information on (i) health-related behavior; (ii) utilization of health services; (iii) health expenditures; (iv) insurance status; and (v) access to health services. The level of detail of the health section has, however, varied across surveys. Complementary data are typically collected through community and price questionnaires. In addition, detailed service provider (health facility or school) data have been collected in some LSMS surveys. The facility surveys have been included to provide complementary data primarily on prices of health care and medicines and health care quality.

Further information, including a list of past and ongoing surveys, survey reports, questionnaires, and information on how to access the data, can be found at http://www.worldbank.org/lsms/.

UNICEF multiple indicator cluster surveys

The multiple indicator cluster surveys (MICS) were developed by UNICEF and others in 1998 to monitor the goals of the World Summit for Children. By 1996, sixty developing countries had carried out stand-alone MICS and another 40 had incorporated some of the MICS modules into other surveys.

The early experience with MICS resulted in revisions of the methodology and questionnaires. These revisions drew on the expertise and experience of many organizations, including WHO, UNESCO, ILO, UNAIDS, the United Nations Statistical Division, CDC Atlanta, MEASURE (USAID), and academic institutions.

The MICS typically include three components: a household questionnaire, a women's questionnaire (15–49 years), and a child (under 5 years) questionnaire. The precise content of questionnaires has varied somewhat across countries. Household questionnaires often cover education, child labor, maternal mortality, child disability, water and sanitation, and salt iodization. The women's questionnaires have tended to include sections on child mortality, tetanus toxoid, maternal health, contraceptive use, and HIV/AIDS. Finally, the child questionnaire covers birth registration, vitamin A, breast-feeding, treatment of illness, malaria, immunizations, and anthropometry.

Further information, including a list of past and ongoing surveys, survey reports, questionnaires, and information on how to access the data can be found at http://www.childinfo.org/index2.htm.

WHO World Health Survey

WHO has developed a World Health Survey (WHS) to compile comprehensive baseline information on the health of populations and on the outcomes associated with the investment in health systems. These surveys have been implemented in 70 countries across the full range of development in collaboration with the people involved in routine HIS. The overall aims of the WHS are to examine the way populations report their health, understand how people value health states, and measure the performance of health systems in relation to responsiveness. In addition, it addresses various issues such as health care expenditures, adult mortality, birth history, various risk factors, and the like.

In the first stage, the WHS targets adult individuals living in private households (18 years or older). A nationally representative sample of households is drawn, and adult individuals are selected randomly from the household roster. Sample sizes vary from 1,000 to 10,000 individuals.

The content of the questionnaires varies across countries but, in general, covers general household information, geocoding, malaria prevention, home care, health insurance, income indicators, and household expenditure (including on health). In addition, a specific module is administered to household members who are trained or are working as health professionals. This module covers a limited set of issues, including occupation, location of work, hours of work, main activities in work, forms and amount of payment, second employment, reasons for not working (if applicable), and professional training. The individual questionnaire includes sections on sociodemographic characteristics, health state descriptions, health state valuations, risk factors, mortality, coverage, health system responsiveness, and health goals and social capital.

Further information, including country reports and questionnaires can be found at http://www.who.int/healthinfo/survey/en/index.html.

WHO multicountry evaluation of the integrated management of childhood illnesses

Currently, WHO is coordinating a multicountry evaluation (MCE) of the integrated management of childhood illnesses (IMCI).[6] Integrated survey instruments for costs and quality have been developed and implemented (or are being implemented) in Bangladesh, Tanzania, Peru, and Uganda. The purpose of the MCEs is to (i) document the effects of IMCI interventions on health workers' performance, health systems, and family behaviors; (ii) determine whether, and to what extent, the IMCI strategy as a whole has a measurable impact on health outcomes (reducing under-5 morbidity and mortality); (iii) describe the cost of IMCI implementation at national, district, and health facility levels; (iv) increase the sustainability of IMCI and other child health strategies by providing a basis for improving implementation; and (v) support planning and advocacy for childhood interventions by ministries of health in developing countries and national and international partners in development. Worldwide there are 30 countries at different stages of implementation of IMCI, among which Uganda, Peru, Bangladesh, and Tanzania will participate in the MCE.

Further information, including country reports, questionnaires, and how to access data can be found at http://www.who.int/imci-mce/.

---

[6]The Integrated Management of Childhood Illnesses (IMCI) Strategy was developed by WHO and UNICEF to address five leading causes of childhood mortality, namely, malaria, pneumonia, diarrhea, measles, and malnutrition. The three main components addressed by the strategy are improved case management, improved health systems, and improved family and community practices.

RAND surveys

RAND has supported the design and implementation of Family Life Surveys (FLS) in developing countries since the 1970s. Currently available country surveys include Indonesia (1993, 1997, 1998, 2000), Malaysia (1976–7, 1988–9), Guatemala (1995), and Bangladesh (1996). Further information about these surveys and information on how to access the data can be found at http://www.rand.org.

INDONESIA FAMILY LIFE SURVEY   The Indonesia Family Life Survey (IFLS) is an ongoing, multitopic longitudinal survey. It aims to provide data for the measurement and analysis of a range of individual- and household-level behaviors and outcomes. It includes indicators of economic well-being, education, migration, labor market outcomes, fertility and contraceptive use, health status, use of health care and health insurance, intrahousehold relationships, and participation in community activities. In addition, community-level data are collected. These include detailed surveys of service providers (schools and health care providers) in the selected communities. The first wave of the survey (IFSL1) was conducted in 1993/4, covering approximately 7,000 households. The IFLS2 and IFLS2+ were conducted in 1997 and 1998, and a further wave (IFLS3) in 2000.

MALAYSIAN FAMILY LIFE SURVEYS   The Malaysian Family Life Surveys were conducted in 1976/7 and 1988. The surveys contain extensive histories on employment, marriage, fertility, and migration. Respondents in the first wave were followed in a second wave, and a refreshment sample was added.

MATLAB HEALTH AND SOCIOECONOMIC SURVEY   The Matlab Health and Socioeconomic Survey was implemented in 1996 in Matlab, a rural region in Bangladesh in which there is an ongoing prospective demographic surveillance system. The general focus of the survey was on issues relating to health and well-being for rural adults and the elderly, including the effects of socioeconomic characteristics on health status and health care utilization; health status, social and kin network characteristics, and resource flows; and community services and infrastructure. The study included a survey of individuals and households, a specialized out-migrant survey (sample of individuals who had left the households of the primary sample since 1982), and a community provider survey.

GUATEMALAN SURVEY OF FAMILY HEALTH   The Guatemalan Survey of Family Health is a single cross-section survey that was conducted in rural communities in 4 of Guatemala's 22 departments. The survey was fielded in 1995.

University of North Carolina surveys

The Carolina Population Center at the University of North Carolina at Chapel Hill has been involved in a range of different data collection exercises. Much of the data are publicly available. Information can be found at http://www.cpc.unc.edu/projects/projects.php.

CEBU LONGITUDINAL HEALTH AND NUTRITION SURVEYS   The Cebu Longitudinal Health and Nutrition Survey is a study of a cohort of Filipino women who gave birth between May 1, 1983, and April 30, 1984, and were reinterviewed, with their children, at three subsequent points in time until 1998/9.

CHINA HEALTH AND NUTRITION SURVEY   The China Health and Nutrition Survey is a six-wave longitudinal survey conducted in eight provinces of China between 1989 and 2004. It provides a wealth of detailed information on health and nutrition of adults and children, including physical examinations.

NANG RONG (THAILAND) PROJECTS   The Nang Rong projects represent a major data collection effort that was started in 1984 with a census of households in 51 villages. The villages were resurveyed in 1988 and again in 1994/5. New entrants were interviewed, and a subsample of out-migrants was followed.

Sample design and the analysis of survey data

Survey data provide information on a subset of a population—a sample. If the sample is appropriately selected, it provides the basis for drawing inferences about the target population, for example, all children under five in a particular country. A sample is selected from a sampling frame, which is a list of sampling units (e.g., households).[7] In a probability sampling design, every element in the sampling frame has a known, nonzero chance of being selected into the survey sample. This is not true with nonprobability methods, such as quota or convenience sampling and random walks.

The most straightforward way of selecting a sample is by simple random sampling–sampling units are selected from the sampling frame with equal probability.[8] In many cases, a single-stage random sampling design is impractical. This may be so because of the difficulty in drawing up a complete list for the entire target population, because of concern that the sample would contain "too few" members of some subpopulations, or because of high costs and logistical constraints in visiting a randomly selected sample. Because of these and other concerns, many surveys have what is referred to as a complex survey design. Three factors that arise from the sample design have important implications for data analysis (Deaton 1997).

- **Stratification**   Stratification is the process by which the population is divided into subgroups or subpopulations, and sampling is then done separately for each subpopulation. Stratification can be done on the basis of geography, level of urbanization, socioeconomic zones or administrative areas, and so forth. Stratification is used when there is an expectation of heterogeneity between different subpopulations. It can then reduce sampling error and ensures that representative estimates can be produced for each strata.

---

[7]The sampling units are often the same as the members of the target population, but that is not always the case. For example, because it would be very difficult to construct a list of all children under 5 in any country, it may be more convenient to consider households as the sampling units and then to include all children under 5 from the selected households in the sample.

[8]In theory, simple random sampling is done with replacement of units after each draw. In practice, sampling is usually without replacement, and there should be a slight adjustment to the standard errors to correct for this (see, for example, Deaton [1997]).

- **Cluster sampling** A cluster is a naturally occurring unit or grouping within the population (e.g., enumeration areas). Cluster sampling entails randomly selecting a number of clusters and then including all or a random selection of units within the cluster. In multistage cluster sampling, further clusters are selected from within the first cluster. For example, enumeration areas may be the primary sampling unit, followed by households as secondary sampling units, and individuals as the final unit. Cluster sampling is useful because it reduces the informational requirement in the sampling process (a complete list of sampling units is required only for selected clusters) and because it can significantly reduce the costs of survey implementation. However, if there is a great deal of homogeneity within clusters, but heterogeneity between clusters, cluster sampling can substantially increase standard errors.
- **Unequal selection probabilities** In many surveys, different observations may have different probabilities of selection. This may be the consequence of stratification or other sample design decisions. In this case, it is necessary to weight each observation in the analysis to generate unbiased estimates of parameters of interest. The weights are equal (or proportional) to the inverse of the probability of being sampled. As a consequence, the weight for a specific observation can be interpreted as the number of elements in the population that the observation represents. In other words, if an element has a very small probability of selection relative to other elements, it should be weighted more heavily in the analysis.

The importance of taking sample design into account: an illustration

Many software packages have preprogrammed features for the analysis of complex survey data. That is the case, for example, with Stata, SPSS, and EpiInfo. For example, in Stata, survey commands can be used for descriptive analysis (e.g., svydes, svymean, svyprop, svytotal, svytab), estimation (e.g. svyreg, svyprobit, svylogit, svymlogit, svyoprobit, svypois), and postestimation testing (e.g., svytest).[9] Issues in the multivariate analysis of complex survey data are discussed in greater detail in chapter 10. Here, we simply illustrate the importance of taking sample design into account when making inferences about a population mean.

The following example is based on the 1997 Mozambique Living Standards and Measurement Survey. The survey sample was selected through a three-stage process, with stratification by province (11 provinces—the variable province) and area (urban/rural—urban), primary sampling at the locality level (locality), followed by sampling of households within each locality. Sampling weights are recorded in the variable wgt. In surveys in which samples are stratified along more than one dimension, a stratification variable (with a unique value for each strata) typically has to be constructed by the analyst. For example in the Mozambique data,

---

[9]For most Stata commands, adjustment for unequal sampling probabilities can be made by applying the weights option, for example, [pw=weight]. Standard errors can also be adjusted for cluster design by the option cluster(). Nonsurvey commands do not handle stratified sampling, however.

there are 21 separate strata (two strata (urban/rural) for each of the 11 provinces, except for Maputo City Province, which is only urban). This stratification variable can be easily constructed in Stata using the group function of the egen command.

```
egen strata = group(province urban)
```

We now have the three variables—wgt, strata, and locality—required to take sample design fully into account in the analysis. Here, we consider how child immunization rates, estimated from a dummy variable vacc indicating whether

Table 2.4 *Child Immunization Rates by Household Consumption Quintile, Mozambique, 1997*

Effect on Point Estimates and Standard Errors of Taking Sample Design into Account

A				B			
pweight: -				pweight: *wgt*			
strata: -				strata: -			
psu: -				psu: -			
Quintile	*Mean*	*s.e.*	*Deff*	*Quintile*	*Mean*	*s.e.*	*Deff*
Poorest	0.545	0.014	1.000	Poorest	0.531	0.017	1.694
2	0.659	0.014	1.000	2	0.629	0.019	2.196
3	0.708	0.013	1.000	3	0.621	0.019	2.117
4	0.805	0.011	1.000	4	0.708	0.024	3.416
Richest	0.892	0.008	1.000	Richest	0.843	0.014	1.488
Total	**0.728**	**0.006**	**1.000**	**Total**	**0.654**	**0.009**	**2.138**
n	6,447			*n*	6,447		
No. strata	1			*No. strata*	1		
No. PSUs	6,447			*No. PSUs*	6,447		

C				D			
pweight: *wgt*				pweight: *wgt*			
strata: *strata*				strata: *strata*			
psu: -				psu: *locality*			
Quintile	*Mean*	*s.e.*	*Deff*	*Quintile*	*Mean*	*s.e.*	*Deff*
Poorest	0.531	0.017	1.630	Poorest	0.531	0.028	4.469
2	0.629	0.019	2.164	2	0.629	0.033	6.577
3	0.621	0.019	2.075	3	0.621	0.026	4.014
4	0.708	0.024	3.366	4	0.708	0.029	5.092
Richest	0.843	0.014	1.456	Richest	0.843	0.018	2.485
Total	**0.654**	**0.008**	**1.942**	**Total**	**0.654**	**0.017**	**8.313**
n	6,447			*n*	6,447		
No. strata	21			*No. strata*	21		
No. PSUs	6,447			*No. PSUs*	273		

Source: Authors.

a child is immunized, vary across consumption quintiles (quint). Four different cases are considered:

A. sample design not taken into account

```
svyset
```

B. sample weights taken into account

```
svyset [pw=wgt]
```

C. sample weights and stratification taken into account

```
svyset [pw=wgt], strata(strata)
```

D. sample weights, stratification, and clustering taken into account

```
svyset locality [pw=wgt], strata(strata)
```

In each case, the svyset command is followed by

```
svy: mean vacc, over(quint)
```

As can be seen from table 2.4, the application of weights has a substantial impact on both point estimates and standard errors. In this application, taking stratification into account reduces the standard errors only slightly, whereas taking clustering into account increases the standard errors substantially. This illustrates that application of weights is not sufficient to correct for the sample design. It corrects the point estimates, but not the standard errors, confidence intervals, and test statistics.

These effects are described by the design effect (deff), which is a measure of how the survey design affects variance estimates. deff is calculated as the design-based variance estimate divided by an estimate of the variance that would have been obtained if a similar survey had been carried out using simple random sampling. It is obtained from the command estat effects following svy.

References

Deaton, A. 1997. *The Analysis of Household Surveys: A Microeconometric Approach to Development Policy.* Baltimore, MD: Published for the World Bank [by] Johns Hopkins University Press.

Grosh, M. E., P. Glewwe, and World Bank. 2000. *Designing Household Survey Questionnaires for Developing Countries : Lessons from 15 Years of the Living Standards Measurement Study.* Washington, DC: World Bank.

Murray, C., and L. Chen. 1992. "Understanding Morbidity Change." *Population and Development Review* 18(3): 481–503.

3

Health Outcome #1: Child Survival

Child mortality is a commonly used measure of average population health (International Monetary Fund et al. 2000; UNICEF 2001) and has been used in studies of the gaps in health outcomes between the poor and the better-off (Gwatkin et al. 2000; Wagstaff 2000). The infant mortality rate (IMR) is the number of deaths occurring in the first year of life per 1,000 live births and measures the probability of a child dying before the child's first birthday. The under-five mortality rate (U5MR) measures the probability of death before a child's fifth birthday. Although the IMR and U5MR can be estimated from vital registration statistics and demographic surveillance systems, these are not widely used in the developing world. In instances in which vital registration systems do exist, their comprehensiveness and reliability are often doubted. Furthermore, even where they exist, it is uncommon for any socioeconomic information to be recorded, making the analysis of socioeconomic inequalities in mortality impossible.

The alternative source of data on child mortality is a household survey. Estimating mortality rates from survey data involves the use of fertility histories. These are constructed from responses to questions posed to women of fertile age about births and deaths of children born to them. A complete fertility history uncovers the dates of birth, and if applicable the deaths, of all children born to the interviewed woman. An incomplete fertility history uncovers only the number of children born to the interviewed woman and the number still alive (or equivalently the number who have died).

Complete and incomplete fertility histories call for two different methods of mortality estimation, the direct method and the indirect method, respectively. Each method has advantages and disadvantages. The complete fertility history places greater informational demands on the survey and the interviewed woman, but generates more information and permits the estimation of standard errors for the mortality estimates. The incomplete history is less demanding in regard to information, but requires that the survey data be supplemented with data from a model life table, and it is not possible to compute standard errors for the mortality estimates.

This chapter describes how to compute mortality rates from household survey data by the direct and indirect methods using two statistical packages. It also explains how survey data can be used to undertake disaggregated mortality estimation, for example, across socioeconomic groups.

Complete fertility history and direct mortality estimation

The direct method of estimating child mortality involves taking the data from the complete fertility history and estimating a life table. This section outlines the steps involved and sets out the Stata code using a worked example from the 1998 Vietnam Living Standards Survey (VLSS) (Wagstaff and Nguyen 2003).

Preparing the data: example from the Living Standards Measurement Study

The complete fertility history allows a child-level data set to be assembled containing data for each child on the date of the mother's interview, the date of birth of the child, a binary variable indicating the child's status (alive or dead), and the survival time. Mortality estimation is based on deaths over a specific period of time—usually the 5 or 10 years before the survey date. It is useful therefore to have a variable indicating how old the child was at the interview date in the case of a still-living child and, in the case of a child who had died, how old the child would have been at the interview date if the child had still been alive at that time. This variable, called hypage below, allows one to easily select only those cases in which the child was born in the past 5 (or 10) years.

The first step is to generate the interview date—or more precisely the date the fertility history was collected. In a typical living standards measurement study (LSMS) survey (for Demographic and Health Surveys [DHS] see below) this date is recorded in the file preceding the household roster. In the first line of code below date2 is the variable recording the date the fertility history was collected. In this particular example it was recorded as a numeric variable in the form *ddmmyy*, where *dd* is the day, *mm* the month, and *yy* the last two digits of the year. The month, *mm*, is entered as two digits (e.g., April was entered as 04 rather than 4), but the day, *dd*, had no trailing zero (e.g., 1 April is entered as 104 rather than 0104). The first few commands generate three new numeric variables corresponding to the day, the month, and the year (in full—i.e., as 1997, rather than 97) when the fertility history was collected. The mdy function puts this into the date variable intrvdate2. The data are then sorted by household ID (househol), in anticipation of a merge with the fertility history data, and saved.

```
gen intrvdate = date2
tostring intrvdate
gen str2 year = substr(intrvdate,-2,.)
gen str2 mnth = substr(intrvdate,-4,.)
destring year , replace
replace year = 1900+year
destring mnth , replace
gen day = int(date2/10000)
gen intrvdate2 = mdy(mnth,day,year)
format %d intrvdate2
sort househol
save filename, replace
```

The next step is to generate each child's date of birth (dob) in the fertility history data file. In the commands below, s8aq05y denotes the last two digits of the year of birth of the child, s8aq05d is the day of the month the child was born, and s8aq05m is the month. In all fertility histories, there is the problem of what to do with cases in which some information in the date of birth is missing. One option is to drop such cases, but this reduces the sample size. Moreover, because it is likely that these cases are more often than not children who have died, dropping them will bias downward the estimated mortality rate. An alternative (the procedure adopted below) is to drop cases in which the year of birth is missing, but to replace missing months by 6 and missing days by 15. The mdy command creates a date variable corresponding to the dob.

```
gen yob = 1900+s8aq05y
gen daybrth = s8aq05d
replace daybrth = 15 if s8aq05d==.
gen mob = s8aq05m
replace mob = 6 if s8aq05m==.
gen dob = mdy(mob,daybrth,yob)
format %d dob
sort househol
```

Next the fertility history data (the open file, or master file) and the interview data (the using data set) are merged using merge, and variables that measure the child's hypothetical age in days (hypagedays) and years (hypageyrs) are computed.

```
merge househol using filename
gen hypagedays = intrvdate2 - dob
gen hypageyrs = hypagedays/365
```

The next step is to generate a status variable, dead, taking a value of 1 if the child has died and zero otherwise. In the commands below s8aq07 is the relevant question (Is child *x* still living with your household?), 1 being "yes", 2 being "no, living in another place," and 3 being "no, died."

```
gen dead =(s8aq07==3)
```

Finally, we need to generate a variable measuring the survival time. This is equal to the time elapsed since birth in the case of children who are still alive and equal to time between birth and death in the case of children who have died. In the 1998 VLSS, s8aq09t measures the survival time of children who have died, and s8aq09u indicates the units in which the survival time is measured (minutes, hours, days, weeks, months, quarters, half years, or years). Here we have computed two variables—timedays and timeyears.

```
gen timedays = hypagedays
replace timedays = s8aq09t/1440 if dead==1 & s8aq09u==1
replace timedays = s8aq09t/24 if dead==1 & s8aq09u==2
replace timedays = s8aq09t if dead==1 & s8aq09u==3
replace timedays = s8aq09t*7 if dead==1 & s8aq09u==4
replace timedays = s8aq09t*30.42 if dead==1 & s8aq09u==5
replace timedays = s8aq09t*91.25 if dead==1 & s8aq09u==6
replace timedays = s8aq09t*182.5 if dead==1 & s8aq09u==7
replace timedays = s8aq09t*365 if dead==1 & s8aq09u==8
gen timeyears = timedays / 365
```

Preparing the data: Demographic and Health Survey

The DHS uses a century month code (CMC) for some of its date variables. A CMC is the number of the month since the start of the century. For example, January 1900 is CMC 1; January 1901 is CMC 13. The variables needed for direct mortality estimation in DHS are

```
V008: date of interview (CMC)
B3: date of birth (CMC)
B7: age at death (month imputed)
B5: whether the child is still alive
```

The age at interview variable, hypage, can be calculated for children alive and children dead in Stata as follows:

```
gen hypage=(v008-b3)/12
```

Then, we can generate the surviving time (in years), timeyears, for each child in the survey and an indicator of whether the child is dead

```
gen timeyears=.
replace timeyears=hypage
replace timeyears=b7/12 if b5==0
gen dead=(b5==0)
```

Computing mortality rates and standard errors

The IMR and U5MR are computed using a life table, produced using the command ltable. The command below selects only those children born in the previous 10 years, including those born exactly 10 years ago. Stata allows one to specify the interval width, which can vary through the life table.[1] In the case below, a fixed half-yearly interval is used.

```
ltable timeyears dead if hypageyrs <=10 , int(.5) gr
```

Stata produces a life table along the lines of table 3.1. The lack of decimals in the intervals makes interpretation somewhat difficult—the first row refers to the first half-year of life, the second row to the second half-year of life, and so on. There were 5,316 children born during the previous 10 years, of whom 114 died during the first six months of life, and 194 were "lost" or censored—that is, they were born within six months of the interview date and were therefore not fully exposed to the risk of death. The assumption made in the life table is that these 194 children were exposed for only half of the interval—in this case three months rather than six. The total number of children exposed during the first six months is thus 5,316 less half of 194, or 5,219. The survival rate for the first six months is therefore (5,316 – 114) divided by 5,219, or 0.9782. The survival rate for each of the subsequent half-years is computed in the same way, and from these the cumulative survival function (labeled simply "survival" in table 3.1) is formed. The IMR is the complement of the cumulative survival function at the end of the first year—that is, 1 – 0.9752, or equivalently 24.8 per 1,000 live births. The U5MR is equal to 1 – 0.9642, or 35.8

---

[1]For example, one could divide the first year into months using int(0.08333, 0.1666, …, 0.9167, 1.5, 2, 2.5, …, 10).

Table 3.1 *Life Table, Vietnam, 1988–98*

Interval		Total	Deaths	Lost	Survival	Error	[95% Conf. Int.]	
0	1	5316	114	194	0.9782	0.0020	0.9738	0.9818
1	1	5008	15	161	0.9752	0.0022	0.9706	0.9791
1	2	4832	12	176	0.9727	0.0023	0.9679	0.9768
2	2	4644	4	190	0.9719	0.0023	0.9670	0.9760
2	3	4450	15	198	0.9685	0.0025	0.9633	0.9730
3	3	4237	0	188	0.9685	0.0025	0.9633	0.9730
3	4	4049	13	227	0.9653	0.0026	0.9598	0.9701
4	4	3809	0	227	0.9653	0.0026	0.9598	0.9701
4	5	3582	4	231	0.9642	0.0027	0.9586	0.9690
5	5	3347	0	284	0.9642	0.0027	0.9586	0.9690
5	6	3063	7	314	0.9619	0.0028	0.9560	0.9670
6	6	2742	0	262	0.9619	0.0028	0.9560	0.9670
6	7	2480	3	263	0.9606	0.0029	0.9546	0.9659
7	7	2214	0	288	0.9606	0.0029	0.9546	0.9659
7	8	1926	3	297	0.9590	0.0030	0.9527	0.9645
8	8	1626	0	323	0.9590	0.0030	0.9527	0.9645
8	9	1303	0	331	0.9590	0.0030	0.9527	0.9645
9	9	972	0	349	0.9590	0.0030	0.9527	0.9645
9	10	623	1	298	0.9570	0.0036	0.9493	0.9636
10	10	324	0	323	0.9570	0.0036	0.9493	0.9636
10	11	1	0	1	0.9570	0.0036	0.9493	0.9636

Source: Authors.

per 1,000. Stata also produces standard errors for the cumulative survival function, which are the standard errors for the IMR and U5MR. For example, the standard error for the IMR is 2.2 per 1,000, or 8.9 percent of the IMR (known in this form as the relative standard error). Figure 3.1 is the chart produced by the gr option in the ltable command above—it shows the cumulative survival function and the 95 percent confidence intervals around the point estimates.

Disaggregated analysis and sample weights

Disaggregated analysis—e.g., mortality rates for different wealth groups—is easily undertaken simply by adding to the ltable command a by(*variable name*) option. This produces as many life tables as there are categories in the stratifying variable.

Sampling weights cannot be used with ltable. Weighted samples can be handled using Stata's st commands. When the data are declared to be survival data with the stset command, pweights can be specified. The sts list command can be used to generate the life table from which the IMR and U5MR can be read.[2]

---

[2]For a brief discussion of the difference between ltable and sts list, see http://www.stata.com/support/faqs/stat/ltable.html.

Figure 3.1 *Survival Function with 95 Percent Confidence Intervals, Vietnam, 1988–98*

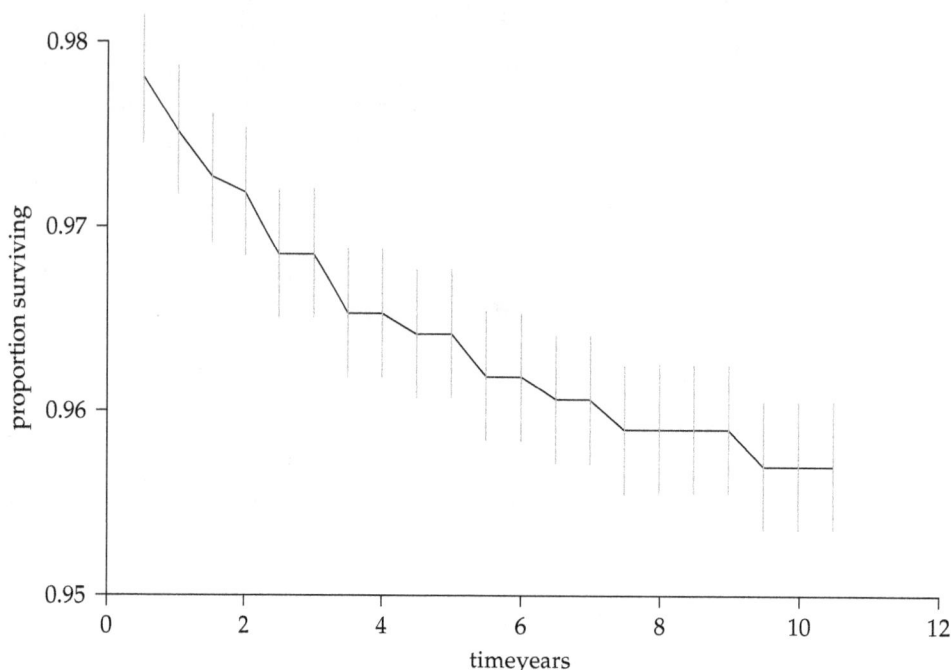

Source: Authors.

Incomplete fertility history and indirect mortality estimation

The incomplete fertility history necessitates the use of the indirect method of mortality estimation (United Nations 1983). This involves superimposing a model life table on data from the incomplete fertility history identifying (i) the number of children born to each woman and (ii) the number surviving. Computation can be done using the DOS program QFIVE (United Nations 1983). This section outlines the steps involved using a worked example based on the 1993 South Africa LSMS (Wagstaff 2000).

Preparing the data for QFIVE

QFIVE requires data for each of seven age groups on (i) the number of women in the sample, (ii) the number of children born, and (iii) the number of children surviving. The age groups are: 15–19, 20–24, 25–29, 30–34, 35–39, 40–44, and 45–49. These summary data can be computed in Stata, but then need to be placed into a text file that can be read into QFIVE. Typically, the age of the women from whom the fertility history is collected is not recorded in the fertility module but needs to be merged from the household roster. The first step is to sort the household roster by the individual ID. In the commands immediately below `filename` is the name of the household roster file; `hhid` is the household ID, and `pcode` is the personal ID in the household.

```
use filename
sort hhid pcode
save filename , replace
```

The next step is to merge the age data from the household roster into the fertility data file. In the use command below `filename` is the name of the fertility data file; in the `merge` command `filename` is the name of the household roster data file. The cases from the household roster for which there are no fertility histories (men, children, and women not interviewed) are dropped using the keep command. Cases outside the seven age categories used in QFIVE are dropped, as are any men inexplicably left in the data file.

```
clear
use filename
sort hhid pcode
merge hhid pcode using filename
keep if _merge==3
gen agecat=age
recode agecat 0/14=0 15/19=1 20/24=2 25/29=3 30/34=4 35/39=5
40/44=6 45/49=7 50/max=8
drop if agecat<1
drop if agecat>7
drop if gender_n ~=2
```

In the South Africa LSMS, women reporting no pregnancies are assigned a value of –2 for the number of births, no_birth, and for the number of children alive, no_alive. These are recoded zero. The tabstat commands then summarize, for each age group, the number of women, the number of children born, and the number of children alive.

```
gen numbrths = no_birth
recode numbrths -2=0
gen numalive = no_alive
recode numalive -2=0
tabstat numbrths numalive , by(agecat) stats(co)
tabstat numbrths numalive , by(agecat) stats(su)
```

The results then need to be inserted into a text file. This can be done manually or by pasting the Stata output into Microsoft Excel, transposing the data (using Paste Special), and copying the transposed data into Microsoft Word. The file needs to be saved as text (txt) file and set out along the lines indicated below. The first row of numbers represents the number of births in each age category, the second the number of children surviving, and the third the number of women. The spacing between the numbers is crucial. It is easiest to check the tab characters and spaces boxes on the View menu under the Tools Options menu in Word, replace the tabs with spaces, and manually line up the numbers by inserting the appropriate number of spaces. Some trial and error is inevitable here, and it is essential to check that QFIVE is reading the data correctly. The "6" in the first line refers to the month in which the data were collected; "1993" is the year; "3" indicates both boys and girls; and "1" indicates that the data refer to the number of women, the number of children born, and the number of children surviving.

Input text file for QFIVE

```
S Africa
 6 1993 3     1
           312    1608    2841    3948    4294    4391    3734
           290    1469    2554    3490    3744    3794    3186
          2034    2063    1683    1479    1250    1099     853
```

Obtaining and interpreting output from QFIVE

Select option 1 (Enter or modify input data) in QFIVE, read in the data, and check that they are being read correctly (use PageDown to see the data). Then select option 2 (Run Q5), and ask for the data to be directed to the printer, screen, or file, as desired. If the latter option is selected, the output needs reformatting to be legible: read the output file into Microsoft Word (select Plain Text as encoding if prompted), select the entire file (Ctl-A), choose a size 8 font, select landscape as the orientation from Page Setup, and select Page Width as the zoom level. This will allow the output to be viewed without wrapping on both screen and paper.

In its output, QFIVE first reproduces the input data (see table 3.2). Then it produces estimates of the IMR, U5MR, and child mortality (mortality between the ages of 1 and 5). It produces separate estimates for each age group and for each of eight different model life tables. The four shown in table 3.3 are based on the popular Coale-Demeny life tables.[3] The estimates indicate how mortality rates vary with the age of the cohort—mostly rates are higher the older the cohort. QFIVE indicates the estimated date to which the mortality rate refers, so the estimated rates for different years (see figure 3.2) can be reported (and graphed). Or an average over cohorts can be calculated. If this is done, it is usual to ignore the rates for the two youngest and two oldest age groups on the grounds that they reflect births to young women who are unrepresentative and births that took place more than 10 years before the survey. One option is to take a simple average of the rates occurring in the age groups 25–29, 30–34, and 35–39, though sometimes it may make sense to include at least the rate for the 20–24 age group as well. If the latter group is ignored, the results in

Table 3.2 *QFIVE's Reproduction of Input Data for South Africa*

INPUT DATA FOR S Africa

BOTH SEXES

ENUMERATION DATE: JUN 1993

Age Group of Women	Number of Women	Number of Children Ever Born	Number of Children Surviving
15–19	2034.	312.	290.
20–24	2063.	1608.	1469.
25–29	1683.	2841.	2554.
30–34	1479.	3948.	3490.
35–39	1250.	4294.	3744.
40–44	1099.	4391.	3794.
45–49	853.	3734.	3186.

MEAN AGE AT MATERNITY WAS NOT GIVEN. THE DEFAULT VALUE OF 27.0 WILL BE USED.

Source: Authors.

---

[3] QFIVE also produces mortality rates for the UN's own life tables; the results are not shown here.

Table 3.3 *Indirect Estimates of Child Mortality, South Africa*

COALE-DEMENY:	NORTH			SOUTH			EAST			WEST	
AGE OF WOMAN	REFERENCE DATE	q		REFERENCE DATE	q		REFERENCE DATE	q		REFERENCE DATE	q
INFANT MORTALITY RATE: q(1)											
15–19	1992.2	.065		1992.2	.063		1992.2	.070		1992.2	.068
20–24	1991.0	.069		1991.0	.076		1990.9	.079		1990.9	.075
25–29	1989.3	.071		1989.2	.081		1989.1	.085		1989.2	.079
30–34	1987.4	.074		1987.2	.087		1987.0	.092		1987.1	.084
35–39	1985.2	.075		1984.9	.091		1984.7	.097		1984.9	.086
40–44	1982.8	.073		1982.3	.092		1982.1	.097		1982.4	.085
45–49	1980.0	.071		1979.2	.092		1978.9	.097		1979.5	.084
PROBABILITY OF DYING BETWEEN AGES 1 AND 5: $_4q_1$											
15–19	1992.2	.039		1992.2	.018		1992.2	.018		1992.2	.027
20–24	1991.0	.042		1991.0	.026		1990.9	.022		1990.9	.031
25–29	1989.3	.043		1989.2	.031		1989.1	.025		1989.2	.034
30–34	1987.4	.046		1987.2	.036		1987.0	.029		1987.1	.038
35–39	1985.2	.047		1984.9	.040		1984.7	.031		1984.9	.039
40–44	1982.8	.045		1982.3	.041		1982.1	.031		1982.4	.039
45–49	1980.0	.043		1979.2	.041		1978.9	.031		1979.5	.038
PROBABILITY OF DYING BY AGE 5: q(5)											
15–19	1992.2	.101		1992.2	.079		1992.2	.086		1992.2	.093
20–24	1991.0	.108		1991.0	.100		1990.9	.099		1990.9	.104
25–29	1989.3	.111		1989.2	.109		1989.1	.108		1989.2	.110
30–34	1987.4	.116		1987.2	.120		1987.0	.118		1987.1	.118
35–39	1985.2	.119		1984.9	.128		1984.7	.124		1984.9	.122
40–44	1982.8	.115		1982.3	.128		1982.1	.125		1982.4	.121
45–49	1980.0	.112		1979.2	.130		1978.9	.125		1979.5	.119

NOTE: A q VALUE OF .999 DENOTES VALUE BELOW A LEVEL 1 MODEL LIFE TABLE.
 "   .000   "   ABOVE A LEVEL 25   "

Source: Authors.

table 3.3 point toward a U5MR for South Africa of 115–119 per 1,000 for 1987. Hill and Yazbeck (1994) and Hill et al. (1999) provide guidance for a large number of developing countries on which one of the Coale-Demeny life tables is most appropriate. In this case, if the North model is used, a U5MR (for 1987) of 115 per 1,000 is obtained.

Disaggregated analysis—for example, mortality rates for different wealth groups—is easily undertaken by computing the necessary input data for QFIVE separately for each subgroup. Sample weights can be handled by specifying the sample weighting scheme when obtaining the data in Stata for the QFIVE input.

Figure 3.2 *Indirect Estimates of U5MR, South Africa*

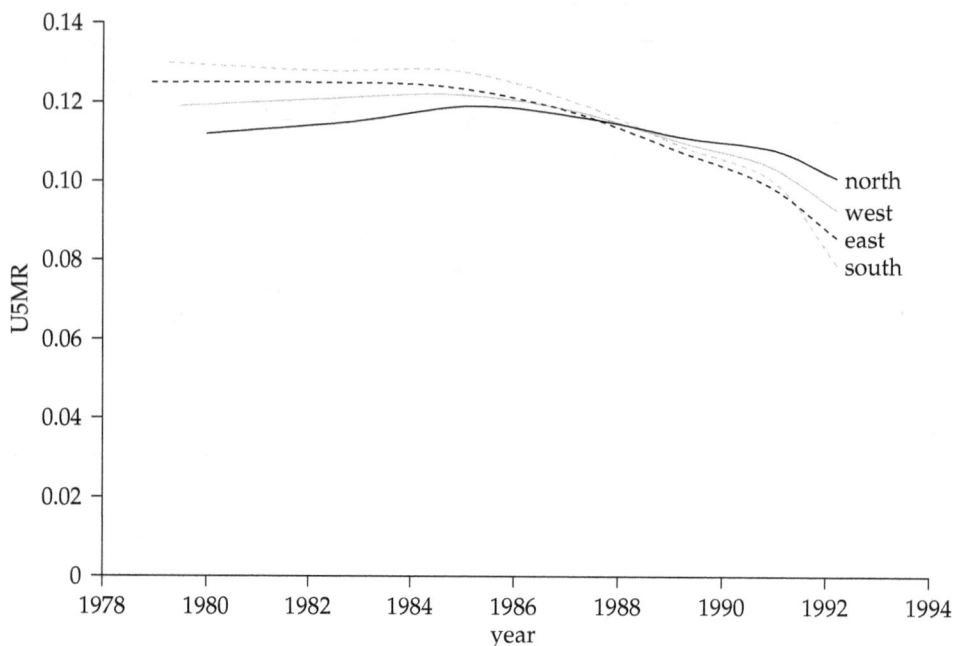

Source: Authors.

References

Gwatkin, D. R., S. Rustein, K. Johnson, R. Pande, and A. Wagstaff. 2000. "Socioeconomic Differences in Health, Nutrition and Population." World Bank Health, Nutrition and Population discussion paper. World Bank, Washington, DC.

Hill, K., and A. Yazbeck. 1994. "Trends in Child Mortality, 1960–90: Estimates for 84 Developing Countries." World Development Report 1993, Background Paper No. 6. World Bank, Washington, DC.

Hill, K., R. Pande, M. Mahy, and G. Jones. 1999. *Trends in Child Mortality in the Developing World: 1960 to 1996.* New York: UNICEF.

International Monetary Fund, OECD, United Nations, and World Bank. 2000. *A Better World for All: Progress Towards the International Development Goals.* Washington, DC: International Monetary Fund, OECD, United Nations, and the World Bank.

UNICEF. 2001. *Progress Since the World Summit for Children: A Statistical Review.* New York: UNICEF.

United Nations. 1983. *Indirect Techniques for Demographic Estimation.* New York: United Nations.

Wagstaff, A. 2000. Socioeconomic Inequalities in Child Mortality: Comparisons across Nine Developing Countries. *Bulletin of the World Health Organization* 78(1): 19–29.

Wagstaff, A., and N. N. Nguyen. 2003. "Poverty and Survival Prospects of Vietnamese Children under Doi Moi." In *Economic Growth, Poverty and Household Welfare: Policy Lessons from Vietnam,* ed. P. Glewwe, N. Agrawal, and D. Dollar. Washington, DC: World Bank.

4

Health Outcome #2: Anthropometrics

Malnutrition remains a widespread problem in developing countries, in particular among the poorest and most vulnerable segments of the population. Typically, malnutrition is caused by a combination of inadequate food intake and infection that impairs the body's ability to absorb or assimilate food. It is an important cause of low birth weight, brain damage, and other birth defects and contributes to developmental (physical and cognitive) retardation, increased risk of infection and death, and other problems in infants and children.

One approach to studying nutrition is to assess nutritional status on the basis of anthropometric indicators. These are based on physical body measurements such as height or weight (related to the age and sex) and have the benefit of being both inexpensive and nonintrusive to collect. Nutritional status can be seen as the output of a health production function in which nutrient intake is one input, but in which other individual, household, and community variables also feature.

Anthropometric indicators are useful both at an individual and at a population level. At an individual level, anthropometric indicators can be used to assess compromised health or nutrition well-being. This information can be valuable for screening children for interventions and for assessing the response to interventions. At the population level, anthropometry can be used to assess the nutrition status within a country, region, community, or socioeconomic group and to study both the determinants and the consequences of malnutrition. This form of monitoring is valuable for both the design and the targeting of health and nutrition interventions.

This chapter discusses the construction, interpretation, and use of anthropometric indicators, with an emphasis on infants and children. The first section provides an overview of anthropometric indicators. The second discusses practical and conceptual issues in constructing anthropometric indicators from physical measurements and illustrates these issues with examples based on household data from Mozambique. Finally, the third section highlights some key issues and approaches to analyzing anthropometric data.

Overview of anthropometric indicators

Survey data often contain measures of weight and height, in particular for children. Weight and height do not indicate malnutrition directly. Besides age and sex, they are affected by many intervening factors other than nutrient intake, in particular genetic variation. However, even in the presence of such natural variation, it is possible to use physical measurements to assess the adequacy of diet and growth, in particular in infants and children. This is done by comparing indicators with the distribution of the same indicator for a "healthy" reference group and identifying "extreme" or "abnormal" departures from this distribution. For example, three of the most commonly used anthropometric indicators for infants and children—weight-for-height, height-for-age, and weight-for-age—can be constructed by comparing indicators based on weight, height, age, and gender with reference data for "healthy" children (Alderman 2000; World Health Organization 1995).[1]

Weight-for-height

Weight-for-height (W/H) measures body weight relative to height and has the advantage of not requiring age data. Normally, W/H is used as an indicator of current nutritional status and can be useful for screening children at risk and for measuring short-term changes in nutritional status. At the other end of the spectrum, W/H can also be used to construct indicators of obesity. Low W/H relative to a child of the same sex and age in a reference population is referred to as "thinness." Extreme cases of low W/H are commonly referred to as "wasting." Wasting may be the consequence of starvation or severe disease (in particular, diarrhea). Low W/H can also be due to chronic conditions, although height-for-age is a better indicator for monitoring such problems. It is important to note that a lack of evidence of wasting in a population does not imply the absence of current nutritional problems such as low height-for-age.

Height-for-age

Height-for-age (H/A) reflects cumulative linear growth. H/A deficits indicate past or chronic inadequacies of nutrition and/or chronic or frequent illness, but cannot measure short-term changes in malnutrition. Low H/A relative to a child of the same sex and age in the reference population is referred to as "shortness." Extreme cases of low H/A, in which shortness is interpreted as pathological, are referred to as "stunting." H/A is used primarily as a population indicator rather than for individual growth monitoring.

Weight-for-age

Weight-for-age (W/A) reflects body mass relative to age. W/A is, in effect, a composite measure of height-for-age and weight-for-height, making interpretation difficult. Low W/A relative to a child of the same sex and age in the reference population is

---

[1] In what follows, we do not distinguish between indexes and indicators. In principle, however, there are important conceptual differences. An index is simply a combination of different measurements. In contrast, an indicator relates to the use or application of an index to measure (or indicate) a specific phenomenon or outcome. For example, typically, anthropometric indexes are used as indicators for nutritional status. However, the extent to which the anthropometric index is an appropriate indicator depends on the nature of the relationship between nutrition and the index in question (formally, the sensitivity and specificity of the indicator). For a more detailed discussion, see WHO (1995).

referred to as "lightness," whereas the term "underweight" is commonly used to refer to severe or pathological deficits in W/A. W/A is commonly used for monitoring growth and to assess changes in the magnitude of malnutrition over time. However, W/A confounds the effects of short- and long-term health and nutrition problems.

Standardization on a reference population

As noted, the construction of anthropometric indicators is based on comparisons with a "healthy" reference population. For a long time, the international reference standard that was most commonly used (and recommended by the World Health Organization [WHO]) was based on data on weight and height from a statistically valid sample of infants and children in the United States.[2] The validity of this reference standard stems from the empirical observation that well-nourished and healthy children will have a distribution of height and weight very similar to the U.S. reference population, regardless of their ethnic background or where they live (Habicht et al. 1974). In other words, although there are some differences in growth patterns across ethnic groups, the largest part of worldwide variation in anthropometric indicators can be attributed to differences in socioeconomic factors.

Notwithstanding this empirical regularity, there is a long-standing debate about the appropriateness of the U.S. reference standard for children in developing countries, in particular concerning the extent to which growth paths will depend on feeding practices. Reflecting these concerns, in 1993 the WHO undertook a comprehensive review of the uses and interpretation of anthropometric references, concluding that the National Center for Health Statistics (NCHS)/WHO growth reference did not adequately represent early childhood growth. Since then, a multicenter growth reference study has been undertaken to develop new growth curves for assessing the growth and development of children, and in April 2006, the WHO issued new standards for children from birth to five years of age (WHO 2006).[3] These new standards capture the growth and development process of children from widely diverse ethnic backgrounds and cultural settings, with mothers engaged in fundamental health-promoting practices (breastfeeding and not smoking).[4] The new growth standards have been shown to have important implications for the monitoring and assessment of child growth and development (de Onis et al. 2006). Nonetheless, the new standards have not yet been routinely incorporated in standard statistical packages. For this reason, the empirical illustrations used in this chapter are not based on the new reference data.[5]

---

[2]This is referred to as the U.S. National Center for Health Statistics (NCHS) reference group. Reference standards are available for children and adolescents up to 16 years of age, but are most accurate for children up to the age of 10.

[3]For a detailed discussion of the rationale, implementation, and findings from this work, see de Onis et al. (2004, 2006) and Garza and de Onis (2004).

[4]Some of the differences between the NCHS/WHO and the new WHO growth reference are also due to the methodologies applied to construct the two sets of growth curves, in particular in the treatment of skewed or kurtotic distributions.

[5]Currently, only the software package ANTRHO has incorporated the new standards. Further details on software packages for anthropometric analysis are provided later in this chapter.

Regardless of what particular reference data are used, anthropometric indices are constructed by comparing relevant measures with those of comparable individuals (in regard to age and sex) in the reference populations. There are three ways of expressing these comparisons:

a. *z-score (standard deviation score):* the difference between the value for an individual and the median value of the reference population for the same sex and age (or height), divided by the standard deviation of the reference population.

b. *Percent of median:* ratio of measured value for an individual to the median value of the reference data for the same sex and age (or height).

c. *Percentile:* rank position of an individual on a given reference distribution, stated in regard to what percentage of the group the individual equals or exceeds.

Box 4.1 *Example Computation of Anthropometric Indices*

For example, consider a 12-month-old girl who weighs 9.1 kg. On the basis of the reference standard weight-for-age for girls, it can be established that the median weight for healthy girls of this age is 9.5 and that the standard deviation in the reference population is 1.0. On this basis, the following calculation can be made:

$$\text{z-score}\,(W/A) = \frac{9.1 - 9.5}{1} = -0.4$$

$$\text{Percent of median}\,(W/A) = \left(\frac{9.1}{9.5}\right) = 95.8\%$$

On the basis of aggregated tables, we can establish only that 9.1 falls between the 30th and 40th percentile.

Source: Authors.

The preferred and most common way of expressing anthropometric indices is in the form of z-scores. That approach has a number of advantages. Most important, z-scores can be used to estimate summary statistics (e.g., mean and standard deviation) for the population or subpopulations. This cannot be meaningfully done with percentiles. Moreover, at the extreme of the distribution, large changes in height or weight are not necessarily reflected in changes in percentile values. The percent of median is deficient relative to the z-score in that it expresses deviation from the reference median without standardizing for the variability in the reference population.

What criterion do we use to determine whether an individual is malnourished or not? Using z-scores, the most commonly used cutoff to define abnormal anthropometry is a value of –2, that is, two standard deviations below the reference median, irrespective of the indicator used.[6] For example, a child whose height-for-age z-score is less than –2 is considered stunted. This provides the basis for estimating prevalence of malnutrition in populations or subpopulations (see table 4.1).[7] The WHO has also proposed a classification scheme for population-level malnutrition.

---

[6] Using this criterion, approximately 2.3 percent of "healthy" children would be classified as having an abnormal deficit in any particular anthropometric indicator.

[7] WHO has also proposed a more general malnutrition classification that distinguishes between mild (z-score ≤1), moderate (z-score ≤2), and severe malnutrition (z-score ≤3).

Table 4.1 WHO Classification Scheme for Degree of Population Malnutrition

Degree of malnutrition	Prevalence of malnutrition (% of children <60 months, below −2 z-scores)	
	W/A and H/A	W/H
Low	<10	<5
Medium	10–19	5–9
High	20–29	10–14
Very high	≥30	≥15

Source: WHO 1995.

Other anthropometric indicators

Although weight-for-height, height-for-age, and weight-for-age are the most commonly used anthropometric indicators for infants and children, they are by no means the only ones that have been used.[8]

MID-UPPER ARM CIRCUMFERENCE   Mid-upper arm circumference (MUAC) is a measure of the diameter of the upper arm and gauges both fat reserves and muscle mass. It is used primarily for children, but can also be applied to pregnant women to assess nutritional status. Measurement is simple and requires minimal equipment. MUAC has therefore been proposed as an alternative index of nutritional status, in particular in situations in which data on height, weight, and age are difficult to collect. For children, a fixed (age-independent) cutoff point has sometimes been used to determine malnutrition. However, this risks overdiagnosing young children and underdiagnosing older children. Reference data based on U.S. children 6 to 60 months of age have been incorporated in recent versions of some anthropometric software packages.

BODY MASS INDEX   Body mass index (BMI) is a measure used to define overweight and thinness. BMI is defined as the weight in kilos divided by the square of height in meters. In developing countries, the BMI is used primarily with age-independent cutoffs to identify chronic energy deficiencies (or obesity) in adults (see table 4.2). Although there is some scope for using BMI for adolescents, the index

Table 4.2 BMI Cutoffs for Adults over 20 (proposed by WHO expert committee)

BMI range	Diagnosis
<16	Underweight (grade 3 thinness)
16–16.99	Underweight (grade 2 thinness)
17–18.49	Underweight (grade 1 thinness)
18.5–24.99	Normal range
25.0–29.99	Overweight (preobese)
>30	Obese

Source: Authors.

---

[8]For further discussion of alternative anthropometric indicators, including indicators for adolescents and adults, see WHO (1995).

Figure 4.1 *BMI for Adults in Vietnam, 1998*

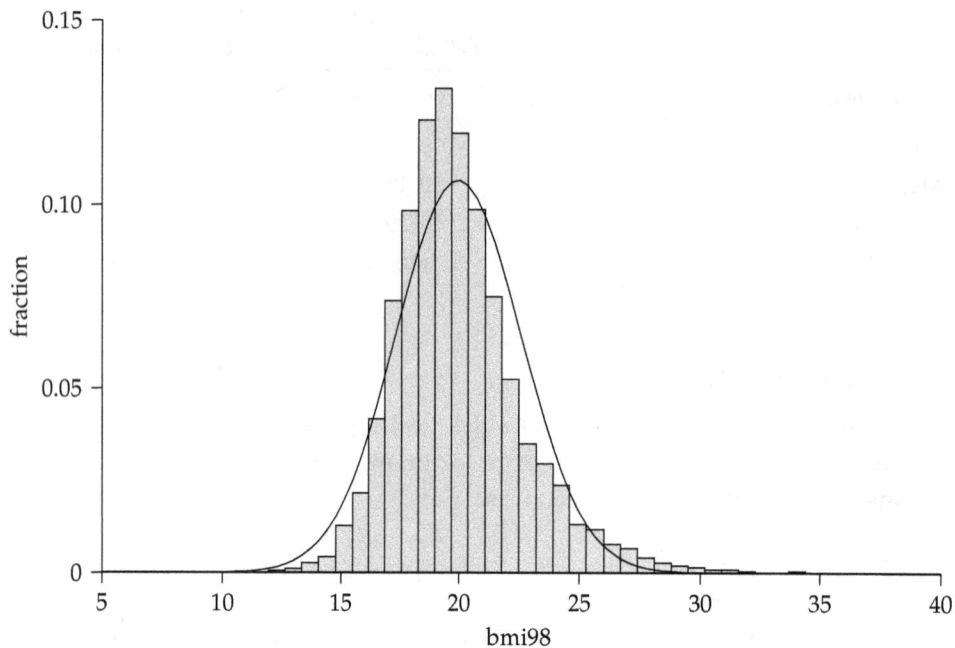

Source: Authors.

varies with age for children and teenagers and must therefore be interpreted in relation to BMI-for-age reference charts.

The incidence of overweight and obesity is a growing problem in many developing countries. In some regions of the world, in particular South and East Asia, prevalence remains relatively low. For example, in figure 4.1, a histogram of BMI for adults (over 20 years of age) in Vietnam illustrates that although nearly 45 percent of individuals are underweight, overweight and obesity are rare (less than 4 percent). However, in other regions of the world, the prevalence of overweight and obesity is high and rising.

Computation of anthropometric indicators

Anthropometric indicators can be computed either by using dedicated anthropometric software, which contains the relevant reference data and has easy procedures for constructing the indicators of interest, or by using a Stata add-in called zanthro.[9] This section provides a brief overview of the most popular anthropometric software packages and a step-by-step guide to either using one of them (EPI-INFO) or using Stata to compute indicators.

Software for anthropometric analysis

At the simplest level, anthropometric software uses raw measurement data in combination with reference data to calculate the corresponding anthropometric indicators. Many of the available software packages also have more advanced functions,

---

[9] zanthro is an ado-file developed by Suzanna Vidmar and Tim Cole. It can be installed in Stata be typing webseek zanthro and following the instructions.

including statistical and graphical analysis. The two most popular software packages for anthropometric analysis are ANTHRO and EPI-INFO. Both can be downloaded without charge.

ANTHRO is a program that can be used to compare the growth of individual children with the growth patterns of the new 2006 WHO growth standards. It requires the sex, height, weight, and age of children to calculate normalized anthropometric z-values, percentiles, and percent-of-median. It can use dBase files for batch processing and has an anthropometric calculator. Recently, beta-versions of macros (`igrowup`) based on ANTHRO have been released for Stata and other statistical software.[10]

EPI INFO is a series of programs for Microsoft Windows. It contains a special-purpose module called NutStat, which can be used to compare data on height, weight, age, sex, and arm circumference with the international reference standards. The program calculates percentiles, z-scores and, depending on the reference data used, percent of median. EPI-INFO uses the Microsoft Access file format as a database standard, but many other file types can be analyzed, imported, or exported.[11]

From physical measurement to anthropometric indicators: a step-by-step guide using EPI INFO

One way to calculate z-scores for anthropometric analysis is to use dedicated software. Broadly speaking, this entails four steps: (i) setting up the data in a general statistical package, (ii) reading and processing the data in the anthropometrics package, (iii) reexporting the constructed variables to the general statistical package, and (iv) performing basic data cleaning. Each of these steps is described below for transitions between Stata and EPI-INFO, with an illustration based on data from a living standards survey from Mozambique.[12]

1. Preparing data for loading into EPI-INFO

The variables that must be loaded into EPI-INFO for the computation of anthropometric indicators depend on the indicators desired and also to some extent on the reference data that are used in the analysis (see table 4.3). The data do not need to contain all the listed fields.

There are a couple of important points to note in relation to the variables used in EPI-INFO. First, for many anthropometric indicators, age-specific reference data are used. When the data permit it, it is always preferable to calculate age as the difference between date of measurement and date of birth. This is almost always more

---

[10]ANTHRO program files and supporting documentation can be downloaded from http://www.who.int/childgrowth/software/en/.

[11]EPI-INFO programs, documentation, and teaching materials can be downloaded from http://www.cdc.gov/epiinfo/index.htm. EPI-INFO is a CDC trademark, but may be freely copied, distributed, or translated.

[12]The 1996/97 Mozambique National Household Survey on Living Conditions (*Inquérito Nacional aos Agregados Familiares Sobre as Condições de Vida*) was designed and implemented by the National Statistics Institute in Mozambique and was conducted from February 1996 to April 1997. The sample covers approximately 43,000 individuals in 8,250 households. It was selected in three stages and is geographically stratified to ensure representativeness at the provincial level and for urban/rural areas.

Table 4.3 *Variables That Can Be Used in EPI-INFO*

Variable	Description and required format
Sex	1 or M for male, 2 or F for female
Age	Months or years
Birth date	Not necessary if age data are available
Date of measurement	Not necessary if age data are available
ID number	Unique individual identifier
First name	
Last name	
Height	In centimeters or inches
Recumbent	Boolean or 1/2; whether child is lying down
Weight	In kilos or pounds
Edema[13]	Boolean or 1/2; excessive amounts of fluid
Arm circumference	In centimeters or inches
Head circumference	In centimeters or inches
Notes	

Source: Authors.

accurate than age reported by survey respondents. The reference curves are based on "biologic" age rather than calendar age. Biologic age in months divides the year into 12 equal segments as opposed to calendar age in which months have from 28 to 31 days. Although this makes little difference in older children, it can have an effect on the anthropometric calculations for infants. Moreover, entering age by rounding to the nearest month and/or the most recently attained month can have a substantial effect on the anthropometric calculations, especially for infants. To calculate biologic age, anthropometric software calculates the number of days between the two dates. The age in days is divided by 365.25 and then multiplied by 12.

Second, for younger children, normally height is measured with the child in a recumbent position. This measurement is sometimes referred to as "length," which is contrasted with standing height measurements, referred to as "stature."[14] In some cases, this distinction is not important from the point of view of the analyst. For example, when the recommended 1978 CDC/WHO reference in EPI-INFO is used, recumbent length is assumed from birth to age 24 months, and standing height for 24 months and older. However, in EPI-INFO it is also possible to use a 2000 CDC reference standard. If this option is chosen, the user must indicate whether the measurements are recumbent length or standing height for children in the age group of

---

[13]Edema refers to the presence of excessive amounts of fluid in the intracellular tissue. There is a strong association between edema and mortality. The presence of edema is therefore important for screening and surveillance purposes and can be used to flag children as severely malnourished, independently of their wasting, stunting, or underweight status. However, although edema is included as a variable in many anthropometric software programs for that reason, it is not generally used for evaluation purposes.

[14]For details on measurement, see WHO (1995) or http://www.cdc.gov/nccdphp/dnpa/bmi/meas-height.htm.

24 to 36 months (for younger and older children, recumbent and standing measurements are assumed, respectively).

Turning to the Mozambique illustration, the first step is to construct a data set with all the relevant variables in the appropriate format. In this case, we have data on the birth date, measurement date, sex, weight, and height of children under five years old. In the following code, the dates are used to construct the age in months and, before the relevant variables are saved in a new data file, weight is adjusted to account for the fact that a minority of children were weighed with their clothes on. At this stage it is also important to ensure that all variables are appropriately coded and in the correct units (see table 4.3).

```
generate birthdate = mdy(birth_mnth, birth_day, birth_yr)
generate measuredate = mdy(visit_mnth, visit_day, visit_year)
generate age_days = measuredate - birthdate
generate age_months = (age_days/365.25) * 12

replace weight_grams = weight_grams - weight_cloth if how_
weighed==1
generate weight_kilos = weight_grams / 1000
keep id sexo age_months weight_kilos height_cm
drop if sexo==. | age_months==. | weight_kilos==. | height_
cm==.
save filename, replace
```

2. Reading and processing the data in EPI-INFO

The NutStat module of EPI-INFO uses data in Access database format.[15] There are two ways of importing external data into NutStat. The Add Statistics feature simply processes the data from a Microsoft Access data file and adds the results of calculations to the file. In contrast, the Import Data feature can be used to import data from an existing table into a new table that has the data structure required by Nutstat. The table can be an EPI-INFO table or a table from Microsoft Access. Both the Add Statistics and Import Data features can be accessed from the File menu. Under either alternative, the user is first required to choose between the two alternative reference standards (1978 CDC/WHO or 2000 CDC). The user must thereafter link variables in the imported data file with fields that EPI-INFO requires to calculate the anthropometric indicators and, for some fields, select the unit of measurement. Finally, the user selects the statistics or indicators to calculate—for example, z-scores, percentiles, and percent of median for W/A, H/A, and W/H.[16] The selection of indicators to be calculated is restricted by the variables that were imported. When the data are then processed, the new variables are either added to the original file (Add Statistics option) or saved in a new data file (Import option) (see table 4.4).

---

[15]Stata or SPSS data can be converted into Access format using conversion software such as DMBScopy or StatTransfer. Alternatively, data can be exported from Stata using the outsheet command, which can then be read into Access. It is also possible to copy data from the Stata browser and paste it in Access.

[16]Further anthropometric indicators can be calculated on the basis of specific WHO reference data (MUAC-for-age) or 2000 CDC reference (head circumference-for-age and BMI-for-age).

Table 4.4 Key Variables Calculated by EPI-INFO

Anthropometric indicator	Variable names 1978 CDC/WHO reference	Variable names 2000 CDC reference[a]
H/A z-score	fldWHOHAZ	fldCDCLAZ, fldCDCSAZ
H/A centile	fldWHOHAC	fldCDCLAC, fldCDCSAC
H/A percent of median	fldWHOHAPM	
W/A z-score	fldWHOWAZ	fldCDCWAZ
W/A centile	fldWHOWAC	fldCDCWAC
W/A percent of median	fldWHOWAPM	
W/H z-score	fldWHOWHZ	fldCDCLAZ, fldCDCSAZ
W/H centile	fldWHOWHC	fldCDCLAC, fldCDCSAC
W/H percent of median	fldWHOWHPM	
MUAC-for-age	MUACAZ[b]	MUACAZ

a. If stature and length are processed separately, two variables are created for each indicator.
b. Based on 2000 CDC reference.
Source: Authors.

3. Exporting the data for analysis

After the variables of interest have been constructed, the Microsoft Access database must be converted into a format that can be read by the general statistical package before the variables can be merged with the original data. In our example, z-scores, percentiles, and percent of median for W/A, H/A, and W/H were saved in a file named `anthro_data.dta`, which can now be merged with the main Statadata file.

```
use anthro_data.dta, clear
sort id
save, replace
use main_data.dta, clear
sort id
merge id using anthro_data.dta
```

4. Performing basic data cleaning

In the previous steps, we have added a set of anthropometric indicators to our original data. Before we proceed with the analysis of these indicators, there are a number of data-cleaning issues and potential sources of bias that analysts must be aware of.

The first issue to contend with concerns the problem of missing values. In most surveys, enumerators are not able to obtain all the relevant data for all sampled individuals. The most common problem concerns the age of the child, in cases in which the parent may not know the precise birth date and birth records are not available. Data may also be missing for weight or height, for example, because some parents do not agree to having their children weighed, or there may have been problems with the measuring equipment. A second problem concerns the calculated z-scores; errors in measurement, reporting of age, coding, or data entry sometimes result in biologically implausible values. The WHO (1995) recommends that, for the purpose of analysis, values outside a certain range should be treated as missing values (see table 4.5).

Table 4.5 *Exclusion Ranges for "Implausible" z-Scores*

Indicator	Exclusion range for z-scores
Height-for-age	<5.0 and >+3.0
Weight-for-height	<4.0 and >+5.0
Weight-for-age	<5.0 and >+5.0

Note: If observed mean z-score is below –1.5, the WHO recommends that a flexible exclusion range be used. For details, see WHO (1995).
Source: Authors.

These problems can be explored by looking at descriptive statistics, scatter plots, and histograms. In the Mozambique data, we construct indicator variables for missing and implausible values in the variables of interest.

```
generate missing = (age_months==. | haz==. | whz==. | waz==.)
generate outrange_haz = (haz < -5 | haz > 3)
replace outrange_haz = . if haz==.
... code for whz and waz
drop if missing==1 | outrange_haz==1 | outrange_whz==1 | out-
range_waz==1
```

In this example, nearly 20 percent of observations have missing values for age, weight, or height. In addition, approximately 3 percent of observations have values for one or more of the anthropometric indicators that are outside the plausible range. This is quite high and casts some doubt on the quality of the data. At this point, it is difficult to correct the problems that gave rise to missing and implausible values. However, before dropping these observations, it is important to assess whether doing so is likely to result in biases in subsequent estimates. This depends both on the proportion of the sample that is being dropped and on the extent to which the true values for the variables of interest are systematically different from the rest of the sample. Of course, with missing data values for the relevant variables, we cannot provide a precise answer to this question. That said, we can look at other characteristics of the observations that we are dropping and draw some conclusions on that basis. For example, in the Mozambique data, both average income and maternal education are significantly lower for the observations that will be dropped, and they are disproportionately from rural areas. Hence, we are dropping observations that most likely have a poorer nutritional status than the population average. Besides such problems of non-sampling bias, sampling bias, whereby the sample that we are analyzing is not representative of the target population, can sometimes be important for anthropometric data.[17] For example, data may be collected through schools or clinics that are not attended by all segments of the population.

Constructing anthropometric indicators using Stata

Some analysts prefer not going through dedicated software for anthropometric analysis. Provided relevant macros or add-ins (i.e., zanthro or igrowup) have been installed, anthropometric indicators can be constructed in Stata.

---

[17]See chapter 2 on sampling and non-sampling bias.

For example, using the zanthro, the following command lines would generate indicator variables for low W/A, H/A, and W/H.

```
egen haz = zanthro(height_cm, ha, US), xvar(age_months)
gender(sexo) gencode(male=1, female=2) ageunit(month)

egen whz_stata = zanthro(weight_kilos, wh, US), xvar(height_
cm) gender(sexo) gencode(male=1, female=2)

egen waz_stata = zanthro(weight_kilos, wa, US), xvar(age_
months) gender(sexo) gencode(male=1, female=2) ageunit(month)
```

In this case, the variables are created using the 2000 CDC reference (US option in the zanthro command). If we had instead specified UK as an option, the 1990 British Growth Reference would have been used instead. The command automatically generates missing values if the absolute value of the z-score is greater than 5. By specifying the option nocutoff, calculation of all z-scores is forced.

Analyzing anthropometric data

At the most basic level, the analysis of anthropometric data concerns the identification of malnourishment in a population or subpopulation. However, in many cases analysts want to go beyond merely establishing prevalence to try to understand the causes of malnourishment and how can they be addressed.

A first step is to look at the distribution of the z-scores and the overall prevalence of malnourishment. When compared with the distribution of z-scores in the reference population, this provides a first impression of different dimensions of nutritional status in the population. In Stata, such descriptive analysis can be carried out as follows:

```
global zscores "haz waz whz"
foreach x of global zscores {
      graph twoway histogram `x' || function normden(x,0,1),
range(`x') title("`x'") xtitle("z-score") ytitle("Density")
legend(off)
      gen below2_`x' = (`x' < -2)
      gen below3_`x' = (`x' < -3)
}
tabstat $zscores below_* [aw=weight], stat(mean sd) col(stat)
```

where below2_haz is a dummy indicating a height-for-age z-score less than –2, and so forth. The results of this analysis of the Mozambique data are reported below. As can be seen from the graphs in figure 4.2 and from table 4.6, there are deficits in both H/A and W/A, but only limited evidence of wasting. More detailed histograms could be drawn by kernel density estimation (kdensity).

It is also useful to look graphically at the relationship between different anthropometric indicators. In general, weight-for-height and height-for-age are not correlated, whereas there tends to be a positive correlation between weight-for-height and weight-for-age and between weight-for-age and height-for-age (see figure 4.3). This pattern is confirmed in the Mozambique data.

```
twoway (scatter whz haz), ylabel(-6 0 5) xlabel(-6 0 5)
twoway (scatter whz waz), ylabel(-6 0 5) xlabel(-6 0 5)
twoway (scatter waz haz), ylabel(-6 0 5) xlabel(-6 0 5)
```

Figure 4.2 *Distribution of z-Scores in Mozambique, 1996/97*

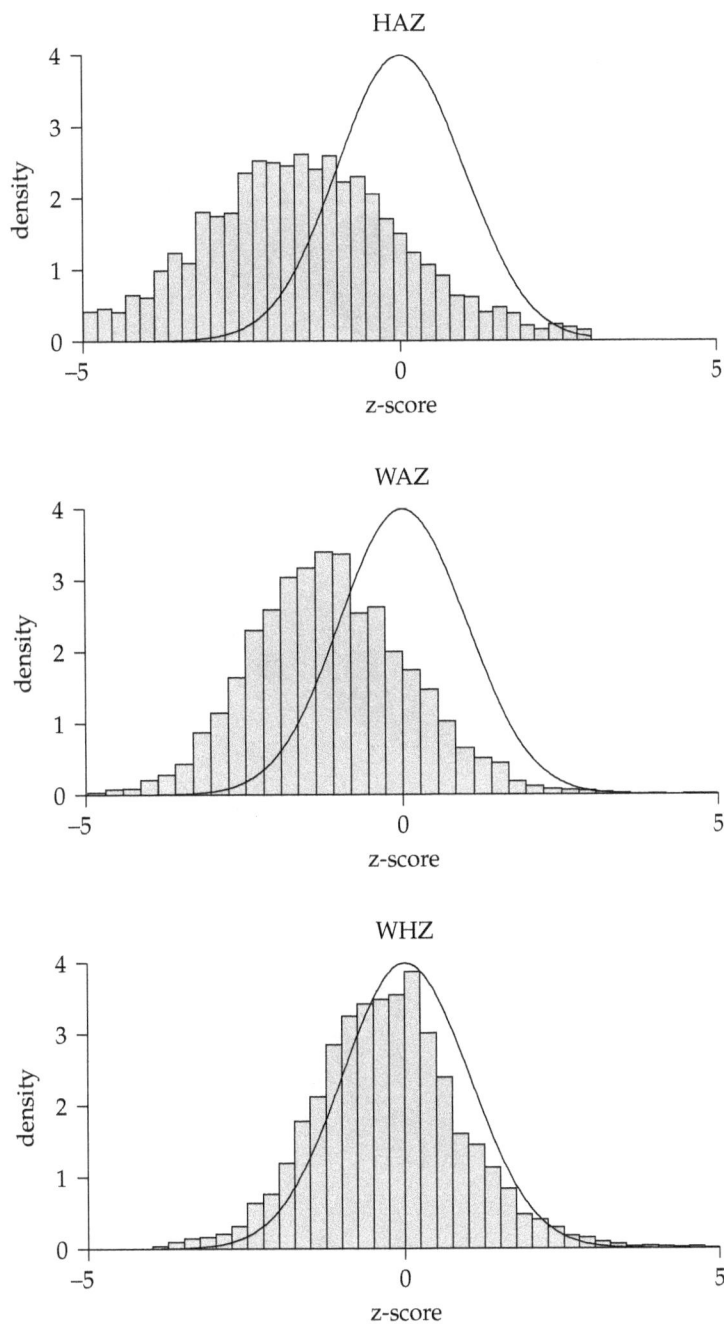

HAZ

WAZ

WHZ

Source: Authors.

Table 4.6 *Descriptive Statistics for Child Anthropometric Indicators in Mozambique, 1996/97*

	HAZ	*WAZ*	*WHZ*	*n*
Mean	−1.88	−1.28	−0.15	4,514
S.D.	1.74	1.31	1.34	4,514
% below −2 S.D.	46.1	28.8	6.4	4,514
% below −3 S.D.	25.4	8.4	1.1	4,514

Source: Authors.

Figure 4.3 *Correlation between Different Anthropometric Indicators in Mozambique*

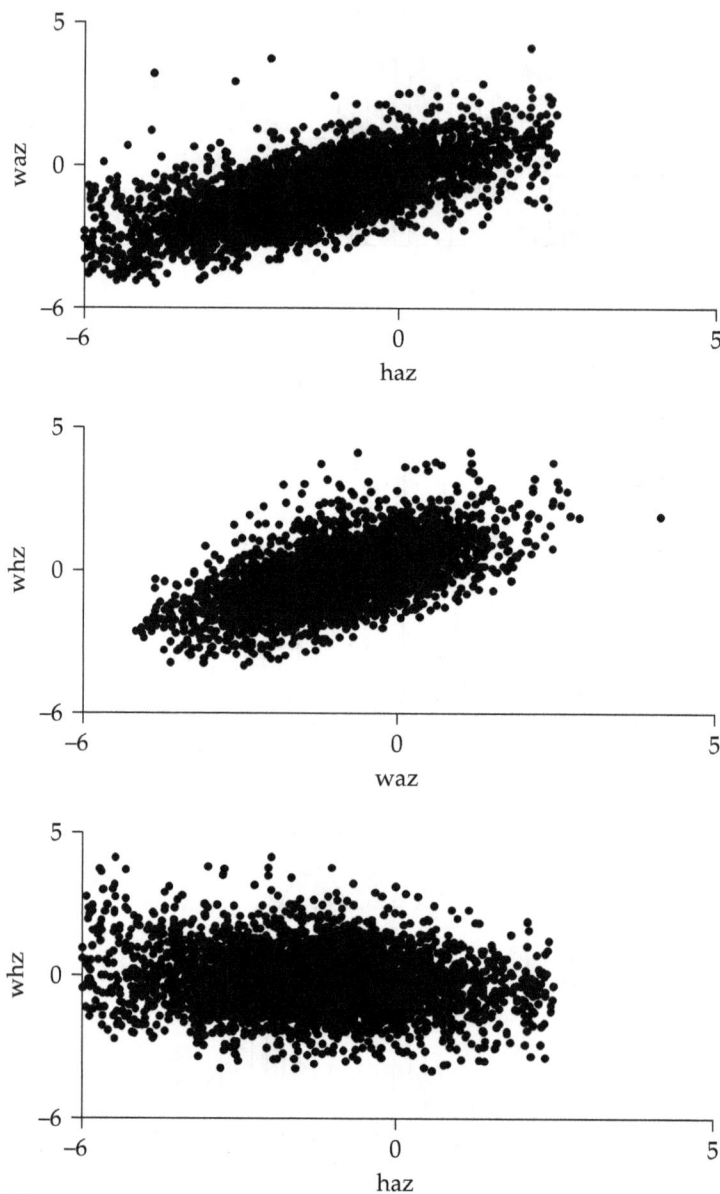

Source: Authors.

For many purposes, anthropometric data should be presented according to age and sex groups. The reason is that (i) patterns of growth failure vary with age, (ii) the identification of determinants of malnutrition is facilitated, and (iii) as a consequence of irregularities in the reference curves, wasting tends to be exaggerated for children in the 12- to 24-month age group. WHO (1995) recommends that at least two age disaggregations be used—under 24 months and 24 months and over—but for some purposes a more detailed disaggregation may be advisable.

```
tabstat below2* [aw=weight] if age_months < 24, stat(mean)
by(sex)
tabstat below2* [aw=weight] if age_months >= 24, stat(mean)
by(sex)
```

Table 4.7 *Stunting, Underweight, Wasting by Age and Gender in Mozambique*

Age (months)	Group	HAZ<–2	WAZ<–2	WHZ<–2	n
0–23	Boys	44.6	35.8	11.2	1,025
	Girls	36.0	23.5	5.7	1,072
	Combined	40.0	29.2	8.3	2,097
24–60	Boys	53.6	28.0	5.0	1,207
	Girls	49.3	29.2	4.4	1,210
	Combined	51.5	28.6	4.7	2,417

Source: Authors.

Of course, a simple disaggregation of children under five into two age groups still hides a great deal of detail. To better understand the nature of malnutrition, it can be useful to look at the mean z-score for smaller age groups (e.g., by month). To do so, the age variable, which is often continuous, needs to be transformed into a categorical variable. The mean z-score for different anthropometric indicators can then be tabulated and graphed. For example, figure 4.4 illustrates how the z-score weight-for-age in children in Mozambique reaches very low levels already by the age of 10 months.

```
recode age_months (0/0.999=0) (1/1.999=1) (2/2.999=2) ///
  (3/3.999=3) (4/4.999=4) (5/5.999=5) ///
  (6/6.999=6) (7/7.999=7) (8/8.999=8) ///
  (9/9.999=9) (10/10.999=10) (11/11.999=11) ///
  (12/12.999=12) (13/13.999=13) (14/14.999=14) ///
  (15/15.999=15) (16/16.999=16) (17/17.999=17) ///
  (18/18.999=18) (19/19.999=19) (20/20.999=20) ///
  (21/21.999=21) (22/22.999=22) (23/23.999=23) ///
  (24/24.999=25), gen(age_months_cat2)
tabstat waz if age_months<=24, by(age_months_cat)
```

Figure 4.4 *Mean z-Score (weight-for-age) by Age in Months*

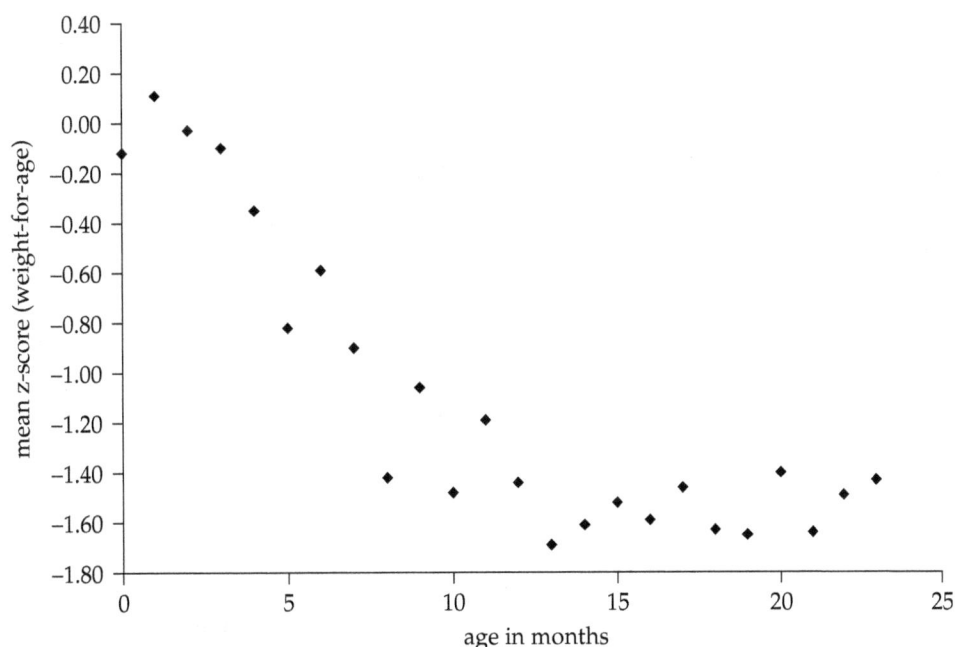

Source: Data from 1997 Mozambique Living Standards Survey.

It is also useful to explore how anthropometric indicators are related to different individual, household, and community characteristics. An important perspective in this regard is to assess socioeconomic inequalities in nutritional status. A simple way of looking at this issue is to examine the prevalence of malnutrition across income or wealth quintiles.

Prevalence rates of stunting, underweight, and wasting for different consumption quintiles in Mozambique are graphed in figure 4.5a, with a disaggregation by sex for stunting in figure 4.5b. The graphs show the expected tendency for malnutrition to be worse in poorer quintiles. But analysts should avoid drawing unwarranted conclusions about socioeconomic inequalities. In particular, it is important to look beyond the simple means by quintiles to assess whether the observed differences are significant. For example, in the case of stunting, a more detailed analysis of the Mozambique data reveals that the only statistically significant difference in prevalence between consumption quintiles is between the richest quintile and the rest. Moreover, although comparing means by quintiles is a useful place to start, it is quite a crude approach to assessing socioeconomic inequalities, and analysts should consider using concentration curves and indices discussed in chapters 7 and 8.

It is important that descriptive analysis of anthropometric data be accompanied by information to assist in the interpretation of findings. This includes information such as general characteristics of the population, sample design and size, method of determining age, and proportion of data missing or excluded. For some purposes it is also important to report standard errors or confidence intervals for estimates.

Analysts may wish to go beyond descriptive analysis and use anthropometric indicators to examine determinants of malnutrition. In that regard, it is customary to distinguish between distant and proximate determinants of malnutrition (Mosley and Chen 1984). Proximal factors are inadequate dietary intake and disease. Distant factors do not influence malnutrition directly, but rather through their impact on proximate determinants. They include, for example, poverty, education, cultural factors (e.g., duration of breast feeding, hygiene practices), and community and environmental characteristics (e.g., availability and quality of health services,

Figure 4.5 *Prevalence Rates of Stunting, Underweight, and Wasting for Different Consumption Quintiles in Mozambique and a Disaggregation by Sex for Stunting*

Figure 4.5a *By quintile*

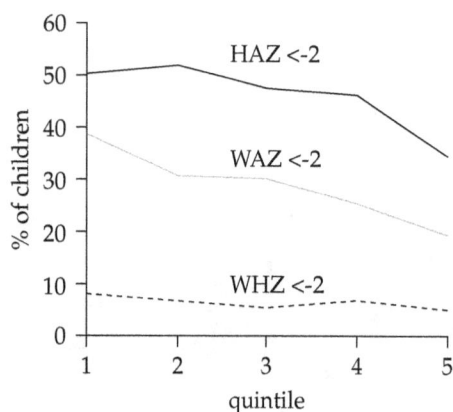

Figure 4.5b *By quintile, disaggregated by sex*

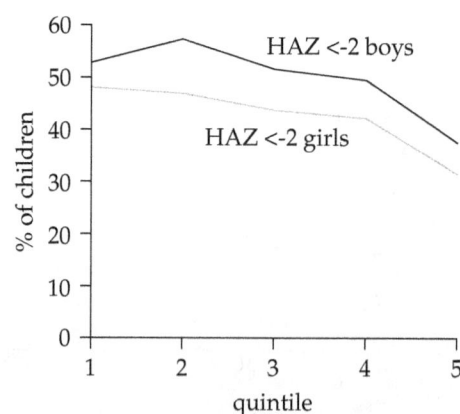

Source: Authors.

epidemiological profile).[18] The identification of socioeconomic inequalities should therefore be considered just the starting point for further analysis. A socioeconomic gradient most likely confounds the influence of many complex factors. To understand the contribution of different factors in determining nutritional status, a multivariate modeling framework is required. This type of analysis also has to contend with difficult conceptual and empirical issues, which are considered in chapter 10.[19]

Useful sources of further information

WHO global database on child growth and malnutrition: http://www.who.int/nutgrowthdb/.

Food Nutrition Technical Assistance Project: http://www.fantaproject.org/publications/anthropom.shtml.

Practical Analysis of Nutritional Data (PANDA): http://www.tulane.edu/~panda2/.

References

Alderman, H. 2000. "Anthropometry." In *Designing Household Survey Questionnaires for Developing Countries: Lessons from 15 Years of the Living Standards Measurement Study,* ed. M. Grosh and P. Glewwe. Washington, DC: World Bank.

Behrman, J. R., and A. B. Deolalikar. 1988. "Health and Nutrition." In *Handbook of Development Economics. Volume 1. Handbooks in Economics,* vol. 9, ed. H. Chenery and T. N. Srinivasan, 631–711. Amsterdam, Netherlands; New York; and Oxford, England: Elsevier Science.

de Onis, M., C. Garza, D. G. Victora, A. W. Onyango, E. A. Frongillo, and J. Martines. 2004. "The WHO Multicentre Growth Reference Study: Planning, Study Design, and Methodology." *Food Nutr Bull* 25(1): S15–26.

de Onis, M., A. W. Onyango, E. Borghi, C. Garza, and H. Yang. 2006. "Comparison of the World Health Organization (WHO) Child Growth Standards and the National Center for Health Statistics/WHO International Growth Reference: Implications for Child Health Programmes." *Public Health Nutr* 9(7): 942–47.

Garza, C., and M. de Onis. 2004. "Rationale for Developing a New International Growth Reference." *Food Nutr Bull* 25(1): S5–14.

Habicht, J. P., R. Martorell, C. Yarbrough, R. M. Malina, and R. E. Klein. 1974. "Height and Weight Standards for Preschool Children. How Relevant Are Ethnic Differences in Growth Potential?" *Lancet* 1(7858): 611–14.

Mosley, W. H., and L. C. Chen. 1984. "An Analytical Framework for the Study of Child Survival in Developing Countries." *Population and Development Review* 10 (Supplement): 25–45.

Strauss, J., and D. Thomas. 1995. "Human Resources: Empirical Modeling of Household and Family Decisions." In *Handbook of Development Economics,* Volume 3A. *Handbooks in Economics,* vol. 9, ed. J. Behrman and T. N. Srinivasan, 1883–2023. Amsterdam, Netherlands; New York, and Oxford, England: Elsevier Science.

---

[18]In some contexts, the distinction between *classifying* and *determining* variables is used; determining variables is used to refer to distal or proximate determinants that are amenable to being changed through interventions (e.g., feeding practices, sanitation, immunization, etc.). UNICEF has also proposed a conceptual framework on the causes of malnutrition, which distinguishes between immediate, underlying, and basic causes of malnutrition.

[19]For a detailed discussion, see Behrman and Deolalikar (1988) and Strauss and Thomas (1995).

WHO (World Health Organization). 1995. "Physical Status: The Use and Interpretation of Anthropometry. Report of a WHO Expert Committee." *World Health Organ Tech Rep Ser* 854: 1–452.

———. 2006. *WHO Child Growth Standards: Length/Height-for-Age, Weight-for-Age, Weight-for-Length, Weight-for-Height, and Body Mass Index-for-Age: Methods and Development*. Geneva, Switzerland: World Health Organization.

5

Health Outcome #3: Adult Health

Child mortality and nutrition status, considered in chapters 3 and 4, respectively, are important indicators of population health. But they provide only a partial picture of the level and distribution of health in a population. Survival is a rather crude indicator of health that ignores all aspects of health-related quality of life. Anthropometrics do indicate quality of life but only in a very partial manner. They are not sensitive to many health problems and are of relatively limited use as indicators of adult health status. To examine inequalities in general health in a population, a measure of health is required that is sensitive to a wide range of health problems and is informative about the health of adults. The literature on health status or health-related quality of life measurement is vast (see, e.g., Patrick and Chiang [2000]). In this chapter, we restrict attention to the measurement of self-reported adult health in the context of general population health inequalities.

Although health is intrinsically a multidimensional concept, for many purposes the interest is in an overall measure that collapses the separate dimensions into one construct. Several index-scoring algorithms have been developed for a number of generic health profiles, such as the SF-36 (Brazier et al. 1998), the Euroqol-5D (Busschbach et al. 1999), the McMaster health utility index (HUI) (Feeny et al. 2002), and more recently, the index fielded in the World Health Organization (WHO) World Health Surveys (Salomon et al. 2002). Such aggregated measures are preferable to others that either treat health as unidimensional or restrict attention to a single dimension, but their availability is usually restricted to health interview surveys, which have very limited information on living standards and so are often not suitable for the analysis of socioeconomic inequalities in health.

Besides the distinction between self-perceived and observed health indicators introduced in chapter 2, the types of indicators typically available for health equity analysis can be categorized under the headings medical, functional, and subjective (Wagstaff et al. 1991). Self-perceived indicators could fall into all three categories; observed indicators are either medical or functional. Medical indicators measure health as defined in relation to deviation from medical norms, such as the presence of certain diseases, conditions, or handicaps. Examples are lists on which the respondent indicates the presence of chronic or acute conditions, possibly diagnosed by a physician. There may be an indication of the duration of the condition. Functional indicators define health in relation to a lack of ability to perform "normal" tasks or roles. Examples include lists of impaired activities of daily living (ADL) or the number of days in a certain period that activities were restricted. According to a subjective model, health is defined in relation to the individual's overall perception of his or her health or the changes therein, possibly relative to that of other people of a similar age. Typical examples here include the question, "How do you rate your health in general—excellent, good, fair, or poor?" or a question asking whether respondents feel that their health has improved or deteriorated during the past year. It is advisable to use these various measures alongside one another to obtain a better picture of the distribution of health in a population.

In the next section of this chapter, we illustrate the use of different types of adult health indicators—medical, functional, and subjective—to describe the distribution of health in relation to socioeconomic status (SES). One may wish to examine the distribution of health in relation to SES conditional on third factors, such as age and sex, which are correlated with both health and SES. In the third section, we demonstrate how to standardize health distributions for differences in demographic composition of SES groups and so provide a more refined description of socioeconomic inequality in health. The final section considers the extent to which the measurement of health inequality is biased by socioeconomic differences in the reporting of health.

Describing health inequalities with categorical data

Some health survey questions demand simple yes or no responses. From these, samples can be divided into fractions of ill and not ill and inequalities in illness rates analyzed. But many questions have ordered response categories, for instance, self-assessed health (SAH) is (i) very good, (ii) good, (iii) fair, (iv) poor, or (v) very poor. Such answers cannot simply be scored as for example, 1,2,3,4,5 because the true scale will not be equidistant between categories. Several methods of scaling SAH for the purpose of inequality measurement have been tried:

a. Dichotomize the multiple-category responses and measure health as the percentage of individuals with that characteristic, that is, those who report their health to be "less than good." This practice avoids the imposition of some scale that is assumed to indicate how much more health is enjoyed in one category compared with another for any one individual. But it obviously results in a loss of information and requires the introduction of an arbitrary cutoff point (Wagstaff and van Doorslaer 1994). If the threshold at which "less than good health" is reported varies across cultures and/or population subgroups, then the dichotomous indicator will not indicate variation in prevalence of a given level of health across countries and/or socioeconomic groups (c.f. Salomon et al 2004).

b. Use a scoring algorithm to construct a scale that has been validated in another context (e.g., Hays et al. 1998). One example is the indicator of functional limitations or ADL index as proposed by the RAND-MOS researchers (Hays et al. 1998). It is defined simply as the sum of all activities scored as 0 if "unable to do," 50 if "able with difficulty," and 100 if "able without any difficulty." This sum ranges between 0 and k*100, where k is the number of activities, but can be rescaled to (0,1) using ADL index = (max-sum)/(max-min), where max and min are the sample maximum and minimum sums, respectively. Direct use of generic index scores (such as the HUI, the SF-36, or the WHO index) is also based on the use of a "scoring" algorithm derived from a (multi-attribute utility) valuation exercise (Brazier et al. 1998; Feeny et al. 2002; Salomon et al. 2002). The relative weights of the various health dimensions and items are then derived from (possibly other) respondents' answers to health (utility) valuation questions. One option is to attribute to each SAH category the mean, or median, scores of the index value (e.g., mean SF-36 score) calculated for the same SAH categories from some other data source in which both types of health measures are available.

c. If no other information on the distribution of health across response categories is available, one can proceed by arbitrarily assuming a functional form for the distribution. The aim is to exploit the full range of categories in the SAH question without imposing the unrealistic assumption of equal distances between categories. One proposed (but arbitrary) procedure is to assume that the observed frequency distribution across the SAH categories is generated by a latent health variable following a standard lognormal distribution (Wagstaff and van Doorslaer 1994). Then, the inverse of the cumulative lognormal distribution gives the cut points corresponding to the observed frequency distribution. Category scores can then be obtained as the expected values within each of the intervals defined by the cut points.

d. An alternative to method c is to generate predictions of an underlying latent variable using an ordered probit/logit or an interval regression model (see chapter 11) and to rescale these predictions to a 0-1 interval using index = (max-sum)/(max-min). If (external) information on the actual distribution of a continuous health measure is available (e.g., from another survey), then this can be used to scale the responses (van Doorslaer and Jones 2003). This has the same aim as method c but estimates the expected values of a latent health index given SAH responses and covariates and an assumed distribution of the error term (normal or logistic). A problem with that approach is that the measures then become highly dependent on the variables included in the prediction equation.

Allison and Foster (2004) introduce a method of obtaining a partial inequality ordering of SAH distributions that is invariant to the scaling of SAH. This is a significant advance in the literature, but it does have two limitations. First, the inequality of two SAH distributions can be compared only when their median categories coincide. Second, the method allows comparison of total inequality in SAH and not in socioeconomic-related inequality in SAH.

Table 5.1 shows the distributions of adult health across quintiles of equivalent expenditure in Jamaica derived from the 1989 Survey of Living Conditions (SLC) for 12 different indicators. All of the medical model indicators are dichotomous except the number of illness days. Two of the functional model indicators are dichotomous, the third is a count (number of restricted-activity days), and the fourth is the ADL index transformed to a (0,1) scale as described in procedure b above. The subjective indicator is SAH with five response categories. From that, two dichotomous indicators of less than good health and poor health are created. A third indicator (SAH index [lognormal]) is constructed following procedure c above, assuming a lognormal distribution for latent health. The final indicator (SAH index [HUI]) is derived by assigning the mean SAH-category-specific McMaster HUI values estimated from Canadian data to the corresponding SAH categories in the Jamaican SLC. While avoiding the assumption of lognormality, this involves imposing the obviously strong assumption that within SAH categories, health is on average equal in Jamaica and Canada.

Table 5.1 Indicators of Adult Health, Jamaica, 1989
Population and Household Expenditure Quintile Means

		Household expenditure quintiles				
	Total	Poorest	2	3	4	Richest
Medical model: 4-week illness						
Any illness or injury?	0.144	0.163	0.135	0.141	0.143	0.140
Number of illness days	1.675	2.279	1.643	1.715	1.550	1.218
Any acute illness (<4 weeks)	0.088	0.080	0.085	0.087	0.094	0.093
Any chronic illness (>4 weeks)	0.055	0.083	0.049	0.055	0.047	0.044
Functional model: activity limitations						
Any major limitation	0.147	0.203	0.169	0.153	0.101	0.115
Any minor limitation	0.260	0.334	0.314	0.255	0.199	0.205
Num. of restricted activity days	0.825	1.307	0.818	0.807	0.752	0.461
ADL index	0.898	0.852	0.885	0.899	0.930	0.924
Subjective model: self-perceived						
Less than good SAH	0.170	0.238	0.193	0.169	0.134	0.120
Poor SAH	0.058	0.097	0.066	0.061	0.035	0.034
SAH index (lognormal)[a]	1.576	1.948	1.621	1.594	1.404	1.331
SAH index (HUI)[b]	0.877	0.856	0.874	0.876	0.887	0.891

Note: a. Larger values indicate worse health.
　　　b. Larger values indicate better health.
Source: Authors.

All indicators show health to be lower among poorer quintiles, but relative differences in health between the richest and poorest quintiles vary across the indicators.

Demographic standardization of the health distribution

In the analysis of health inequality, the basic aim of standardization is to describe the distribution of health by SES conditional on other factors, such as age and sex. This will be referred to as the age-sex standardized health distribution. It is interesting only in the case in which two conditions are satisfied: (i) the standardizing variables are correlated with SES and (ii) they are correlated with health. It is important to realize that the purpose is not to build a causal, or structural, model of health determination. The analysis remains descriptive, but we simply seek a more refined description of the relationship between health and SES.

There are two fundamentally different ways of standardizing, direct and indirect. Direct standardization provides the distribution of health across SES groups that would be observed if all groups had the same age structure, for example, but had group-specific intercepts and age effects. Indirect standardization, however, "corrects" the actual distribution by comparing it with the distribution that would be observed if all individuals had their own age but the same mean age effect as the entire population.

Both methods of standardization can be implemented through regression analysis. In each case, one can standardize for either the full or the partial correlations of the variable of interest with the standardizing variables. In the former case, only the standardizing, or confounding, variables are included in the regression analysis. In the latter case, nonconfounding variables are also included, not to standardize on these variables but to estimate the correlation of the confounding variables with health conditional on these additional variables. For example, take the case in which age is correlated with education and both are correlated with both health and income. If one includes only age in a health regression, then the estimated coefficient on age will reflect the joint correlations with education and, inadvertently, one would be standardizing for education, in addition to age, differences by income. One may avoid this, if so desired, by estimating the age correlation conditional on education.

Indirect standardization

The most natural way to standardize is by the indirect method, which proceeds by estimating a health regression such as the following:

$$(5.1) \qquad y_i = \alpha + \sum_j \beta_j x_{ji} + \sum_k \gamma_k z_{ki} + \varepsilon_i,$$

where y_i is some indicator of health; i denotes the individual; and α, β, and γ are parameter vectors. The x_j are confounding variables for which we want to standardize (e.g., age and sex), and the z_k are nonconfounding variables for which we do *not* want to standardize but to control for in order to estimate partial correlations with the confounding variables. In the instance that we want to standardize for the full correlations with the confounding variables, the z_k variables are left out of the regression. Ordinary least squares (OLS) parameter estimates ($\hat{\alpha}$, $\hat{\beta}_j$, $\hat{\gamma}_k$), individual values of the confounding variables (x_{ji}), and sample means of the nonconfounding variables ($\bar{z}_k$) are then used to obtain the predicted, or "x-expected," values of the health indicator $\hat{y}_i^X$:

$$(5.2) \qquad \hat{y}_i^X = \hat{\alpha} + \sum_j \hat{\beta}_j x_{ji} + \sum_k \hat{\gamma}_k \bar{z}_k.$$

Estimates of indirectly standardized health, $\hat{y}_i^{IS}$, are then given by the difference between actual and x-expected health, plus the overall sample mean ($\bar{y}$),

$$(5.3) \qquad \hat{y}_i^{IS} = y_i - \hat{y}_i^X + \bar{y}.$$

The distribution of $\hat{y}_i^{IS}$ (e.g., across income) can be interpreted as the distribution of health that would be expected to be observed, irrespective of differences in the distribution of the x's across income. A standardized distribution of health across quintiles could be generated, for instance, by averaging $\hat{y}_i^{IS}$ within quintiles.

Direct standardization

The regression-based variant of direct standardization proceeds by estimating, for each SES group g, an equation such as the following:

$$(5.4) \qquad y_i = \alpha_g + \sum_j \beta_{jg} x_{ji} + \sum_k \gamma_{kg} z_{ki} + \varepsilon_i,$$

which is a group-specific version of equation 5.1. OLS estimates of the group-specific parameters ($\hat{\alpha}_g, \hat{\beta}_{jg}, \hat{\gamma}_{kg}$), sample means of the confounding variables ($\overline{x}_j$), and group-specific means of the nonconfounding variables ($\overline{z}_{kg}$) are then used to generate directly standardized estimates of the health variable $\hat{y}_i^{DS}$ as follows:

$$(5.5) \qquad \hat{y}_i^{DS} = \hat{y}_g^{DS} = \hat{\alpha}_g + \sum_j \hat{\beta}_{jg} \overline{x}_j + \sum_k \hat{\gamma}_k \overline{z}_{kg}.$$

Note that this method immediately gives the standardized health distribution across groups because there is no intragroup variation in the standardized values.

For grouped data, both the direct and indirect methods answer the question, "What would the health distribution across groups be if there were no correlation between health and demographics?" But their means of controlling for this correlation is different. The direct method uses the demographic distribution of the population as a whole (the $\overline{x}_j$), but the behavior of the groups (as embodied in the $\hat{\beta}_{jg}$'s and $\hat{\gamma}_{kg}$'s). The indirect method employs the group-specific demographic characteristics (the $\overline{x}_{jg}$), but the populationwide demographic effects (in $\hat{\beta}_j$ and $\hat{\gamma}_k$). The advantage of the indirect method, however, is that it does not require any grouping and is equally feasible at the individual level. The results of the two methods will differ to the extent that there is heterogeneity in the coefficients of x variables across groups because the indirect methods impose homogeneity and the difference will depend on the grouping used in the direct method.

Example—age-sex standardization of an SAH distribution, Jamaica 1989

Table 5.2 shows household expenditure quintile means of SAH in Jamaica with categories coded according to mean HUI values for corresponding SAH categories from Canadian data. Results are presented for nonstandardized means and for means standardized for age and sex by both direct and indirect methods. For each method, results are given with and without control for household expenditure when estimating the age/sex effects on SAH. In the former case, household expenditure is being treated as a z variable in equations 5.1 and 5.4. Without doing this, the age-sex effects will pick up the omitted expenditure effects and there is a danger that standardization will not only correct for differences in demographic composition but will also remove part of the "effect" of household expenditure on

Table 5.2 *Direct and Indirect Standardized Distributions of Self-Assessed Health Household Expenditure Quintile Means of SAH Index (HUI)*

		Standardized			
		Indirect		Direct	
Quintiles	Observed	Excl. expenditure	Incl. expenditure	Excl. expenditure	Incl. expenditure
Poorest	0.8564	0.8683	0.8682	0.8669	0.8668
2	0.8742	0.8739	0.8738	0.8777	0.8777
3	0.8763	0.8772	0.8772	0.8756	0.8756
4	0.8870	0.8804	0.8805	0.8816	0.8816
Richest	0.8913	0.8859	0.8860	0.8862	0.8862

Source: Authors.

SAH. In fact, the four standardized distributions are very similar in this example, suggesting that there is little heterogeneity in the age-sex effects across quintiles and that omitting expenditure from the SAH regressions does not bias these effects. However, standardization, by whichever method, does reduce the measured rich-poor disparities in SAH.

Computation for demographic standardization

Computation of standardized quintile means such as those in table 5.2 is straightforward in a package such as Stata. Demographics can be represented by age-sex specific dummies. In the example above, we use five age groups (18–34, 35–44, 45–64, 65–74, 75+) for each gender to give 10 dummies (fage1, fage2, etc.). Label the health variable y; in the example it is SAH index (HUI). For illustration, (log of) household expenditure (lnhhexp) will be included in the standardizing regression as a control (z) variable along with years of education (education) and a dummy for employment (works).[1] Let there be a sample weight variable, weight.[2]

INDIRECT STANDARDIZATION   First, estimate equation 5.1.

```
global xvar "mage2 mage3 mage4 mage5 fage1 fage2 fage3 fage4
fage5"
global zvar "lnhhexp education works"
regress y $xvar $zvar [pw=weight]
```

If control (z) variables were not included in the regression, then predicted values (equation 5.2) would be obtained immediately using,

```
predict yhat
```

When control variables are included, as above, they must be set to their mean values before predictions are obtained. This can be done by using loops, as follows:

```
foreach z of global zvar {
    quietly sum `z' [aw=weight]
    gen `z'_mean = r(mean)
    gen `z'_copy = `z'
    replace `z' = `z'_mean
}
predict yhat
foreach z of global zvar {
    replace `z' = `z'_copy
    drop `z'_copy `z'_mean
}
```

Standardized values (equation 5.3) are then computed by the following:

```
qui sum y [aw=weight]
gen yis = y-yhat + r(mean)
```

---

[1] In the Jamaican example, lnhhexp was the only z variable. We include others here to make the computation more generally applicable.
[2] The Jamaican sample was self-weighting, but we illustrate a more general case with weights.

DIRECT STANDARDIZATION   Direct standardization requires group-specific estimates of the regression coefficients. We illustrate the procedure when groups are defined as expenditure (hhexp) quintiles. Compute a categorical variable identifying quintiles, as follows:

```
xtile quintile=hhexp [pw=weight], nq(5)
```

Use a loop to obtain estimates of population means of the standardizing variables to be used in the prediction equation (equation 5.5):

```
foreach x of global xvar {
        qui sum `x' [aw=weight]
        gen `x'_mean = r(mean)
        gen `x'_copy = `x'
}
```

Now loop through each quintile group, running a regression for each one and obtaining predicted values with standardizing variables at population means and control variables at group means, as in equation 5.5:

```
gen yds=.
forvalues i=1/5 {
    qui regr y $xvar $zvar [pw=weight] if quintile==`i'
    foreach x of global xvar {
        replace `x' = `x'_mean
    }
    foreach z of global zvar {
        qui sum `z' [aw=weight] if quintile==`i'
        gen `z'_mean = r(mean)
        gen `z'_copy = `z'
        replace `z' = `z'_mean
    }
    predict yds`i' if e(sample)
    replace yds=yds`i' if quintile==`i'
    foreach z of global zvar {
        replace `z'=`z'_copy
        drop `z'_mean `z'_copy
    }
    foreach x of global xvar {
        replace `x'=`x'_copy
    }
}
```

The predicted variable, yds, is the directly standardized mean health for each quintile. The quintile means of nonstandardized and indirectly and directly standardized health can be compared using the following:

```
tabstat y yis yds [aw=weight], by(quintile)
```

Conclusion

Most of the health indicators obtained from surveys are self-reported. Besides being convenient, these indicators have been demonstrated to be effective in capturing health variation in a population. Self-assessed health, in particular, has been shown to predict mortality even conditional on detailed physiological measures of health (Idler and Benyamini 1997; van Doorslaer and Gerdtham 2003). Inevitably, however, there is heterogeneity in the reporting of health. Perceptions of health depend on expectations about health. If these expectations differ systematically across the population, comparison across subgroups becomes problematic. If, for instance, the poor systematically understate their true health, then the self-reported measures will not reflect the full extent of health inequalities.

Differences in health disparities derived from self-reported and more objective indicators are suggestive of systematic variation in reporting behavior. In Australia, Aboriginals tend to report better health despite being seriously disadvantaged according to more objective health indicators, such as mortality (Mathers and Douglas 1998). In India, the state of Kerala consistently shows the highest rates of reported morbidity, despite having the lowest rates of infant and child mortality (Murray 1996). Wagstaff (2002) notes that income-related inequalities in objective indicators of ill health, such as malnutrition and mortality, tend to be higher than those in subjective health. Moreover, the use of subjective health measures has led to some improbable health gradients in developing countries, with the rich reporting worse health than the poor (Baker and Van der Gaag 1993), which seems quite inconsistent with substantial pro-rich inequality in infant and child mortality rate and in anthropometric indicators (Gwatkin et al. 2003).

Formal testing has found evidence of reporting differences across age-sex groups but not across socioeconomic groups in Sweden and Canada (Lindeboom and van Doorslaer 2004; van Doorslaer and Gerdtham 2003). Milcent and Etile (2006) find some evidence of reporting differences by income in the middle categories of SAH and suggest that bias in the measurement of health inequality can be minimized by dichotomizing SAH into an indicator of poor health. This evidence is encouraging for the measurement of health inequality in developed countries, but one may worry that the bias is greater in developing countries where differences in the conception of illness by education and income levels may be greater. A promising solution to the reporting heterogeneity problem is to identify reporting differences from evaluations of given health states represented by hypothetical case vignettes and then to purge these reporting differences from individuals' evaluations of their own health (Salomon et al. 2004; Tandon et al. 2003). Case vignettes have been collected in the WHO World Health Surveys. Bago d'Uva et al. (2006) use vignettes to test for reporting heterogeneity by demographic and socioeconomic factors in data from China, India, and Indonesia. They find that reporting differences by sociodemographic groups are significant, but that, in general, the size of the reporting bias in measures of health disparities is not large.[3]

---

[3]Reporting bias is likely to be larger in response to questions about illness in the past four weeks, a common question in the World Bank Living Standards Measurement Surveys. The answer to that question may be influenced by conceptions of illness, access to health care, and work activity (Makinen et al. 2000).

References

Allison, R. A., and J. E. Foster. 2004. "Measuring Health Inequality Using Qualitative Data." *Journal of Health Economics* 23(3): 505–24.

Bago d'Uva, T., E. van Doorslaer, M. Lindeboom, O. O'Donnell, and S. Chatterji. 2007. "Does Reporting Heterogeneity Bias the Measurement of Health Disparities?" *Health Economics* (forthcoming).

Baker, J. L., and J. Van der Gaag. 1993. "Equity in Health Care and Health Care Financing: Evidence from Five Developing Countries." In *Equity in the Finance and Delivery of Health Care*, ed. E. van Doorslaer, A. Wagstaff, and F. Rutten. Oxford, United Kingdom: Oxford University Press.

Brazier, J., T. Usherwood, R. Harper, and K. Thomas. 1998. "Deriving a Preference-Based Single Index from the UK SF-36 Health Survey." *J Clin Epidemiol* 51(11): 1115–28.

Busschbach, J. J. V., J. McDonnell, M. L. Essink-Bot, and B. A. van Hout. 1999. "Estimating Parametric Relationships Between Health Description and Health Valuation with an Application to the EuroQol EQ-5D." *Journal of Health Economics* 18(5): 551–71.

Feeny, D., W. Furlong, G. W. Torrance, C. H. Goldsmith, Z. Zhu, S. DePauw, M. Denton, and M. Boyle. 2002. "Multiattribute and Single-Attribute Utility Functions for the Health Utilities Index Mark 3 System." *Med Care* 40(2): 113–28.

Gwatkin, D. R., S. Rustein, K. Johnson, R. Pande, and A. Wagstaff. 2003. *Initial Country-Level Information about Socio-Economic Differentials in Health, Nutrition, and Population*, Volumes I and II. Washington, DC: World Bank Health, Population and Nutrition.

Hays, R. D., C. D. Sherbourne, and R. M. Mazel. 1998. *User's Manual for the Medical Outcomes Study (MOS) Core Measures of Health-Related Quality of Life*. Santa Monica: RAND Corporation.

Idler, E., and Y. Benyamini. 1997. "Self-Rated Health and Mortality: A Review of Twenty-Seven Community Studies." *Journal of Health and Social Behavior* 38(1): 21–37.

Lindeboom, M., and E. van Doorslaer. 2004. "Cut-Point Shift and Index Shift in Self-Reported Health." *Journal of Health Economics* 23(6): 1083–99.

Makinen, M., H. Waters, S. Ram, R. Bitran, D. MacIntyre, M. Rauch, and L. Gilson. 2000. "An Analysis of Equity in Morbidity, Health Care Use, and Health Care Expenditures in Selected Developing and Transitional Countries." *Bulletin of the World Health Organization* 78(1).

Mathers, C. D., and R. M. Douglas. 1998. "Measuring Progress in Population Health and Well-Being." In *Measuring Progress: Is Life Getting Better?* ed. R. Eckersley, 125–55. Collingwood, Ontario, Canada: CSIRO Publishing.

Milcent, C., and F. Etile. 2006. "Income-Related Reporting Heterogeneity in Self-Assessed Health: Evidence from France." *Health Economics* 15(9): 965–81.

Murray, C. J. L. 1996. "Epidemiology and Morbidity Transitions in India." In *Health, Poverty and Development in India*, ed. M. Dasgupta, L. Chen, and T. N. Krishnan, 122–47. Delhi, India: Oxford University Press.

Patrick, D. L., and Y.-P. Chiang. 2000. "Health Outcomes Methodology: Symposium Proceedings." *Medical Care* 38(9) (Supplem. II): II1–II209.

Salomon, J. A., C. J. L. Murray, T. B. Ustun, and S. Chatterji. 2002. "Health Stata Valuations in Summary Measures of Population Health." In *Health Systems Performance Assessment: Debates, Methods and Empiricism*, ed. C. J. L. Murray and D. B. Evans. Geneva, Switzerland: World Health Organization.

Salomon, J., A. Tandon, and C. J. L. Murray. World Health Survey Pilot Study Collaborating Group. 2004. "Comparability of Self-Rated Health: Cross Sectional Multi-Country Survey Using Anchoring Vignettes." *British Medical Journal* (328): 258.

Tandon, A., C. J. L. Murray, J. A. Salomon, and G. King. 2003. "Statistical Models for Enhancing Cross-Population Comparability." In *Health Systems Performance Assessment: Debates, Methods and Empiricisms,* ed. C. J. L. Murray and D. B. Evans, 727–46. Geneva, Switzerland: World Health Organization.

van Doorslaer, E., and U.-G. Gerdtham. 2003. "Does Inequality in Self-Assessed Health Predict Inequality in Survival by Income? Evidence from Swedish Data." *Social Science and Medicine* 57(9): 1621–29.

van Doorslaer, E., and A. M. Jones. 2003. "Inequalities in Self-Reported Health: Validation of a New Approach to Measurement." *Journal of Health Economics* 22.

Wagstaff, A. 2002. "Poverty and Health Sector Inequalities." *Bulletin of the World Health Organization* 80(2): 97–105.

Wagstaff, A., P. Paci, and E. van Doorslaer. 1991. "On the Measurement of Inequalities in Health." *Soc Sci Med* 33(5): 545–57.

Wagstaff, A., and E. van Doorslaer. 1994. "Measuring Inequalities in Health in the Presence of Multiple-Category Morbidity Indicators." *Health Economics* 3: 281–91.

6

Measurement of Living Standards

The common theme throughout this book is the examination of disparities in a particular health variable (be it health status, health service utilization, or payments for health care) across people with different standards of living. For example, the concern might be to see whether gaps in health outcomes between the poor and the better off have grown or whether they are larger in one country than another. This raises the question of how best to measure living standards. One approach is to use "direct" measures, such as income, expenditure, or consumption. Another is to use a "proxy" measure, making the best use of available data. One popular approach in this vein is to use principal components analysis to construct an index of "wealth" from information on household ownership of durable goods and housing characteristics.

In approaching the issue of living standards measurement, it is important to be aware of the limitations and potential problems of alternative measures. This requires an understanding not only of the conceptual differences between different approaches, but also of the problems that can arise in the construction of living standards variables. With this in mind, this chapter has four purposes: (i) to outline different approaches to living standards measurement, (ii) to discuss the relationship between and merits of different living standards measures, (iii) to discuss briefly how different measures can be constructed from survey data, and (iv) to provide guidance on where further information on living standards measurement can be obtained.

An overview of living standards measures

Direct measures of material living standards

The most direct (and popular) measures of living standards are income and consumption. In general terms, income refers to the earnings from productive activities and current transfers. It can be seen as comprising claims on goods and services by individuals or households.

In contrast, consumption refers to resources actually consumed. Although many components of consumption are measured by looking at household expenditures, there are important differences between the two concepts. First, expenditure excludes consumption that is not based on market transactions. Given the importance of home production in many developing countries, this can be an important distinction. Second, expenditure refers to the purchase of a particular good or service. However, the good or service may not be immediately consumed, or at least

---

Box 6.1 *Brief Definitions of Direct Measures of Living Standards*

Income. The amount of money received during a period of time in exchange
for labor or services, from the sale of goods or property, or as a profit
from financial investments.

Expenditure. Money payments or the incurrence of a liability to obtain goods
or services.

Consumption. Final use of goods and services, excluding the intermediate
use of some goods and services in the production of others.

Source: Authors.

---

there may be lasting benefits. This is the case, for example, with consumer durables.
Ideally, in this case, consumption should capture the benefits that come from the
use of the good, rather than the value of the purchase itself (see box 6.1).

Measured income often diverges substantially from measured consumption (see figure 6.1). In part, this is due to conceptual differences in the respective
terms—it is possible to save from income and to finance consumption from bor-
rowing. Moreover, although this is not inherent in the definition of income, income
surveys often exclude household production. There is a long-standing and vigor-
ous debate about which is the better measure of standards of living. For developing
countries, a strong case can be made for preferring consumption, based on both
conceptual and practical considerations (Deaton and Grosh 2000).

1. Income is received only intermittently, whereas consumption can be "smoothed"
over time. As a consequence, it is reasonable to expect that consumption will be
more directly related to current living standards than will current income, at
least for short reference periods. In other words, although the flow of consump-

Figure 6.1 *The Relationship between Income and Consumption*

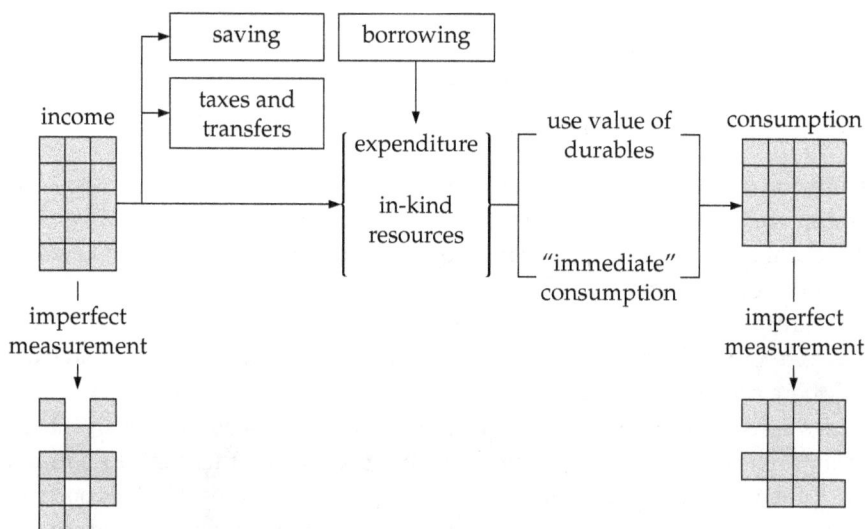

Source: Authors.

tion over a period of, say, a week or a month, may provide a good indication of the level of consumption during a full year, measured income over the same period is most likely an inaccurate measure of income for a full year.

2. Income and expenditure data are both difficult to collect. In developed countries, in which a large proportion of the population works in the formal sector and in which consumption patterns are very complex, the balance often tips in favor of measuring income rather than consumption. Even so, these surveys often have considerable problems dealing with self-employment, informal economic activities, and widespread reluctance to disclose information on income to survey enumerators. In developing countries, formal employment is less common, many households have multiple and continually changing sources of income, and home production is more widespread. In these contexts, it is generally far easier to measure consumption than income.

Proxy measures of living standards

Both income and consumption data are expensive and difficult to collect, and many otherwise useful data sources lack direct measures of living standards (e.g., the demographic and health surveys [DHS]). On the face of it, this precludes the analysis of socioeconomic inequalities of health, as well as testing of hypotheses relating to the impact of living standards on health and health service outcomes. Moreover, the exclusion of living standards measures in multivariate analysis raises the possibility that other coefficient estimates are rendered biased. These concerns have prompted researchers to use data on household assets and other characteristics to construct alternative measures of welfare or living standards (Bollen et al. 2001; Filmer and Pritchett 2001; Montgomery et al. 2000; Sahn and Stifel 2000). This approach has the considerable merit of requiring only data that can be easily and quickly collected in a single household interview and, although lacking somewhat in theoretical foundations, can provide a convenient way to summarize the living standards of a household. There are three primary approaches to constructing welfare indices, which differ in how different household assets and characteristics are weighted in the overall index.[1]

- **"Arbitrary" approach:** Some studies have used what may be referred to as "naïve" indices to proxy or control for living standards, often constructed as the sum of indicator or dummy variables for whether a household possesses certain assets (Case et al. 2004; Montgomery et al. 2000; Morris et al. 2000). For example, a simple "asset score," constructed by assigning equal weight to each of 10 assets, has been proposed as a "convenient proxy" in the context of the new core welfare indicator questionnaire (CWIQ) surveys.[2]
- **Principal components and factor analysis:** As an alternative to a simple sum of asset variables that are available in the data, it is possible to use statistical techniques to determine the weights in the index. The two most common

---

[1]In regression analysis, it is also possible to include assets and other living standards proxies separately in the analysis. Although that may provide adequate control for living standards, it does not permit a ranking of households or individuals.

[2]See http://www4.worldbank.org/afr/stats/cwiq.cfm. The CWIQ methodology also suggests that assets can be selected and weighted on the basis of a consumption regression in cases in which the requisite data are available.

approaches for doing that are principal components analysis and factor analysis.[3] These are essentially tools for summarizing variability among a set of variables. Specifically, principal components analysis seeks to describe the variation of a set of variables as a set of linear combinations of the original variables, in which each consecutive linear combination is derived so as to explain as much as possible of the variation in the original data, while being uncorrelated with other linear combinations. Typically, the asset index is assumed to be the first principal component—that is, the first linear combination.[4] Principal components analysis suffers from an underlying lack of theory to motivate either the choice of variables or the appropriateness of the weights.

- **Predicting consumption:** In cases in which complementary consumption data are available—from a past or parallel survey—it may be possible to derive weights for a living standards index through a "consumption regression." In other words, consumption data are regressed on a set of household assets and characteristics that are common to the two surveys, and coefficient estimates are used as weights. This approach draws on the techniques from the targeting literature, which seek to identify a set of variables that predict consumption and use this information to channel services or benefits (e.g., cash transfers) to the poorer segments of the population (Coady et al. 2004; Grosh and Baker 1995). Consumption regressions have also been implemented in other contexts, for example, to link survey and census data for the purposes of poverty mapping. In many cases, the estimated models have considerable predictive power. However, in both of these cases, the set of household and asset characteristics has been broader than has typically been the case for assets constructed through principal components or factor analysis, including for example, educational status, language, location, and ethnic affiliation. In other words, many of the attempts to predict consumption have included not only indicators but also determinants of income and consumption.

Some practical issues in constructing living standards variables

Measuring income

Broadly speaking, income is composed of earnings from productive activities and transfers. It is customary to distinguish four main components in the measurement of income: (i) wage income from labor services; (ii) rental income from the supply of land, capital, or other assets; (iii) self-employment income; and (iv) current transfers from government or nongovernment agencies or other households. There is, however, some disagreement about what exactly should be considered "productive

---

[3]For a detailed discussion of the statistical techniques, see Bartholomew et al. (2002).
[4]In contrast to the principal components approach proposed by Filmer and Pritchett (1999), Sahn and Stifel (2000) construct a welfare index on the basis of factor analysis. They argue that factor analysis is preferable to the principal component method because it does not force all of the components to accurately and completely explain the correlation structure between the assets. Despite the perceived advantages, they note that the Spearman rank correlation between the principal components and factor analysis asset indices is about 0.98 for each of the samples considered.

activities," and hence, what should be included in income measures (McKay 2000). In particular, many attempts to measure income have not considered home production, although this can be conceived as a form of income. In cases in which home production is considered, practical considerations often limit the scope. For example, some income measures seek to include subsistence agricultural production in the calculation of household income. In contrast, "service activities" such as child minding performed in the household are generally excluded. For home-produced goods that are either exchanged by barter or consumed directly in the household, and for any income received in-kind, values have to be imputed.[5]

Although some surveys in developing countries—for example, in Latin America—have collected detailed income data, attention is often restricted to employment income. That is the case, for example, in most Living Standards Measurement Study (LSMS) surveys. Moreover, the quality of the data has often been poor. As a consequence, income data from these surveys have rarely been used as a proxy for living standards. If reasonably complete income data are available, a measure of total income may be a useful proxy for living standards, in particular if consumption data are not available. In cases in which consumption data are available, it is always advisable to try to assess the validity of the relative measures. That entails comparing household income with consumption aggregates, but it also requires a detailed analysis of the questionnaire and the data collection process.

Measuring consumption and constructing consumption aggregates

As noted, consumption is seen by many as the preferred measure of living standards. Surveys have differed a great deal in the level of detail of their consumption modules. Some surveys have included comprehensive and detailed lists of consumption items. For example, the Brazilian budget survey uses a list of 1,300 items. Most surveys, however, are less detailed. The LSMS surveys, which have been designed and implemented with the explicit objective of measuring living standards, have included somewhere in the region of 20 to 40 food items and a similar number of nonfood items.[6] Because of this heterogeneity, it is not possible to provide general guidelines on how to construct consumption aggregates or to fully account for the methodological challenges and pitfalls in this process.[7] Here, we restrict ourselves to a general overview of the steps of the process.

Most surveys collect data on four main classes of consumption: (i) food items, (ii) nonfood, nondurable items, (iii) consumer durables, and (iv) housing.[8] Consumption is measured with a particular reference period in mind. Although the reference

---

[5] The imputation of values for home production is discussed in more detail below.

[6] Morris et al. (2000) have suggested that in many contexts, aggregate consumption can be proxied by a reduced list of consumption items. They report results in which a proxy constructed from 10 items was correlated with total household consumption at the $r = 0.74$ level.

[7] There are, however, good sources of information on these issues. For example, Deaton and Zaidi (2002) provide a detailed review and offer many examples of Stata code.

[8] Because of the difficulty in defining meaningful shadow prices, most consumption measures exclude publicly supplied goods and services, even though these services can have a big impact on material living standards. Similarly, conceptual problems in establishing the value of leisure, in particular in contexts in which un- or underemployment is widespread, often make it impractical to include leisure as a component of consumption.

period varies, many surveys aim to accurately measure the total consumption of the household in the past year. In this way, temporary drops in consumption are ignored, and it is still possible to capture changes in living standards of a single individual or household over time. In some contexts—for example, where there are important seasonal variations in living standards—it may be appropriate to focus on time periods shorter than a year. The reference period should be distinguished from the recall period, which refers to the time period for which respondents are asked to report consumption in the survey. Recall periods tend to differ for different types of goods, such that reporting on goods that tend to be purchased infrequently is based on a longer time period. The balance has to be struck between capturing a sufficiently long period so that the consumption during the period is representative of the reference period (year) as a whole and making it sufficiently short such that households can remember expenditures and consumption with reasonable accuracy. Surveys have taken different approaches to striking that balance.

In general, there are three steps in the construction of a consumption-based living standards measure: (i) construct an aggregate of different components of consumption, (ii) make adjustments for cost of living differences, and (iii) make adjustments for household size and composition. These steps are discussed in turn.

AGGREGATING DIFFERENT COMPONENTS OF CONSUMPTION   The first step in constructing a consumption aggregate is to simply add up the values of different types of consumption. However, before this can be done, a common reference period has to be established for all items, and values have to be imputed in cases in which they are not available.

Food consumption: A food consumption subaggregate is constructed through the aggregation of (i) food purchased in the marketplace, (ii) food that is home-produced, (iii) food items received as gifts or remittances from other households, and (iv) food received as in-kind payment from employers.

1. All data on food expenditures or consumption must be converted to a uniform reference period—for example, a year. Some care is required in this because the recall periods can sometimes vary for different types of food items. For example, some nonperishable food items are consumed infrequently. In these cases, "food consumed" during a recall period may be different from "food purchased." Ideally, that should be reflected in the questionnaire design by extending the recall period for these items.

2. In some surveys, data may be available for more than one reference period. For example, some LSMS surveys collect data both on food expenditures in the "past two weeks" and on food expenditures in a "usual month." In these cases, a choice has to be made, taking into account the benefits and problems of alternative designs.

3. Many households, in addition to consuming goods and services procured in the market, also produce goods for the market or home consumption. Home production presents both theoretical and practical challenges that relate to determining the appropriate value of home-produced goods and services.[9]

---

[9]In situations in which a large proportion of consumption comes from home production, there is a real risk that the measures of living standards reflect assumptions about the value of different goods and services, rather than some theoretically appealing measure of welfare.

In most surveys, attention is restricted to home-produced food, which typically is captured in a separate questionnaire module. The survey may collect data only on the value of different home-produced food items, or on both value and quantity. If data on the value of these items are not available, it is possible to impute the value by using quantities and estimates of "farm-gate" prices.

4. Information on food received as in-kind payment may not be collected in all surveys, or it may be collected in a different part of the questionnaire from other food-related questions. If the data are available, the values should be added to other food consumption for a subaggregate.

Nonfood consumption: Most surveys collect data only on purchased nonfood items and do not consider home-production. Data generally are collected on a wide range of items. However, because values rather than quantities typically are reported, the aggregation is straightforward.

1. Similarly to food consumption, the recall period may vary for different nonfood consumption items. It may be a month for daily-use items, but considerably longer for items that are purchased less frequently. It is therefore important to ensure that the data are converted to a common reference period.

2. It may also be advisable to exclude some nonfood expenditures—for example, tax payments, gifts, and transfers to other households as well as lumpy expenditures (marriages, funerals, etc.). However, there are no general rules in this regard, and it will require a judgment based on considerations of the particular context and on how the data will be used.

Consumer durables: We have noted that in the case of durable goods, it is not appropriate to measure consumption by expenditure on the item. Rather, consumption refers to the "rental equivalent" or "user cost" of the good. This can be thought of as comprising two components: (i) the opportunity cost of funds tied up in the durable good and (ii) the depreciation of the good. Generally, these values must be imputed. For this reason, most surveys collect data on the stock and characteristics of durables, rather than on expenditures on these items.

1. Generally, the most important "durable good" is housing. In this case, rental data are sometimes available. For households that do not report rent, a value can be imputed by using the relationship between rent and housing characteristics in the subset of households that report rent (a "hedonic regression").[10] However, this approach can be tenuous in contexts in which this subset is a small proportion of all households or in which these households are "unrepresentative" in respect to the relationship between paid rent and housing characteristics.

2. For other household durables, the imputation of values is normally done on the basis of data on date of purchase and cost of acquisition, combined with assumptions about the lifetime of the good. Alternatively, depreciation rates can be calculated using reported "current values." Procedures are described in detail by Deaton and Zaidi (2002).

---

[10] A "hedonic regression" simply refers to the regression of rental value on a number of housing characteristics (e.g., number of rooms, type of floor, type of roof, access to water, type of toilet, etc.). The estimated relationship can be used to predict values for households in cases in which rent is not observed (but housing characteristics are).

ADJUSTING FOR COST-OF-LIVING DIFFERENCES   Monetary estimates of total consumption must be adjusted to reflect differences in prices. This concerns mainly regional differences in prices. For example, prices tend to be lower in rural than in urban areas, at least for some goods and services. However, if the fieldwork was carried out during an extensive period, it may also be necessary to take into account temporal variation in prices, even in a simple cross-section survey.

Price adjustments raise both practical and conceptual issues (Deaton and Grosh 2000; Deaton and Zaidi 2002). At a practical level, a decision has to be made about the source of price data. In general, there are three options: (i) household-level data on the volume and value of purchases, (ii) a dedicated price questionnaire, or (iii) price data from separate price surveys. Although household-level price data have some problems—in particular in relation to the definition of units of consumption and heterogeneity in quality—generally, they are seen as the preferred source. It may, however, be advisable to average prices over households in clusters. Price data from market or community questionnaires have also been used in many surveys. Although these data can be difficult to collect and have limitations, they are a useful substitute. Data from statistical offices or ministries of finance are often based on irregular price surveys, and the spatial disaggregation of the data may be limited. These types of data should hence be used only as a last resort.

In general terms, a price index is constructed as a weighted sum of price ratios of different commodities,

$$PI = \sum_k w_k \left(\frac{p_k^h}{p_k^0} \right),$$

where k is the set of commodities, w is the weight, p^h is the price faced by the household, and p^0 is a reference price (often the median price for the respective commodity). There are different approaches to constructing a price index. The fundamental difference concerns the weights that are used. For a Paasche price index, the weights are simply the share of each household's budget devoted to the particular good. As a consequence, the weights vary across households. In contrast, the Laspeyres price index uses the same weights for all households, based on budget shares of households on or near the poverty line. The results from the different approaches correspond to different theoretical approaches to the measurement of welfare and can sometimes lead to different findings. Although the Laspeyres price index may be more convenient to calculate because the weights are constant, Deaton and Zaidi (2000) suggest that the Paasche index is preferable because it tends to indicate welfare more correctly.

ADJUSTING FOR HOUSEHOLD SIZE AND COMPOSITION   As noted, most surveys use the household as a unit of observation in the measurement of consumption. The reason is that it would be both costly and time-consuming to collect consumption data on an individual basis. It also facilitates the treatment of joint household goods such as housing, where it is not possible to assign consumption to specific individuals. Although this is convenient, we are often interested in *individual* consumption or welfare.[11] To obtain individual-level estimates, it is necessary to adjust household

---

[11] Treating the household as the unit of observation also ignores the possibility that the intra-household distribution of resources can be very uneven.

estimates of aggregate consumption to reflect household size and composition. This is done by using a deflator, or equivalence scale. In the simplest case, we can simply use the number of household members to convert household consumption into individual consumption. However, although per capita household consumption is a convenient measure of living standards, it ignores household economies of scale that arise because some goods and services that are consumed by the household have public good characteristics—that is, they generate benefits for other household members besides the primary consumer. There may also be age- or gender-specific differences in consumption needs (in particular to reflect the consumption needs of children relative to adults).

Reflecting these concerns, equivalence scales can be constructed as some function of the household size and demographic composition provided estimates are available for household economies of scale and the cost of children. A common approach is to define the number of adult equivalents (AE) in the household as

$$AE = (A + \alpha K)^{\theta},$$

where A is the number of adults in the household, K is the number of children, α is the "cost of children," and θ reflects the degree of economies of scale (Cirto and Michael 1995). The challenge is to determine the appropriate values for α and θ. Identifying equivalence scales is notoriously difficult (Deaton 1997). Behavioral (Deaton and Muellbauer 1986; Deaton and Paxson 1998) and subjective (van Praag and Warnaar 1997) approaches have been taken. While recognizing the difficulty of identifying equivalence scales for developing countries, Deaton and Zaidi (2002) propose values in the region of 0.3 to 0.5 for α (higher in developed countries) and 0.75 to 1.0 for θ, given that food accounts for a large proportion of total consumption, and economies of scale are relatively limited.[12]

Constructing an asset index

PRINCIPAL COMPONENTS AND FACTOR ANALYSIS Because asset indices constructed from principal components and factor analysis generally are highly correlated, the choice of technique is mainly a matter of convenience.[13] In the case of principal component analysis, the asset index, A_i, for individual i is defined as follows:

$$A_i = \sum_k \left[f_k \frac{(a_{ik} - \bar{a}_k)}{s_k} \right],$$

---

[12]The selection of values of α and θ is not a strictly technical exercise, but also reflects value judgments. For example, there are no clear technical grounds on which to determine how the value of household public goods declines as it is shared across more household members. Similarly, although the nutritional requirements of children relative to adults can be determined on technical grounds, other child "needs" are more difficult to establish. Given inherent uncertainty about the parameter values and given that the choice of parameter reflects value judgments, it is advisable to construct several individual consumption aggregates and to test the robustness of findings to different assumptions concerning economies of scale and consumption needs. Insofar as findings (e.g., comparisons of inequality over time and across countries) vary on the choice of parameters, analysts need to assess not only the soundness of chosen parameters on technical grounds, but also whether the choice is consistent with the views and values of policy makers and society.

[13]For a detailed discussion of how to construct asset indices, see Vyas and Kumaranayake (2006).

where a_{ik} is the value of asset k for household i, $\bar{a}_k$ is the sample mean, s_k is the sample standard deviation, and f_k are the weights associated with the first principal component.

Such an index can be computed fairly easily in many statistical packages. In Stata, principal components or factors are computed by the following:

```
#delimit ;
global assets "elctrcty radio fridge tv bike motor_bike car
tele water_piped water_pumpwell water_pubwell water_open
water_other wc latrine floor_dirt floor_cement floor_brick floor_
adobe floor_parq floor_other persroom";
#delimit cr
factor $assets [aw=weight], pcf
```

where the list of household assets and characteristics are specified in the global macro assets.[14] Because the option pcf is specified, this command extracts the principal components.[15] The default is to perform ordinary factor analysis. An option factors() can be added to control the number of factors that are extracted. For example, if one is interested only in the first principal component, factors(1) could be added. The command displays a table of components, and it is possible to read off the proportion of variance in the variables that is accounted for by each component.

In the construction of living standards indices on the basis of principal components analysis, it is generally assumed that the first component is an adequate measure of welfare. The index is computed with the following:

```
predict asset_index
```

This is essentially the sum of the asset variables, weighted by the elements of the first eigenvector. If consumption data are available, the correlation with the asset index can be examined. In fact, living standard indices based on principal components analysis often have a weak relationship with consumption, with correlation coefficients often in the region of 0.2 to 0.4. In part, this may be due to a poor selection of asset variables, but there may also be deeper reasons that consumption is only weakly related to asset ownership.[16]

Health variables are often compared across quantiles of some measure of living standards—income, consumption, or an assets index. In Stata, a categorical variable identifying quantiles can be computed by the following:

```
xtile quintile=asset_index [aw = weight], nq(5)
```

Here, we construct quintiles (nq(5)). Note that weights must be applied if the sample is not self-weighted.

---

[14]The command #delimit ; changes the way Stata reads code in a do-file. Rather than executing line by line, the program now treats semicolons as the end of the commands. This means that commands can be spread over several lines to improve readability. The command #delimit cr returns to the default setting of line-by-line processing. An alternative way of spreading a command over multiple lines is to end a command line with ///.

[15]Alternatively, principal components can be computed in Stata using the command pca.

[16]Moser (1998) has argued that the choice of asset indicators needs to be tailored to the circumstances of a particular context.

USING FACTOR WEIGHTS FROM ANOTHER SURVEY   Nationally representative samples do not provide the detailed data required to answer all questions of interest. For example, one might be interested in utilization of a specific health service that is not separately identified in a national survey. Or, one might be interested in the use of a specific provider or in health or health service utilization in a particular locality. In such cases, a detailed but small-scale and nonrepresentative survey may be undertaken to extract the required data on the health variable of interest. For example, an exit survey could be used to collect data directly from the users of a particular service. Given the detailed consideration of health variables in such a study and the limited time available for enumeration, it will not usually be possible to have detailed measurement of income or consumption. Recording assets and housing conditions is easier and offers a more feasible way of assessing living standards. Factor or principal components analysis could be applied to the assets data from the specific survey. But one may worry that the weights derived from such a specialized survey may not be consistent with those that would be obtained from a nationally representative survey and further, one may be interested in where sample observations lie in the national distribution of living standards. If there exists a national survey that collects data on the same assets as those in the specific survey, then the former can be used to compute factor weights and these can be applied to the specific survey assets data to derive assets index scores that can be assessed against the national distribution of the index.

This is the approach adopted by, for example, Thiede et al. (2005) in their study of the use of HIV/AIDS voluntary counseling and testing (VCT) services in South Africa. They collected data on assets from users of public clinics in townships only and computed a wealth score using the principal component factor loadings from an analysis of all urban households in the national demographic and health survey (DHS). From the DHS data, the cutoff points for wealth quintiles in South Africa's whole urban population could be calculated and the fraction of township residents located in each urban wealth quintile identified. Township residents were concentrated in the middle part of the urban wealth distribution—only 14 percent of the township population was located in the poorest urban wealth quintile, and only 8 percent was in the richest quintile (see table 6.1). The fraction of township clinic users could then be compared with the respective population shares in each wealth quintile for the entire urban population. For example, although the poorest urban quintile accounted for 8 percent of the township population, it accounted for 36 percent of township VCT users (table 6.1). The richest urban quintile, although

Table 6.1 *Percentage of Township Population and Users of HIV/AIDS Voluntary Counseling and Testing Services by Urban Wealth Quintile, South Africa*

Urban quintile	Percent of township population	Percent of users of HIV/AIDS VCT services
Poorest 20%	14.0	35.6
2nd	23.7	38.9
3rd	28.8	17.3
4th	25.4	7.2
Richest 20%	8.1	1.0

Source: Thiede et al. 2005.

accounting for 8 percent of the township population, accounted for just 1 percent of township VCT users.

Does the choice of the measure of living standards matter?

So far, we have focused on the construction of different measures of living standards. We have noted that there are both conceptual and practical differences between different measures. But one could reasonably ask which is the "best" measure. Unfortunately, there is not a simple answer to this question. Arguably, income is an inferior measure, not only because of measurement challenges, but also because for most households the fluctuation in income over time does not imply commensurate changes in living standards. In other words, if a household suffers a temporary negative income shock due to illness, but is able to maintain consumption through savings or insurance, it may be misleading to rank the household based on income or to express out-of-pocket payments as a share of income.

On normative grounds, most analysts prefer to assess living standards with reference to some notion of long-term command over resources. This latent variable can be proxied by consumption or an asset index. As mentioned above, most economists prefer consumption because it is rooted in economic theory. Consumption data, however, are expensive to collect and may also be more susceptible to measurement error.[17] In contrast, asset and housing data are easier to collect and potentially less susceptible to measurement error.

In practice, the correlation between consumption and asset indices is often low. But does the choice between these two measures matter for the analysis of health equity? Montgomery et al. (2000) show that although asset indices are often poor predictors of consumption, they may still be useful in testing the hypothesis of whether consumption is a significant determinant of health outcomes, in particular in cases in which sample sizes are large and there is a great deal of variation in consumption.[18] They also find little evidence that the use of asset indices to proxy for consumption results in biased coefficient estimates on other variables of interest. Focusing specifically on health equity, Wagstaff and Watanabe (2003) compare measured inequality in wasting and stunting for 19 countries (based on LSMS data) and find that for most countries the choice between consumption and the asset index as the welfare measure makes little difference to the measured degree of socioeconomic inequality in malnutrition. This finding offers a degree of confidence to analysts who are concerned about the robustness of their results.

But robustness is not a consistent finding. Results have also been shown to be sensitive to the choice of assets and household characteristics that are included in the index (Houweling et al. 2003). Moreover, in some contexts, the choice of welfare indicator can drive conclusions in important ways. This is the case, for example, in Mozambique, where the choice of welfare indicator has a large and significant impact on socioeconomic inequalities in service use and on the incidence of public

---

[17]Although measurement error in consumption has been used as an argument for asset indices (Filmer and Pritchett 2001; Sahn and Stifel 2003), measurement error can also be an important problem in the collection of data on household assets and characteristics. As a result, reliability of asset-based measures of SES may also be low (Onwujekwe et al. 2006).

[18]See also Bollen et al. (2001), Sahn and Stifel (2003), and McKenzie (2005).

spending (Lindelow 2006). For most health services, this study found less inequality in utilization when consumption rather than the assets index was used as the living standards measure. For example, although the poorest quintile ranked by the assets index received only 9.6 percent of all child immunizations, the poorest quintile ranked by consumption received 21.4 percent. For health center visits, inequality moved in the opposite direction—there was inequality favoring the poor using the assets index as the living standards measure but inequality favoring the rich using consumption.[19] Clearly such results suggest that the sensitivity of results to the living standards measure should be checked when it is possible to do so.

References

Bartholomew, D., F. Steele, I. Moustkaki, and J. Galbraith. 2002. *The Analysis and Interpretation of Multivariate Data for Social Scientists.* London, England: Chapman and Hall.

Bollen, K. A., J. L. Glanville, and G. Stecklov. 2001. "Socioeconomic Status and Class in Studies of Fertility and Health in Developing Countries." *Annual Review of Sociology* 27: 153–85.

Case, A., C. Paxson, and J. Ableidinger. 2004. "Orphans in Africa: Parental Death, Poverty, and School Enrollment." *Demography* 41(3): 483–508.

Cirto, C., and R. Michael. 1995. *Measuring Poverty: A New Approach.* Washington, DC: National Academy Press.

Coady, D., M. Grosh, and J. Hoddinott. 2004. *Targeting of Transfers in Developing Countries: Review of Lessons and Experience: Regional and Sectoral Studies.* Washington, DC: World Bank.

Deaton, A. 1997. *The Analysis of Household Surveys: A Microeconometric Approach to Development Policy.* Baltimore, MD: Published for the World Bank [by] Johns Hopkins University Press.

Deaton, A., and M. Grosh. 2000. "Consumption." In *Designing Household Survey Questionnaires for Developing Countries: Lessons from 15 Years of the Living Standards Measurement Study*, ed. M. Grosh and P. Glewwe. Washington, DC: World Bank.

Deaton, A., and J. Muellbauer. 1986. "On Measuring Child Costs: With Applications to Poor Countries." *Journal of Political Economy* 4: 720–44.

Deaton, A., and C. H. Paxson. 1998. "Economies of Scale, Household Size, and the Demand For Food." *Journal of Political Economy* 106: 897–930.

Deaton, A., and S. Zaidi. 2002. "Guidelines for Constructing Consumption Aggregates." LSMS Working Paper No. 135. World Bank, Washington, DC.

Filmer, D., and L. Pritchett. 1999. "The Effect of Household Wealth on Educational Attainment: Evidence from 35 Countries." *Population and Development Review* 25(1): 85–120.

Filmer, D., and L. Pritchett. 2001. "Estimating Wealth Effects without Expenditure Data—or Tears: An Application to Educational Enrollments in States of India." *Demography* 38(1): 115–133.

Grosh, M., and J. Baker. 1995. "Proxy Means Tests for Targeting Social Programs: Simulations and Speculation." LSMS Working Paper No. 118. World Bank, Washington DC.

Houweling, T. A., A. E. Kunst, and J. P. Mackenbach. 2003. "Measuring Health Inequality among Children in Developing Countries: Does the Choice of the Indicator of Economic Status Matter?" *Int J Equity Health* 2(1): 8.

---

[19]See chapter 8 for further discussion of this study.

Lindelow, M. 2006. "Sometimes More Equal Than Others: How Health Inequalities Depend on the Choice of Welfare Indicator." *Health Economics* 15: 263–79.

McKay, A. 2000. "Should the Survey Measure Total Household Income?" In *Designing Household Survey Questionnaires for Developing Countries: Lessons from 15 Years of the Living Standards Measurement Study*, ed. M. Grosh and P. Glewwe. Washington, DC: The World Bank.

McKenzie, D. J. 2005. "Measuring Inequality with Asset Indicators." *Journal of Population Economics* 18(2): 229–60.

Montgomery, M. R., M. Gragnaloti, K. Burke, and E. Paredes. 2000. "Measuring Living Standards with Proxy Variables." *Demography* 37(2): 155–74.

Morris, S. S., C. Calogero, J. Hoddinot, and L. J. M. Christiaensen. 2000. "Validity of Rapid Estimates of Household Wealth and Income for Health Surveys in Rural Africa." *Journal of Epidemiology and Community Health* 54: 381–87.

Moser, C. 1998. "The Asset Vulnerability Framework: Reassessing Urban Poverty Reduction Strategies." *World Development* 26(1): 1–19.

Onwujekwe, O., K. Hanson, and J. Fox-Rushby. 2006. "Some Indicators of Socio-economic Status May Not Be Reliable and Use of Indices with These Data Could Worsen Equity." *Health Economics* 15(6): 639–44.

Sahn, D. E., and D. C. Stifel. 2000. "Poverty Comparisons Over Time and Across Countries in Africa." *World Development* 28(12): 2123–55.

Sahn, D. E., and D. C. Stifel. 2003. "Exploring Alternative Measures of Welfare in the Absence of Expenditure Data." *Review of Income and Wealth* 49(4): 463–89.

Thiede, M., N. Palmer, and S. Mbatsha. 2005. "South Africa: Who Goes to the Public Sector for Voluntary HIV/AIDS Counselling and Testing?" In *Reaching the Poor with Health, Nutrition and Population Services: What Works, What Doesn't, and Why*, ed. D. R. Gwatkin, A. Wagstaff, and A. S. Yazbeck. Washington, DC: World Bank.

van Praag, B. M. S., and M. F. Warnaar. 1997. "The Cost of Children and the Use of Demographic Variables in Consumer Demand." In *Handbook of Population and Family Economics*, ed. M. Rosenzweig and O. Stark, 241–73. Amsterdam, Netherlands: North-Holland.

Vyas, S., and L. Kumaranayake. 2006. "Constructing Socio-Economic Status Indices: How to Use Principal Components Analysis." *Health Policy Plan* 21(6): 459–68.

Wagstaff, A., and N. Watanabe. 2003. "What Difference Does the Choice of SES Make in Health Inequality Measurement?" *Health Economics* 12(10): 885–90.

7

Concentration Curves

In previous chapters, we assessed health inequality through variation in mean health across quintiles of some measure of living standards. Although convenient, such a grouped analysis provides only a partial picture of how health varies across the full distribution of living standards. A complete picture can be provided using a concentration curve, which displays the share of health accounted for by cumulative proportions of individuals in the population ranked from poorest to richest (Kakwani 1977; Kakwani et al. 1997; Wagstaff et al. 1991). The concentration curve can be used to examine inequality not just in health outcomes but in any health sector variable of interest. It can also be used to assess differences in health inequality across time and countries. For example, it has been used to assess whether subsidies to the health sector are targeted toward the poor and whether the targeting is better in some countries than in others (O'Donnell et al. 2007; Sahn and Younger 2000). It has also been used to assess whether child mortality is more unequally distributed to the disadvantage of poor children in one country than in another (Wagstaff 2000) and whether inequalities in adult health are more pronounced in some countries than in others (van Doorslaer et al. 1997). Many other applications are possible.

In this chapter we explain how to compute a concentration curve. We also explain how to test whether a concentration curve departs significantly from an equal distribution and whether there is a statistically significant difference between two concentration curves that may represent different health services, time periods, or countries. This requires computation of standard errors of the concentration curve ordinates.

The concentration curve defined

The two key variables underlying the concentration curve are the health variable, the distribution of which is the subject of interest, and a variable capturing living standards against which the distribution is to be assessed. Measurement of key health sector variables and of household living standards has been considered in earlier chapters. The health variable must be measured in units that can be aggregated across individuals. This is not necessary for the living standards measure, which is used only to rank individuals from richest to poorest.

The data could be at the individual level (e.g., raw household survey data), in which case values of both the health variable and the living standards variable are available for each observation. Alternatively, the data could be grouped, in which case, for each living-standard group (e.g., income quintile), the mean value of the health variable is observed. The ranking of the groups (which group is poorest, which group is second poorest, and so on) and the percentage of the sample falling into each group are known. In the case of grouped data, the only advantage of the concentration curve over a table of group means is that it gives a graphical representation of the data.

The concentration curve plots the cumulative percentage of the health variable (y-axis) against the cumulative percentage of the population, ranked by living standards, beginning with the poorest, and ending with the richest (x-axis). In other words, it plots shares of the health variable against quantiles of the living standards variable. Examples are given in the figure in box 7.1 and in figures 7.1 and 7.2. So, for example, the concentration curve might show the cumulative percentage of health subsidies accruing to the poorest p percent of the population. If everyone, irrespective of his or her living standards, has exactly the same value of the health variable, the concentration curve will be a 45-degree line, running from the bottom left-hand corner to the top right-hand corner. This is known as the line of equality. If, by contrast, the health sector variable takes higher (lower) values among poorer people, the concentration curve will lie above (below) the line of equality. The farther the curve is above the line of equality, the more concentrated the health variable is among the poor.

Concentration curves for the same variable in different countries or time periods can be plotted on the same graph. Similarly, curves for different health sector variables in the same country and time period can be plotted against each other. For example, the analyst may wish to assess whether inpatient care is more unequally distributed than primary care. If the concentration curve for one country (or time period or health service) lies everywhere above that for the other, the first curve is said to dominate the second, and the ranking by degree of inequality is unambiguous.[1] Alternatively, curves may cross, in which case neither distribution dominates the other. It is then still possible to make comparisons of degrees of inequality but only by resorting to a summary index of inequality, which inevitably involves the imposition of value judgments concerning the relative weight given to inequality arising at different points in the distribution (see chapter 8). Rankings by degree of inequality can then differ depending on the inequality index chosen.

Graphing concentration curves—the grouped-data case

In the grouped-data case, the required data and the corresponding charts are easily produced in a spreadsheet program such as Microsoft Excel. The table in box 7.1 is pasted directly from Excel and contains all the data required to plot the concentration curve shown in the box. The curve is constructed in Excel using the XY (scatter) chart-type with the "scatter with data points connected by smoothed lines" option. The first series graphs the line of equality, the x-values and the y-values both being the cumulative percentage of the sample. The no-marker option is selected for the line of equality. The second series graphs the concentration curve, the x-values being the cumulative percentage of the sample, the y-values being the cumulative percentage of the health variable. It is important to include a 0 percent in both series. Both the x-axis and the y-axis need to be restricted to the range 0 to 100 percent.

---

[1] For an introduction to the concept of dominance, its relation to inequality measurement, and the related concept of stochastic dominance, see Deaton (1997).

Box 7.1 Example of a Concentration Curve Derived from Grouped Data

In this example, the sample comprises births, the living standards measure is the assets (wealth) index, and the health variable is deaths of children under five years of age. The data are from the demographic and health surveys of India and Mali. The table shows the number of births in each wealth index quintile during the period 1982–92 in India. Expressing these as percentages of the total number of births and cumulating them gives the cumulative percentage of births, ordered by wealth. That is what is plotted on the *x*-axis in the figure. Also shown are the under-five mortality rates (U5MR) for each of five wealth groups. Multiplying the U5MR by the number of births gives the number of deaths in each wealth group. Expressing these as a percentage of the total number of deaths and cumulating them gives the cumulative percentage of deaths. That is what is plotted on the *y*-axis in the figure. The concentration curve for India lies above (dominates) the line of equality, indicating that child deaths are concentrated among the poor. Also shown in the figure is the concentration curve for under-five deaths for Mali for the period 1985–95. The Mali curve lies everywhere below that of India (i.e., the India curve dominates the Mali curve), indicating there is less inequality in under-five mortality in Mali than in India.

Under-Five Deaths in India, 1982–92

Wealth group	No. of births	Rel % births	Cumul % births	U5MR per 1,000	No. of deaths	Rel % deaths	Cumul % deaths
			0				0
Poorest	29,939	23	23	154.7	4,632	30	30
2nd	28,776	22	45	152.9	4,400	29	59
Middle	26,528	20	66	119.5	3,170	21	79
4th	24,689	19	85	86.9	2,145	14	93
Richest	19,739	15	100	54.3	1,072	7	100
Total/average	129,671			118.8	15,419		

Concentration Curves for Under-Five Deaths in India and Mali

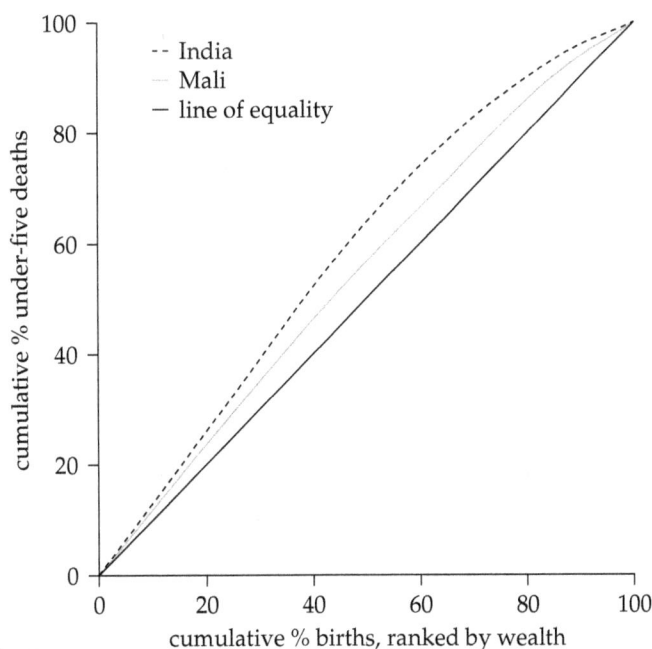

Source: Authors.

Graphing concentration curves—the microdata case

Graphing concentration curves in Stata can be done using the command glcurve (an ado file downloadable from the Stata Web site). However, better-looking charts can be obtained using the twoway command.

In the example that follows, we plot concentration curves for child malnutrition in Vietnam in 1992/93 and 1997/98, with malnutrition measured by the negative of height-for-age, as in Wagstaff et al. (2003). The dataset contains stacked data for the two years (year being 0 for 1992/93 and 1 for 1997/98), neghaz and lnpcexp being, respectively, the negative of height-for-age and the log of per capita expenditure for the year in question. We ignore below-sample weights, but they can be incorporated in both of the approaches below, as will be clear from Stata code elsewhere in the book.

The concentration curve can be produced directly using glcurve as follows:

```
glcurve neghaz, glvar(yord) pvar(rank) sortvar(lnpcexp)
replace by(year) split lorenz
```

The rank variable here is the lnpcexp. glcurve generates three new variables: rank, which is the child's rank in the expenditure distribution in each year, and yord_0 and yord_1, which are respectively the y-ordinates for 1992/93 and 1997/98. Adding the lorenz option requests that y-ordinates be cumulative proportions of the health variable and not the cumulative means, which is the default.

Alternatively, these three variables could have been obtained through the following commands:

```
sort year lnpcexp
forval i = 0/1 {
  sum neghaz if year==`i'
  scalar nobs`i' = r(N)
}
ge rank=.
egen tmp = rank(lnpcexp) if year==0
replace rank=tmp/nobs0 if year==0
drop tmp
egen tmp = rank(lnpcexp) if year==1
replace rank=tmp/nobs1 if year==1

forval i = 0/1 {
  sum neghaz if year==`i'
  scalar s_malnut`i' = r(sum)
}
gen yord_0 = sum(neghaz)/s_malnut0 if year==0
gen yord_1 = sum(neghaz)/s_malnut1 if year==1
```

Whichever way the x-ordinates and y-ordinates are obtained, the concentration curve can be graphed using the full range of the options provided by twoway as follows:

```
ge rank2=rank
lab var yord_0 "1992/93"
lab var yord_1 "1997/98"
```

```
lab var rank "cumul share of children (poorest first)"
lab var rank2 "line of equality"

twoway (line yord_0 rank , sort clwidth(medthin) ///
clpat(solid))(line yord_1 rank, sort clwidth(medthin) ///
clpat(longdash) clcolor("153 204 0"))(line rank2 rank , ///
sort clwidth(medthin) clcolor(gray)), ///
ytitle(cumulative share of malnutrition, size(medsmall)) ///
yscale(titlegap(5))  xtitle(, size(medsmall)) ///
legend(rows(5)) xscale(titlegap(5)) ///
legend(region(lwidth(none))) plotregion(margin(zero)) ///
ysize(5.75) xsize(5) plotregion(lcolor(none))
graph export "$path0\cc curves 1992 and 1997.emf" , replace
```

The first line generates a duplicate rank variable that allows the line of equality to be plotted and labeled. The colors, pattern, and thickness of the concentration curves are controlled in the `twoway` command using the `clcolor`, `clwidth`, and `clpat` options. (The `///` in the code simply allows code to be continued over several lines.) The last line of code exports the graph in Windows Enhanced Meta Format (emf), which allows easy viewing from within Windows Explorer and easy insertion into a Word document or a PowerPoint presentation (using Insert, Picture, From File). Figure 7.1 shows the resultant concentration curve chart, which reveals,

Figure 7.1 *Concentration Curve for Child Malnutrition in Vietnam, 1992/93 and 1997/98*

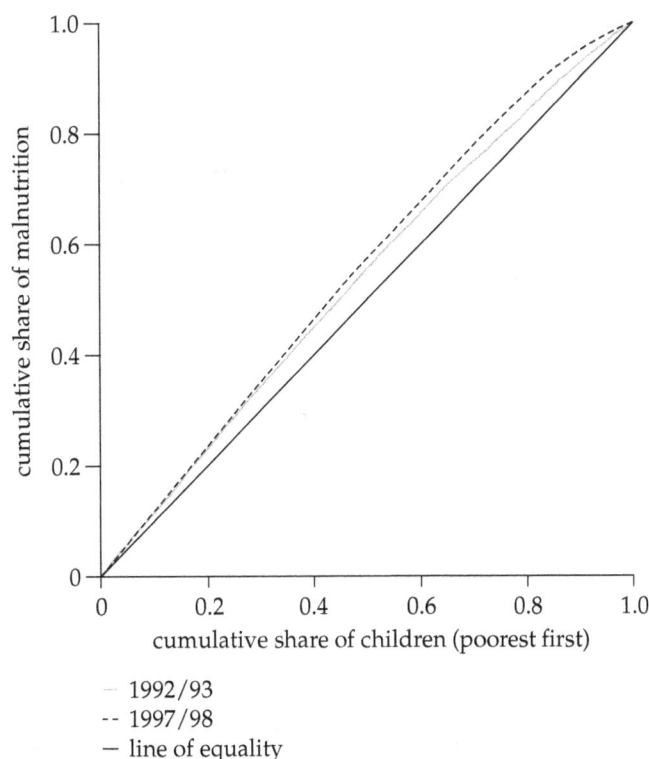

Source: Authors.

as indicated in Wagstaff et al. (2003), that inequality in child malnutrition increased somewhat in Vietnam between 1992/93 and 1997/98.

Testing concentration curve dominance

Concentration curves are estimated from survey data and so are subject to sampling variability. Although visual inspection of a concentration curve in comparison with the 45-degree line or another concentration curve may give an impression of whether there is dominance, obviously this inspection is not sufficient to conclude whether or not dominance is statistically significant. To make inferences about dominance, the standard errors of the concentration curve ordinates must be computed in addition to their point estimates. If the analyst wishes to test dominance of a concentration curve against the Lorenz curve of income/consumption or against another concentration curve estimated from the same sample, then the standard errors for the differences between curve ordinates must be computed. This is complicated by the fact that, in such cases, the curves are dependent. The appropriate variance-covariance matrix, allowing for dependence between curves, has been derived by Bishop et al. (1994) and Davidson and Duclos (1997).

One decision rule that has been used in Lorenz (concentration) dominance tests has been to reject the null of nondominance in favor of dominance if there is at least one significant difference between curves (or a curve and the 45-degree line) in one direction and no significant difference in the other. For example, if there is at least one quantile point at which curve A lies significantly above curve B and there is no quantile point at which curve B lies above curve A, then it is concluded that A dominates B. If conventional critical values are used with such a decision rule, then there will be overrejection of the null because there is no correction for the fact that multiple comparisons are being made (Howes 1996). One solution is to use the same decision rule but to take multiple testing into account by using critical values from the studentized maximum modulus (SMM) distribution (Beach and Richmond 1985; Bishop et al. 1992; Stoline and Ury 1979). This is referred to as *the multiple comparison approach* (Dardanoni and Forcina 1999). An alternative criterion requires significant difference between ordinates at all quantile points to accept dominance (Howes 1996; Sahn and Younger 2000; Sahn et al. 2000). This is consistent with the intersection union principle (Dardanoni and Forcina 1999). Dardanoni and Forcina (1999) present Monte Carlo evidence showing that although this stricter rule reduces the probability of erroneously rejecting nondominance, it has greatly reduced the power of detecting dominance when true. If there is at least one significant difference between ordinates in each direction, then it is concluded that curves cross. If there are no significant differences in either direction, then, with the multiple comparison approach, null of nondominance is not rejected.

Besides the decision rule, the analyst must choose the number of quantile points at which ordinates are to be compared. If the number of comparison points is too restricted, then dominance across the full range of the distribution is not being tested. It is difficult, however, to find dominance at the extremes of distributions (Howes 1996). With reasonably large samples, a popular choice has been to test for differences at 19 evenly spaced quantiles from 0.05 to 0.95 (O'Donnell et al. forthcoming; Sahn and Younger 2000; Sahn et al. 2000).

The best statistical package for dominance testing is DAD, a specialist package for poverty and inequality analysis.[2] We have written our own Stata ado file for dominance testing.[3] The command follows the conventional Stata syntax,

```
dominance varlist [if] [in] [weight] [using filename],
  sortvar() [options]
```

If one variable is included in *varlist*, dominance of the concentration curve for this variable is tested against both the 45-degree line and the Lorenz curve of the living standards variable specified in sortvar(), which must be included. The default uses the multiple comparison approach decision rule, with comparisons at 19 equally spaced quantile points and a 5 percent significance level. The decision criterion can be changed to that of the intersection union principle with the option rule(iup), or results using both decision rules can be requested with rule(both). The number of comparison points can be changed with the option level(#), with 20 being the maximum value. The significance level can be changed from 5 percent to 1 percent with level(1).

Quintile (or decile) cumulative shares of the health variable and the living standards variable can be requested by the option shares(quintiles). This will also report the *p*-value for a test of significant differences between the cumulative shares of the health and living standards variables at each quintile (decile). Differences between the shares of each variable and the population shares are also tested.

To illustrate, we use data from the 1995-6 National Sample Survey to test dominance of the concentration curve for the public health subsidy (totsub) in India against both the 45-degree and the Lorenz curve for equivalent household consumption (hhexp_eq) as follows:[4]

```
dominance totsub [aw=weight], sortvar(hhexp_eq)
shares(quintiles)
```

Results confirm that the concentration curve is dominated by (lies below) the 45-degree line, but there is no dominance between the concentration curve of the subsidy and the Lorenz curve of household consumption. The cumulative quintile shares for the subsidy reported with the output are as follows:

```
Cumulative shares of totsub

Quantile Cum. share std. error Diff. from Diff. from
 pop. share income share

 p-value p-value
------------------------------------------------------------
q20 12.4911% 0.9554 0.0000 0.0366
q40 26.8893% 1.3009 0.0000 0.0979
q60 43.3710% 1.5738 0.0000 0.4922
q80 67.0052% 1.7219 0.0000 0.1175
------------------------------------------------------------
```

---

[2] The program can be downloaded free from http://132.203.59.36/dad/.

[3] The file can be downloaded from the Web site for this book. The program calls two other ados that need to be downloaded from the Stata Web site, glcurve and locpoly.

[4] For details of the application see O'Donnell et al (forthcoming).

The poorest 20 percent of individuals receive only 12.5 percent of the subsidy. The *p*-value in the fourth column confirms that this subsidy share is significantly less than the respective population share, and that is true at all quintiles. The *p*-values in the final column indicate that the subsidy shares are not significantly different from the consumption shares for all quintiles. Although there is a significant difference (at 5 percent) for the first quintile group, that is not inconsistent with the earlier finding of nondominance against the Lorenz curve, because in the dominance test critical values are adjusted for multiple comparisons.

If two variables are included in *varlist*, the program tests for dominance between the concentration curves of the two variables, allowing for dependence between the curves. In this case, the shares() option is not available.

To illustrate, we examine dominance between the concentration curves for the subsidy to nonhospital care (nonhsub) and the subsidy to hospital inpatient care (ipsub) in India (see O'Donnell et al. [forthcoming]). From figure 7.2, it appears that the concentration curve for nonhospital care lies above that for inpatient care.

Figure 7.2 was produced with the following commands:

```
#delimit ;
glcurve nonhsub [aw=weight], sortvar(hhexp_eq) lorenz pvar(rank)
  glvar(nonh) nograph;

glcurve ipsub [aw=weight], sortvar(hhexp_eq) lorenz
  plot(line nonh rank, legend(label(2 "non-hospital"))
  line rank rank, legend(label(3 "45 degree")))
  legend(label(1 "inpatient")) ll(Cumulative subsidy proportion);
```

Figure 7.2 *Concentration Curves of Public Subsidy to Inpatient Care and Subsidy to Nonhospital Care, India, 1995–96*

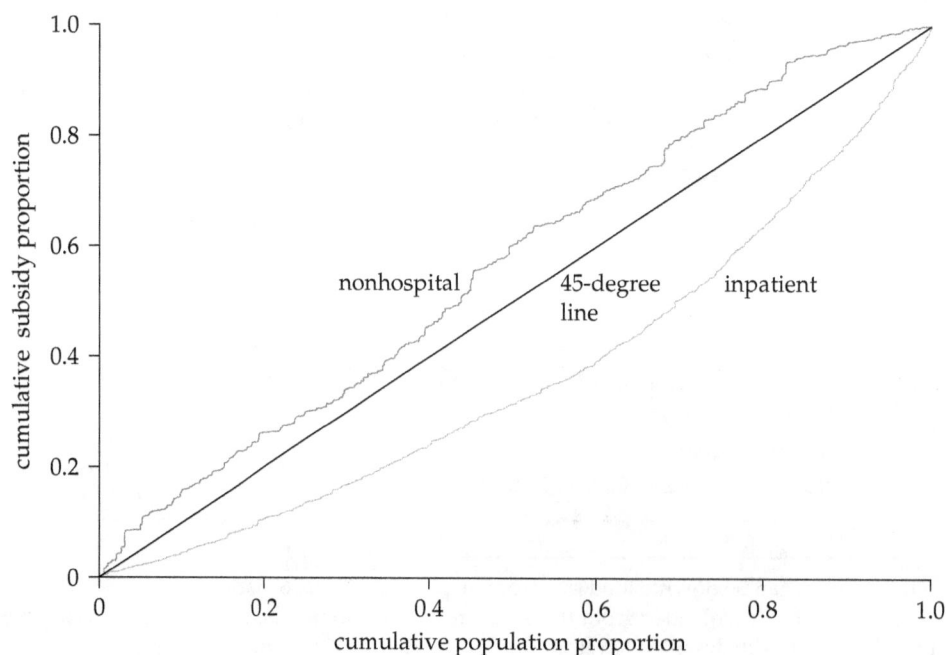

Source: Authors.

where the first `glcurve` command generates the *x* and *y* coordinates of the concentration curve for the nonhospital subsidy, and the second command plots this curve along with that for inpatient care and the 45-degree line.

We test for statistically significant dominance between the curves with

```
dominance nonhsub ipsub [aw=weight], sortvar(hhexp_eq)
```

The result confirms that the subsidy to nonhospital care dominates (is more pro-poor than) the inpatient subsidy.

The analyst may wish to test dominance between two concentration curves of the same variable estimated from independent samples. In this case, dominance testing is more straightforward because the ordinates of the respective concentration curves are independent. An important application is for cross-country comparisons of the distribution of a particular health or health care variable. For example, is the distribution of the public subsidy to health care less pro-poor in India than it is in Vietnam? To answer this question, we use data from the Indian 1995/96 NSS and the 1998 Vietnam Living Standards Survey.[5] The appropriate test can be carried out using the `dominance` command. In this case, the `using` option must be specified, and `varlist` must contain only one variable. Assume that we have the Indian data file loaded in Stata, that the Vietnam data file is named `Vietnam`, and that both files contain the variables `totsub` (total public health subsidy), `hhexp_eq` (equivalent household consumption), and `weight`. The syntax would then be as follows:

```
#delimit ;
dominance totsub [aw=weight] using Vietnam,
  sortvar(hhexp_eq) labels(India Vietnam) ;
```

where the `labels()` option gives labels to the two concentration curves that are used in the output. The result is reported as follows:

```
Test of dominance between concentration curves of totsub for
India and Vietnam

Data 1 Data 2 Sign. level # points Rule
------------------------------------------------------------

India Vietnam 5% 19 mca

 Vietnam dominates India
```

This confirms that the distribution of the public health subsidy is more pro-poor in Vietnam than it is in India.

One other thing the analyst might want to do is to check dominance across years. For example, is it really the case that the 1997/98 concentration curve in Figure 7.2 lies everywhere above that of 1992/93? `dominance` requires the 1992/93 and 1997/98 data to be in two separate data files. The code below first saves the data set with the newly constructed rank variable, then saves the 1997/98 cases separately in the file VN97.dta. The code then loads the original stacked data set

---

[5]See O'Donnell et al. (2007) for details and for more cross-country comparisons of the distribution of public health subsidies in Asia.

containing the data for 1992/93 and 1997/98, drops the observations for 1997/98, and runs the `dominance` routine, requesting that results using both decision rules be reported.

```
save "$path0\ch 7.dta", replace

use "$path0\ch 7.dta", clear
keep if year==1
save "$path0\VN97.dta", replace

use "$path0\ch 7.dta", clear
keep if year==0
dominance neghaz using VN97, sortvar(rank) labels(1993 1997)
  rule(both)
```

The output from Stata in this case is

Test of dominance between concentration curves of neghaz for 1993 and 1997

Data 1	Data 2	Sign. level	# points	Rule
1993	1997	5%	19	mca
1997 dominates 1993				
1993	1997	5%	19	iup
nondominance				

In this case, the 1997/98 concentration curve dominates (lies above) that of 1992/93 according to the less strict mca option, but not according to the stricter iup option. This reflects the fact that the two curves overlap toward the bottom of the income distribution.

References

Beach, C., M., and J. Richmond. 1985. "Joint Confidence Intervals for Income Shares and Lorenz Curves." *International Economic Review* 26: 439–50.

Bishop, J. A., J. P. Formby, and P. D. Thistle. 1992. Convergence of the South and Non-South Income Distributions, 1969–1979. *American Economic Review* 82(1): 262–72.

Bishop, J. A., K. V. Chow, and J. P. Formby. 1994. "Testing for Marginal Changes in Income Distributions with Lorenz and Concentration Curves." *International Economic Review* 35(2): 479–88.

Dardanoni, V., and A. Forcina. 1999. "Inference for Lorenz Curve Orderings." *Econometrics Journal* 2: 49–75.

Davidson, R., and J.-Y. Duclos. 1997. "Statistical Inference for the Measurement of the Incidence of Taxes and Transfers." *Econometrica* 65(6): 1453–65.

Deaton, A. 1997. *The Analysis of Household Surveys: A Microeconometric Approach to Development Policy.* Baltimore, MD: Johns Hopkins University Press.

Howes, S. 1996. "A New Test for Inferring Dominance from Sample Data." Mimeo. World Bank, Washington, DC.

Kakwani, N. C. 1977. "Measurement of Tax Progressivity: An International Comparison." *Economic Journal* 87(345): 71–80.

Kakwani, N. C., A. Wagstaff, and E. van Doorslaer. 1997. "Socioeconomic Inequalities in Health: Measurement, Computation and Statistical Inference." *Journal of Econometrics* 77(1): 87–104.

O'Donnell, O., E. van Doorslaer, R. P. Rannan-Eliya, A. Somanathan, S. R. Adhikari, D. Harbianto, C. G. Garg, P. Hanvoravongchai, M. N. Huq, A. Karan, G. M. Leung, C.-W. Ng, B. R. Pande, K. Tin, L. Trisnantoro, C. Vasavid, Y. Zhang, and Y. Zhao. 2007. "The Incidence of Public Spending on Health Care: Comparative Evidence from Asia." *World Bank Economic Review* 21(1): 93–123.

Sahn, D., and D. Younger. 2000. "Expenditure Incidence in Africa: Microeconomic Evidence." *Fiscal Studies* 21(3): 321–48.

Sahn, D. E., S. D. Younger, and K. R. Simler. 2000. "Dominance Testing of Transfers in Romania." *Review of Income and Wealth* 46(3): 309–27.

Stoline, M. R., and H. K. Ury. 1979. "Tables of the Studentized Maximum Modulus Distribution and an Application to Multiple Comparisons among Means." *Technometrics* 21(1): 87–93.

van Doorslaer, E., A. Wagstaff, H. Bleichrodt, S. Calonge, U. G. Gerdtham, M. Gerfin, J. Geurts, L. Gross, U. Hakkinen, R. E. Leu, O. O'Donnell, C. Propper, F. Puffer, M. Rodriguez, G. Sundberg, and O. Winkelhake. 1997. "Income-Related Inequalities In Health: Some International Comparisons." *J Health Econ* 16(1): 93–112.

Wagstaff, A. 2000. "Socioeconomic Inequalities in Child Mortality: Comparisons across Nine Developing Countries." *Bulletin of the World Health Organization* 78(1): 19–29.

Wagstaff, A., P. Paci, and E. van Doorslaer. 1991. "On the Measurement of Inequalities in Health." *Soc Sci Med* 33(5): 545–57.

Wagstaff, A., E. van Doorslaer, and N. Watanabe. 2003. "On Decomposing the Causes of Health Sector Inequalities, with an Application to Malnutrition Inequalities in Vietnam." *Journal of Econometrics* 112(1): 219–27.

8

The Concentration Index

Concentration curves can be used to identify whether socioeconomic inequality in some health sector variable exists and whether it is more pronounced at one point in time than another or in one country than another. But a concentration curve does not give a measure of the magnitude of inequality that can be compared conveniently across many time periods, countries, regions, or whatever may be chosen for comparison. The concentration index (Kakwani 1977, 1980), which is directly related to the concentration curve, does quantify the degree of socioeconomic-related inequality in a health variable (Kakwani, Wagstaff, and van Doorslaer 1997; Wagstaff, van Doorslaer, and Paci 1989). It has been used, for example, to measure and to compare the degree of socioeconomic-related inequality in child mortality (Wagstaff 2000), child immunization (Gwatkin et al. 2003), child malnutrition (Wagstaff, van Doorslaer, and Watanabe 2003), adult health (van Doorslaer et al. 1997), health subsidies (O'Donnell et al. 2007), and health care utilization (van Doorslaer et al. 2006). Many other applications are possible.

In this chapter we define the concentration index, comment on its properties, and identify the required measurement properties of health sector variables to which it can be applied. We also describe how to compute the concentration index and how to obtain a standard error for it, both for grouped data and for microdata.

Definition and properties

Definition

The concentration index is defined with reference to the concentration curve, introduced in chapter 7. The concentration index is defined as twice the area between the concentration curve and the line of equality (the 45-degree line). So, in the case in which there is no socioeconomic-related inequality, the concentration index is zero. The convention is that the index takes a negative value when the curve lies above the line of equality, indicating disproportionate concentration of the health variable among the poor, and a positive value when it lies below the line of equality. If the health variable is a "bad" such as ill health, a negative value of the concentration index means ill health is higher among the poor.

Formally, the concentration index is defined as

$$(8.1) \qquad C = 1 - 2 \int_0^1 L_h(p)dp.$$

The index is bounded between –1 and 1. For a discrete living standards variable, it can be written as

(8.2)
$$C=\frac{2}{N\mu}\sum_{i=1}^{n}h_i r_i -1-\frac{1}{N},$$

where h_i is the health sector variable, μ is its mean, and $r_i = i/N$ is the fractional rank of individual i in the living standards distribution, with $i = 1$ for the poorest and $i = N$ for the richest.[1] For computation, a more convenient formula for the concentration index defines it in terms of the covariance between the health variable and the fractional rank in the living standards distribution (Jenkins 1988; Kakwani 1980; Lerman and Yitzhaki 1989),

(8.3)
$$C=\frac{2}{\mu}\text{cov}(h,r).$$

Note that the concentration index depends only on the relationship between the health variable and the rank of the living standards variable and not on the variation in the living standards variable itself. A change in the degree of income inequality need not affect the concentration index measure of income-related health inequality.

The concentration index summarizes information from the concentration curve and can do so only through the imposition of value judgments about the weight given to inequality at different points in the distribution. Alternative weighting schemes implying different judgments about attitudes to inequality are considered in the next chapter. Inevitably, the concentration index loses some of the information that is contained in the concentration curve. The index can be zero either because the concentration curve lies everywhere on top of the 45-degree line or because it crosses the line and the (weighted) areas above and below the line cancel out. It is obviously important to distinguish between such cases, and so the summary index should be examined in conjunction with the concentration curve.

The sign of the concentration index indicates the direction of any relationship between the health variable and position in the living standards distribution, and its magnitude reflects both the strength of the relationship and the degree of variability in the health variable. Although this is valuable information, one may also wish to place an intuitive interpretation on the value of the index. Koolman and van Doorslaer (2004) have shown that multiplying the value of the concentration index by 75 gives the percentage of the health variable that would need to be (linearly) redistributed from the richer half to the poorer half of the population (in the case that health inequality favors the rich) to arrive at a distribution with an index value of zero.

Properties

The properties of the concentration index depend on the measurement characteristics of the variable of interest. Strictly, the concentration index is an appropriate measure of socioeconomic-related health (care) inequality when health (care) is measured on a ratio scale with nonnegative values. The concentration index is

---

[1]For large N, the final term in equation 8.3 approaches zero and it is often omitted.

invariant to multiplication of the health sector variable of interest by any scalar (Kakwani 1980). So, for example, if we are measuring inequality in payments for health care, it does not matter whether payments are measured in local currency or in dollars; the concentration index will be the same. Similarly, it does not matter whether health care is analyzed in terms of utilization per month or if monthly data are multiplied by 12 to give yearly figures. However, the concentration index is not invariant to any linear transformation of the variable of interest. Adding a constant to the variable will change the value of the concentration index. In many applications this does not matter because there is no reason to make an additive transformation of the variable of interest. There is one important application in which this does represent a limitation, however. We are often interested in inequality in a health variable that is not measured on a ratio scale. A ratio scale has a true zero, allowing statements such as "A has twice as much X as B." That makes sense for dollars or height. But many aspects of health cannot be measured in this way. Measurement of health inequality often relies on self-reported indicators of health, such as those considered in chapter 5. A concentration index cannot be computed directly from such categorical data. Although the ordinal data can be transformed into some cardinal measure and a concentration index computed for this (van Doorslaer and Jones 2003; Wagstaff and van Doorslaer 1994), the value of the index will depend on the transformation chosen (Erreygers 2005).[2] In cross-country comparisons, even if all countries adopt the same transformation, their ranking by the concentration index could be sensitive to differences in the means of health that are used in the transformation.

A partial solution to this problem would be to dichotomize the categorical health measure. For example, one could examine how the proportion of individuals reporting poor health varies with living standards. Unfortunately, this introduces another problem. Wagstaff (2005) has demonstrated that the bounds of the concentration index for a dichotomous variable are not –1 and 1 but depend on the mean of the variable. For large samples, the lower bound is $\mu - 1$ and the upper bound is $1 - \mu$. So the feasible interval of the index shrinks as the mean rises. One should be cautious, therefore, in using the concentration index to compare inequality in, for example, child mortality and immunization rates across countries with substantial differences in the means of these variables. An obvious response is to normalize the concentration index by dividing through by 1 minus the mean (Wagstaff 2005).

If the health variable of interest takes negative as well as positive values, then its concentration index is not bounded within the range of (–1,1). In the extreme, if the mean of the variable were 0, the concentration index would not be defined.

Bleichrodt and van Doorslaer (2006) have derived the conditions that must hold for the concentration index (and related measures) to be a measure of socioeconomic-related health inequality consistent with a social welfare function. They argue that one condition—the principle of income-related health transfers—is rather restrictive. Erreygers (2006) has derived an alternative measure of socioeconomic-related health inequality that is consistent with this condition and three others argued to be desirable.

---

[2]Erreygers (2005) suggests a couple of alternatives to the concentration index to deal with this problem.

Estimation and inference for grouped data

Point estimate of the concentration index

The concentration index for $t=1,...,T$ groups is easily computed in a spreadsheet program using the following formula (Fuller and Lury 1977):

$$(8.4) \qquad C=\left(p_1 L_2 - p_2 L_1\right)+\left(p_2 L_3 - p_3 L_2\right)+...+\left(p_{T-1} L_T - p_T L_{T-1}\right)$$

where p_t is the cumulative percentage of the sample ranked by economic status in group t, and L_t is the corresponding concentration curve ordinate. To illustrate, consider the distribution of under-five mortality by wealth quintiles in India, 1982–92. We drew the concentration curve for these data in chapter 7. Table 8.1 reproduces table 7.1 with the terms in brackets in the formula above added to the final column. The sum of these terms is –0.1694, which is the concentration index. The negative concentration index reflects the higher mortality rates among poorer children.

Standard error

A standard error of the estimator of C in the grouped data case can be computed using a formula given in Kakwani, Wagstaff, and van Doorslaer (1997). Let f_t be the proportion of the sample in the tth group, and define the fractional rank of group t by

$$(8.5) \qquad R_t = \sum_{k=1}^{t-1} f_k + \tfrac{1}{2} f_t,$$

which is the cumulative proportion of the population up to the midpoint of each group interval. The variance of the estimator of C is given by

$$(8.6) \qquad \mathrm{var}(\hat{C}) = \frac{1}{n}\left[\sum_{t=1}^{T} f_t a_t^2 - \left(1+C\right)^2\right] + \frac{1}{n\mu^2}\sum_{t=1}^{T} f_t \sigma_t^2 \left(2R_t - 1 - C\right)^2,$$

where n is the sample size, σ_t^2 is the variance of the health variable in the tth group, μ is its mean,

$$a_t = \frac{\mu_t}{\mu}\left(2R_t - 1 - C\right) + 2 - q_{t-1} - q_t, \text{ and}$$

$$q_t = \frac{1}{\mu}\sum_{k=1}^{t} \mu_k f_k,$$

which is the ordinate of $L_h(p)$, $q_0 = 0$, and $p_t = \sum_{k=1}^{t} f_k R_k$ (Kakwani, Wagstaff, and van Doorslaer 1997).

Table 8.1 *Under-Five Deaths in India, 1982–92*

Wealth group	No. of births	Rel % births	Cumul % births	U5MR per 1,000	No. of deaths	Rel % deaths	Cumul % deaths	Conc. index
Poorest	29,939	23	23	154.7	4,632	30	30	–0.0008
2nd	28,776	22	45	152.9	4,400	29	59	–0.0267
Middle	26,528	20	66	119.5	3,170	21	79	–0.0592
4th	24,689	19	85	86.9	2,145	14	93	–0.0827
Richest	19,739	15	100	54.3	1,072	7	100	0.0000
Total/average	129,671			118.8	15,419			–0.1694

Source: Authors.

CASE IN WHICH WITHIN-GROUP VARIANCES ARE UNKNOWN In many applications, the within-group variances will be unknown. For example, the data might have been obtained from published tabulations by income quintile. In such cases, it must be assumed that there is no within-group variance and the second term in equation 8.6 is set to zero. However, in addition, n needs to be replaced by T in the denominator of the first term because there are in effect only T observations, not n.

Table 8.2 gives an example using data on under-five mortality (rates per birth, not rates per 1,000 births) from the 1998 Vietnam Living Standards Survey (VLSS). The data were computed directly from the survey, with children being grouped into household per capita consumption quintiles. The assumption made in table 8.2 is that the within-group variances in mortality are not known and are set to zero. Below, we relax this assumption. The table, which is extracted from an Excel file, shows the values for each quintile of R, q, a, and fa^2 computed by substituting estimates for the parameters in the formula above. Also shown is the sum of fa^2 across the five quintiles. Substituting $\Sigma f \cdot a^2 = 0.680$, $C = -0.1841$, and $T = 5$ into equation 8.6 gives 0.0029 for the variance of the estimate of C and hence a standard error equal to 0.0537. The t-statistic for C is therefore −3.43.

CASE IN WHICH WITHIN-GROUP VARIANCES ARE KNOWN In some cases, the within-group variances will be known, and this provides us with more information. In effect, we move from having information only on the T group means to having information on the full sample—albeit with the variation within the groups being picked up only by the group standard deviations. One such scenario is the case in which we are working with mortality data—the rates are defined at the group level only, but the within-group standard deviations are reported.[3]

In such cases, n is used (rather than T) in the denominator of the first term in equation 8.6, and the second term needs to be computed as well. Table 8.3 shows the standard errors for each quintile's under-five mortality rate from the Vietnam data. The final column shows the value for each quintile of the term in the summation operator in the second term of equation 8.6, as well as the sum of these across the five quintiles. Dividing this sum through by $n\mu^2$ gives 1.511e-6, which is the second term of equation 8.6. Dividing Σfa^2 through by n (=5,315) gives 2.717e-6, which is

Table 8.2 Under-Five Deaths in Vietnam, 1989–98 (within-group variance unknown)

Consumption group	No. of births	Cumul % births	R	U5MR	Cumul % deaths	CI	q	a	$f \cdot a^2$
Poorest	1,002	19	0.094	0.060	31	−0.024	0.312	0.648	0.079
2nd	949	37	0.278	0.034	48	−0.013	0.482	0.959	0.164
Middle	1,002	56	0.461	0.041	69	−0.053	0.695	0.944	0.168
4th	1,082	76	0.657	0.028	85	−0.095	0.854	0.842	0.144
Richest	1,280	100	0.880	0.022	100	0.000	1.000	0.719	0.124
Total/average	5,315			0.036		−0.184			0.680

Source: Authors.

---

[3]Or the standard errors of the group means are reported, from which estimates of the variances can be recovered provided group sizes are known.

Table 8.3 *Under-Five Deaths in Vietnam, 1989–98 (within-group variance known)*

Consumption group	No. of births	R	U5MR	CI	q	a	$f \cdot a^2$	Std Error	$f\sigma^2(2R-0.5-0.5C)^2$
Poorest	1,002	0.094	0.060	−0.024	0.312	0.648	0.079	0.008	4.631E-06
2nd	949	0.278	0.034	−0.013	0.482	0.959	0.164	0.006	4.354E-07
Middle	1,002	0.461	0.041	−0.053	0.695	0.944	0.168	0.007	9.085E-08
4th	1,082	0.657	0.028	−0.095	0.854	0.842	0.144	0.005	1.423E-06
Richest	1,280	0.880	0.022	0.000	1.000	0.719	0.124	0.004	3.780E-06
Total/average	5,315		0.036	−0.184			0.680		1.036E-05

Source: Authors.

the first term in equation 8.6. The sum of the two terms is the variance, equal in this case to 4.228e-6, giving a standard error of the estimate of C equal to 0.0021. This, unsurprisingly, is substantially smaller than the standard error obtained assuming no within-group variance.

Estimation and inference for microdata

Point estimate of the concentration index

The concentration index (C) can be computed very easily from microdata by using the "convenient covariance" formula (equation 8.3). If the sample is not self-weighted, weights should be applied in computation of the covariance, the mean of the health variable, and the fractional rank. Given the relationship between covariance and ordinary least squares (OLS) regression, an equivalent estimate of the concentration index can be obtained from a "convenient regression" of a transformation of the health variable of interest on the fractional rank in the living standards distribution (Kakwani, Wagstaff, and van Doorslaer 1997). Specifically,

$$(8.7) \qquad 2\sigma_r^2\left(\frac{h_i}{\mu}\right)=\alpha+\beta r_i+\varepsilon_i,$$

where σ_r^2 is the variance of the fractional rank. The OLS estimate of β is an estimate of the concentration index equivalent to that obtained from equation 8.3. This method gives rise to an alternative interpretation of the concentration index as the slope of a line passing through the heads of a parade of people, ranked by their living standards, with each individual's height proportional to the value of his or her health variable, expressed as a fraction of the mean.

Computation of the concentration index

To illustrate computation, we estimate the concentration index for the public subsidy to hospital outpatient care (subsidy) in Vietnam using data from the 1998 Vietnam Living Standards Survey (see chapter 14 and O'Donnell et al. [2007]). The living standards variable is household consumption per equivalent adult (eqcons), and the sample must be weighted (by variable weight).

By using equation 8.3 or 8.7, an estimate of a concentration index can be computed easily with any statistical package. The only slight complication involves computation of the fractional rank variable in the case that the data must be weighted. The weighted fractional rank is defined as follows:

$$(8.8) \qquad r_i = \sum_{j=0}^{i-1} w_j + \frac{w_i}{2},$$

where w_i is the sample weight scaled to sum to 1, observations are sorting in ascending order of living standards, and $w_0 = 0$. In Stata, this can be computed as follows:

```
egen raw_rank=rank(eqcons), unique
sort raw_rank
quietly sum weight
gen wi=weight/r(sum)
gen cusum=sum(wi)
gen wj=cusum[_n-1]
replace wj=0 if wj==.
gen rank=wj+0.5*wi
```

where `income` is the measure of living standards, `weight` is the original sample weight, `wi` is a scaled version of this that sums to 1, `wj` is the first term in equation 8.8, and `rank` is r_i in equation 8.8. Alternatively, the weighted fractional rank can be generated using `glcurve`,[4]

```
glcurve eqcons [aw=weight], pvar(rank) nograph
```

Because weights are applied, the generated variable `rank` is the weighted fractional rank. The rank variables produced by the two procedures will be perfectly correlated. The (weighted) mean of the rank produced from the first procedure will always be exactly 0.5, and the mean of the rank produced by `glcurve` will differ from 0.5 only at the 4th–5th decimal place.

By using equation 8.3, the concentration index can then be computed using[5]

```
qui sum subsidy [fw=weight]
scalar mean=r(mean)
cor subsidy rank [fw=weight], c
sca c=(2/mean)*r(cov_12)
sca list c
```

By using equation 8.7, the index is computed as follows:

```
qui sum rank [fw=weight]
sca var_rank=r(Var)
gen lhs=2*var_rank*(subsidy/mean)
regr lhs rank [pw=weight]
sca c=_b[rank]
sca list c
```

---

[4]See chapter 7 for an explanation of `glcurve`.

[5]For the `corr` and `sum` commands, frequency weights (`fw`) should be used to get the correct variance of the weighted rank and its covariance with the health variable of interest. The weight variable must be an integer for the frequency weight to be accepted by Stata. If the weight variable is a noninteger, analysts will first need to multiply the weight by 10^k, where k is the largest number of decimal places in any value of the weight variable. A new integer weight variable will then have to be created using the `gen new _ weight = int (weight)`. The alternative is to use analytic weights and accept some imprecision.

Both procedures give an estimate of the concentration index of 0.16700, indicating that the better-off receive more of the public subsidy to hospital outpatient care in Vietnam.

Standard error

Kakwani, Wagstaff, and van Doorslaer (1997) derived the standard error of a concentration estimated from microdata. They did this by noting that the concentration index can be written as a nonlinear function of totals, and so the delta method (Rao 1965) can be applied to obtain the standard error. The resulting formula is essentially a simplified version of equation 8.6 without the second term because at the individual level there is no within-group variation. Specifically,

$$(8.9) \qquad \mathrm{var}\left(\hat{C}\right) = \frac{1}{n}\left[\frac{1}{n}\sum_{i=1}^{n} a_i^2 - \left(1+C\right)^2\right],$$

where
$$a_i = \frac{h_i}{\mu}\left(2r_i - 1 - C\right) + 2 - q_{i-1} - q_i,$$

and
$$q_i = \frac{1}{\mu n}\sum_{j=1}^{i} h_j$$

is the ordinate of the concentration curve $L_h(p)$, and $q_0 = 0$.

Unfortunately, equation 8.9 does not take into account sample weights and other sample design features, such as cluster sampling (see chapters 2 and 9), although in principle it could be adapted to do so. The formula can be computed easily in Stata. We demonstrate this for the Vietnam subsidy example. First, we must recompute the concentration index without the application of weights, as follows:

```
glcurve subsidy, sortvar(eqcons) pvar(ranku) glvar(ccurve)
lorenz nograph;
qui sum ranku
sca var_ranku=r(Var)
qui sum subsidy
sca meanu=r(mean)
gen lhsu=2*var_ranku*(subsidy/meanu)
regr lhsu ranku
sca conindu=_b[rank]
```

The estimate of the concentration index from the unweighted data is 0.16606. Standard errors are then computed using equation 8.9 as follows:

```
sort ranku
gen cclag = ccurve[_n-1]
replace cclag=0 if cclag==.
gen asqr=((subsidy/meanu)*(2*ranku-1-conindu)+2-cclag-
ccurve)^2
qui sum asqr
sca var=(r(mean)-(1+conindu)^2)/r(N)
sca se=sqrt(var)
sca list conindu se
```

That gives a standard error of 0.033976, and so a *t*-ratio of 4.89.

The limitation of equation 8.9 is that it cannot be applied directly to data that are weighted and/or do not have a simple random sample design. To take such sample features into account, one option is simply to use the standard error of the coefficient on the rank variable in the convenient regression. Because this coefficient is an estimate of the concentration index, one might expect its standard error to be that of the concentration index. This is not quite correct because it takes no account of the sampling variability of the estimate of the mean of the health variable that enters the transformation giving the left-hand side of the convenient regression. Note that the variance of the fractional rank, which is also used in the transformation, depends only on the sample size and so has no sampling variability.[6] It can be treated as a constant. One computationally simple way of taking account of the sampling variability of the mean is to run the convenient regression without transforming the left-hand-side variable but (equivalently) transforming the rank coefficient instead. A delta method standard error can then be computed for the transformed coefficient that takes account of the sampling variability of all terms used in the transformation. From the regression

(8.10)
$$h_i = \alpha_1 + \beta_1 r_i + u_i$$

the estimate of the concentration index is given by

(8.11)
$$\hat{\beta} = \left(\frac{2\sigma_r^2}{\hat{\mu}} \right) \hat{\beta}_1.$$

By using the facts that the least squares predicted value has the same mean as the dependent variable and that the mean of the fractional rank variable is 0.5, equation 8.11 can be written as

(8.12)
$$\hat{\beta} = \left(\frac{2\sigma_r^2}{\hat{\alpha}_1 + \dfrac{\hat{\beta}_1}{2}} \right) \hat{\beta}_1.$$

Because the estimate is now written as a function of the regression coefficients, a standard error can be obtained by applying the delta method. In Stata, this procedure can be implemented very easily using nlcom.

```
regr subsidy rank [pw=weight]
nlcom ((2*var_rank)/(_b[_cons]+0.5*_b[rank]))*_b[rank]
```

For the Vietnam outpatient subsidy example, that gives a standard error of 0.034016 for the estimate of the (weighted) concentration index of 0.16700 reported above. The standard error of the rank coefficient from equation 8.7 is 0.034945, and so it appears that taking account of the sampling variability of the mean makes very little difference. Experimentation suggests that this is generally the case, and so standard errors from the convenient regression equation 8.7 can be used without too much concern for inaccuracy.

In Stata, if weights are applied in the regression, then the standard error returned will be robust to heteroskedasticity. If there are no weights, heteroskedasticity robust

---

[6]This is due to the nature of the fractional rank variable. Its weighted mean is always 0.5, and its variance approaches 1/12 as n goes to infinity. For given n, the variance of the fractional rank is always the same.

standard errors can be obtained by adding the option robust to the regression. If this is done, then the delta method standard errors computed by a nlcom command following the regression will also be robust. If the survey has a cluster sampling design, then the standard errors should be corrected for within-cluster correlation. This is achieved by adding the option cluster,

```
regr subsidy rank [pw=wt], cluster(commune)
nlcom ((2*var_rank)/(_b[_cons]+0.5*_b[rank]))*_b[rank]
```

where commune is the variable denoting the primary sampling unit—communes in the VLSS. Allowing for within-cluster correlation raises the standard error in the Vietnam subsidy example from 0.034016 to 0.041988.

Correcting for across-cluster correlation may or may not be necessary, depending on the sample design, but a form of serial correlation is always likely to be present owing to the rank nature of the regressor (Kakwani, Wagstaff, van Doorslaer 1997). To correct the standard errors for this, one can use the Newey-West (Newey and West 1994) variance-covariance matrix, which corrects for autocorrelation, as well as heteroscedasticty. In Stata, the command newey produces OLS regression coefficients with Newey-West standard errors. To use this, the data must be set to a time series format with the time variable being, in this case, the living standards rank. This must be an integer valued variable, and so the fractional rank created above cannot be used. Below, we create the appropriate rank variable (ranki) before running the newey command:

```
egen  ranki=rank(eqcons), unique
tsset ranki
newey subsidy rank [aw=weight], lag(1)
nlcom ((2*var_rank)/(_b[_cons]+0.5*_b[rank]))*_b[rank]
```

Note that the (weighted) fractional rank and not the integer valued rank is still used in the regression. Weights (analytical) are allowed, and the lag(#) option must be included to specify the maximum number of lags to be considered in the autocorrelation structure. For our example, this estimator gives a standard error of 0.034568, slightly larger than if we allow for heteroskedasticity only (0.034016), but smaller than if we allow for within-cluster correlation (0.041988).

Demographic standardization of the concentration index

As discussed in chapter 5, we are often interested in measuring socioeconomic-related inequality in a health variable after controlling for the confounding effect of demographics. In chapter 5 we explained how this can be done using both direct and indirect methods of standardization. To estimate a standardized concentration index, one could use either method of standardization to generate a predicted health variable purged of the influence of demographics across socioeconomic groups, as explained in chapter 5, then compute the concentration index for this standardized variable.

In the case that one wishes to standardize for the full correlation with confounders, and so there are no control (z) variables (see chapter 5), a shortcut method of obtaining an indirectly standardized concentration index is simply to include the standardizing variables directly in the convenient regression. This is precisely what is being done in the literature that makes use of the relative index of inequality (e.g., Mackenbach et al. [1997]). From the regression

$$(8.13) \qquad 2\sigma_r^2\left(\frac{h_i}{\mu}\right) = \alpha_2 + \beta_2 r_i + \sum_j \delta_j x_{ji} + v_i,$$

where x_j are the confounding variables, for example, age, sex, and so on, the OLS estimate $\hat{\beta}_2$ is an estimate of the indirectly standardized concentration index. Computation requires simply adding the confounding variables to the regression commands discussed above.

Sensitivity of the concentration index to the living standards measure

In chapter 6 we described alternative measures of living standards—consumption, expenditure, wealth index—and noted that it is not always possible to establish a clear advantage of one measure over others. It is therefore important to consider whether the chosen measure of living standards influences the measured degree of socioeconomic-related inequality in the health variable of interest. When the concentration index is used as a summary measure of inequality, the question is whether it is sensitive to the living standards measure.

As noted above, the concentration index reflects the relationship between the health variable and living standards rank. It is not influenced by the variance of the living standards measure. In some circumstances, this may be considered a disadvantage. For example, it means that, for a given relationship between income and health, the concentration index cannot discriminate the degree of income-related health inequality in one country in which income is distributed very unevenly from that in another country in which the income distribution is very equal. On the other hand, when one is interested in inequality at a certain place and time, it is reassuring that the differing variances of alternative measures of living standards will not influence the concentration index. However, the concentration index may differ if the ranking of individuals is inconsistent across alternative measures.

Wagstaff and Watanabe (2003) demonstrate that the concentration index will differ across alternative living standards measures if the health variable is correlated with changes in an individual's rank on moving from one measure to another. The difference between two concentration indices C_1 and C_2, where the respective concentration index is calculated on the basis of a given ranking (r_{1i} and r_{2i})—for example, consumption and a wealth index—can be computed by means of the regression

$$(8.14) \qquad 2\sigma_{\Delta r}^2\left(\frac{h_i}{\mu}\right) = \alpha + \gamma \Delta r_i + \varepsilon_i,$$

where $\Delta r_i = r_{1i} - r_{2i}$ is the reranking that results from changing the measure of socioeconomic status, and $\sigma_{\Delta r}^2$ is its variance. The OLS estimate of γ provides an estimate of the difference ($C_1 - C_2$). Significance of the difference between indices can be tested by using the standard error of γ.[7]

For 19 countries, Wagstaff and Watanabe (2003) test the sensitivity of the concentration index for child malnutrition to the use of household consumption and a

---

[7]This ignores the sampling variability of the left-hand-side estimates.

Table 8.4 *Concentration Indices for Health Service Utilization with Household Ranked by Consumption and an Assets Index, Mozambique 1996/97*

	Consumption		Asset index		Difference $CI_C - CI_{AI}$	t-value for difference
	CI	t-value	CI	t-value		
Hospital visits	0.166	8.72	0.231	12.94	−0.065	−3.35
Health center visits	0.066	3.85	−0.136	−8.49	0.202	9.99
Complete immunizations	0.059	8.35	0.194	34.69	−0.135	−19.1
Delivery control	0.063	11.86	0.154	35.01	−0.091	−15.27
Institutional delivery	0.089	11.31	0.266	43.26	−0.176	−20.06

Source: Lindelow 2006.

wealth index as the living standards ranking variable. Malnutrition is measured by a binary indicator of underweight and another for stunting (see chapter 4). For each of underweight and stunting, the difference between the concentration indices is significant (10%) for 6 of 19 comparisons. This suggests that in the majority of countries, child nutritional status is not strongly correlated with inconsistencies in the ranking of households by consumption and wealth.

But there is some evidence that concentration indices for health service utilization are more sensitive to the living standards measure. Table 8.4, reproduced from Lindelow (2006), shows substantial and significant differences between the concentration indices (CI) for a variety of health services in Mozambique using consumption and an asset index as the living standards measure. In the case of consumption, the concentration index indicates statistically significant inequality in favor of richer households for all services. With households ranked by the asset index rather than consumption, the inequality is greater for all services except health center visits, for which the concentration index indicates inequality in utilization in favor of poorer households.

It appears that the choice of welfare indicator *can* have a large and significant impact on measured socioeconomic inequalities in a health variable, but it depends on the variable examined. Differences in measured inequality reflect the fact that consumption and the asset index measure different things, or at least are different proxies for the same underlying variable of interest. But only in cases in which the difference in rankings between the measures is also correlated with the health variable of interest will the choice of indicator have an important impact on the findings. In cases in which both asset and consumption data are available, analysts are in a position to qualify any analysis of these issues by reference to parallel analysis based on alternative measures. However, data on both consumption and assets are often not available. In these cases, the potential sensitivity of the findings should be explicitly recognized.

References

Bleichrodt, H., and E. van Doorslaer. 2006. "A Welfare Economics Foundation for Health Inequality Measurement." *Journal of Health Economics* 25(5): 945–57.

Erreygers, G. 2005. *Beyond the Health Concentration Index: An Atkinson Alternative to the Measurement of Socioeconomic Inequality of Health.* University of Antwerp. Antwerp, Belgium.

Erreygars, G. 2006. *Correcting the Concentration Index.* University of Antwerp. Antwerp, Belgium.

Fuller, M., and D. Lury. 1977. *Statistics Workbook for Social Science Students.* Oxford, United Kingdom: Phillip Allan.

Gwatkin, D. R., S. Rustein, K. Johnson, R. Pande, and A. Wagstaff. 2003. *Initial Country-Level Information about Socio-Economic Differentials in Health, Nutrition and Population,* Volumes I and II. Washington, DC: World Bank Health, Population and Nutrition.

Jenkins, S. 1988. "Calculating Income Distribution Indices from Microdata." *National Tax Journal* 61: 139–42.

Kakwani, N. C. 1977. "Measurement of Tax Progressivity: An International Comparison." *Economic Journal* 87(345): 71–80.

Kakwani, N. C. 1980. *Income Inequality and Poverty: Methods of Estimation and Policy Applications.* New York: Oxford University Press.

Kakwani, N. C., A. Wagstaff, and E. van Doorslaer. 1997. "Socioeconomic Inequalities in Health: Measurement, Computation and Statistical Inference." *Journal of Econometrics* 77(1): 87–104.

Koolman, X., and E. van Doorslaer. 2004. "On the Interpretation of a Concentration Index of Inequality." *Health Economics* 13: 649–56.

Lerman, R. I., and S. Yitzhaki. 1989. "Improving the Accuracy of Estimates of Gini Coefficients." *Journal of Econometrics* 42(1): 43–47.

Lindelow, M. 2006. "Sometimes More Equal Than Others: How Health Inequalities Depend upon the Choice of Welfare Indicator." *Health Economics* 15(3): 263–80.

Mackenbach, J. P., A. E. Kunst, A. E. J. M. Cavelaars, F. Groenhof, and J. J. M.Geurts. 1997. "Socioeconomic Inequalities in Morbidity and Mortality in Western Europe." *Lancet* 349: 1655–59.

Newey, W. K., and K. D. West. 1994. "Automatic Lag Selection in Covariance Matrix Estimation." *Review of Economic Studies* 61(4): 631–53.

O'Donnell, O., E. van Doorslaer, R. P. Rannan-Eliya, A. Somanathan, S. R. Adhikari, D. Harbianto, C. G. Garg, P. Hanvoravongchai, M. N. Huq, A. Karan, G. M. Leung, C-W Ng, B. R. Pande, K. Tin, L. Trisnantoro, C. Vasavid, Y. Zhang, and Y. Zhao. Forthcoming. "The Incidence of Public Spending on Health Care: Comparative Evidence from Asia." *World Bank Economic Review.*

Rao, C. R. 1965. *Linear Statistical Inference and its Applications.* New York: Wiley.

van Doorslaer, E., and A. M. Jones. 2003. "Inequalities in Self-Reported Health: Validation of a New Approach to Measurement." *Journal of Health Economics* 22.

van Doorslaer, E., C. Masseria, X. Koolman, and the OECD Health Equity Research Group. 2006. "Inequalities in Access to Medical Care by Income in Developed Countries." *Canadian Medical Association Journal* 174: 177–83.

van Doorslaer, E., A. Wagstaff, H. Bleichrodt, S. Calonge, U. G. Gerdtham, M. Gerfin, J. Geurts, L. Gross, U. Hakkinen, R. E. Leu, O. O'Donnell, C. Propper, F. Puffer, M. Rodriguez, G. Sundberg, and O. Winkelhake. 1997. "Income-Related Inequalities in Health: Some International Comparisons." *J Health Econ* 16(1): 93–112.

Wagstaff, A. 2000. "Socioeconomic Inequalities in Child Mortality: Comparisons across Nine Developing Countries." *Bulletin of the World Health Organization* 78(1): 19–29.

Wagstaff, A. 2005. "The Bounds of the Concentration Index When the Variable of Interest Is Binary, with an Application to Immunization Inequality." *Health Economics* 14(4): 429–32.

Wagstaff, A., and E. van Doorslaer. 1994. "Measuring Inequalities in Health in the Presence of Multiple-Category Morbidity Indicators." *Health Economics* 3: 281–91.

Wagstaff, A., E. van Doorslaer, and P. Paci. 1989. "Equity in the Finance and Delivery of Health Care: Some Tentative Cross-Country Comparisons." *Oxford Review of Economic Policy* 5(1): 89–112.

Wagstaff, A., E. van Doorslaer, and N. Watanabe. 2003. "On Decomposing the Causes of Health Sector Inequalities, with an Application to Malnutrition Inequalities in Vietnam." *Journal of Econometrics* 112(1): 219–27.

Wagstaff, A., and N. Watanabe. 2003. "What Difference Does the Choice of SES Make in Health Inequality Measurement?" *Health Economics* 12(10): 885–90.

9

Extensions to the Concentration Index: Inequality Aversion and the Health Achievement Index

The concentration index is a useful tool for measuring inequalities in the health sector. It does, however, have limitations.

First, like the Gini coefficient, it has implicit in it a particular set of value judgments about aversion to inequality. This chapter shows how to operationalize Wagstaff's (2002) "extended" concentration index, which allows attitudes to inequality to be made explicit, and to see how measured inequality changes as the attitude to inequality changes.

The second drawback of the concentration index—and the generalization of it—is that it is just a measure of inequality. Although equity is an important goal of health policy, it is not the only one. It is not just health inequality that matters; the average level of health also matters. Policy makers are likely to be willing to trade one off against the other—a little more inequality might be considered acceptable if the average increases substantially. This points to a second extension of the concentration index (Wagstaff 2002): a general measure of health "achievement" that captures inequality in the distribution of health (or some other health sector variable) as well as its mean.

The extended concentration index

The regular concentration index C is equal to (Kakwani, Wagstaff, and van Doorslaer 1997)

$$(9.1) \qquad C = \frac{2}{n \cdot \mu} \sum_{i=1}^{n} h_i R_i - 1,$$

where n is the sample size, h_i is the ill-health indicator for person i, μ is the mean level of ill health, and R_i is the fractional rank in the living-standards distribution of the ith person. The value judgments implicit in C are seen most easily when C is rewritten in an equivalent way as

$$(9.2) \qquad C = 1 - \frac{2}{n \cdot \mu} \sum_{i=1}^{n} h_i (1 - R_i).$$

The quantity $h_i/n\mu$ is the share of health (or ill health) enjoyed (or suffered) by person i. This is then weighted in the summation by twice the complement of the person's fractional rank, that is, $2(1 - R_i)$. So, the poorest person has his or her health share weighted by a number close to two. The weights decline in a stepwise fashion, reaching a number close to zero for the richest person. The concentration index is simply one minus the sum of these weighted health shares.

The *extended* concentration index can be written as follows:

$$(9.3) \qquad C(v) = 1 - \frac{v}{n \cdot \mu} \sum_{i=1}^{n} h_i \left(1 - R_i\right)^{(v-1)} \qquad v > 1.$$

In equation 9.3, v is the inequality-aversion parameter, which will be explained below. The weight attached to the ith person's health share, $h_i/n\mu$, is now equal to $v(1 - R_i)^{(v-1)}$, rather than by $2(1 - R_i)$. When $v = 2$, the weight is the same as in the regular concentration index; so $C(2)$ is the standard concentration index. By contrast, when $v = 1$, everyone's health is weighted equally. This is the case in which the value judgment is that inequalities in health do not matter. So, $C(1) = 0$ however unequally health is distributed across the income distribution. As v is raised above 1, the weight attached to the health of a very poor person rises, and the weight attached to the health of people who are above the 55th percentile decreases. For $v = 6$, the weight attached to the health of persons in the top two quintiles is virtually zero. When v is raised to 8, the weight attached to the health of those in the top *half* of the income distribution is virtually zero (Figure 9.1).

Computing the extended concentration index on microdata

Like the regular concentration index, the extended concentration index can be written as a covariance (cf. equation 8.3). This is an easy way to compute the extended concentration index on microdata. The relevant covariance (Wagstaff 2002) is

$$(9.4) \qquad C(v) = -\frac{v}{\mu} \text{cov}\left(h_i, \left(1 - R_i\right)^{v-1}\right).$$

This can be computed in a straightforward manner for different values of v.

As an example, we compute the extended concentration index for values $v = 1$, $v = 2$, $v = 3$, $v = 4$, and $v = 5$ for (the negative of) height-for-age for children in the 1993 Vietnamese Living Standards Measurement Study. (The negative of the height-for-age variable captures malnutrition, the rate of which is higher among poorer children, so $C < 0$.) These are the same data used by Wagstaff, van Doorslaer, and

Figure 9.1 *Weighting Scheme for Extended Concentration Index*

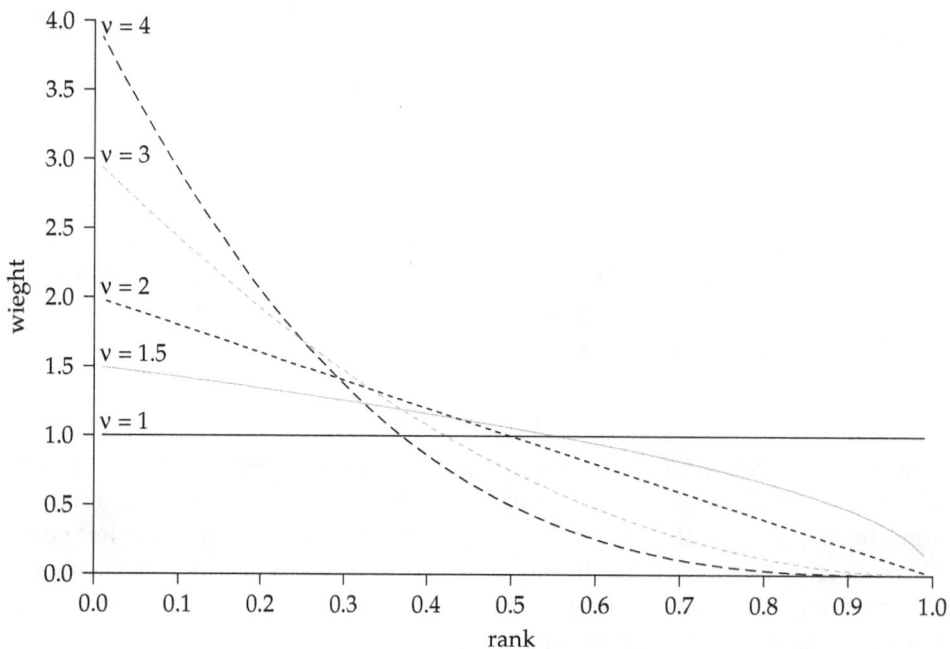

Source: Authors.

Watanabe (2003). We know, of course, that $C(1) = 0$. We also know from Wagstaff, van Doorslaer, and Watanabe (2003) that for the year 1993 $C(2)$ is equal to -0.077 (cf. Wagstaff, van Doorslaer, and Watanabe 2003, p. 213). The Stata code to loop through $v = 1$, $v = 2$, $v = 3$, $v = 4$, and $v = 5$ is

```
sca drop _all
sum neghaz
scalar mean = r(mean)
forval i = 1/5 {
        ge adjrnk`i' = (1-rank)^(`i'-1)
        corr neghaz adjrnk`i' , covar
        sca ci`i' = -`i'*r(cov_12)/mean
}
sca li _all
```

Here neghaz is the negative of the height-for-age score (i.e., y_i), and rank is the fractional rank variable (i.e., R_i). The sum command stores the mean of neghaz in the scalar mean. For each of the values of v, the loop generates an adjusted rank variable, computes the required covariance, calculates the concentration index, and stores $C(v)$ in the scalar ci v. The scalar list command at the end produces the following:

```
sca    li _all
       ci5 = -.14068989
       ci4 = -.12858764
       ci3 = -.11006521
       ci2 = -.0771886
       ci1 = 0
       mean = 2.0298478
```

confirming that $C(1) = 0$ and $C(2) = -0.077$ for these data, and that as v is raised above 2, $C(v)$ becomes increasingly negative, reflecting the increasing weight that is being attached to the (ill-) health scores of poorer people.

Alternatively, the extended concentration index can be computed on microdata by means of a convenient regression (cf. equation 8.7). The appropriate convenient regression is

$$(9.5) \qquad -v \operatorname{var}\left[\left(1-R_i\right)^{v-1}\right] \cdot \left[y_i / \mu\right] = \alpha_1 + \beta_1 \cdot \left(1-R_i\right)^{v-1} + u_i,$$

where β_1 is the extended concentration index. This is straightforward to set up and run once the desired values of v have been selected.

The Stata code to implement the convenient regression and loop through $v = 1$, $v = 2$, $v = 3$, $v = 4$, and $v = 5$ is

```
sum neghaz
scalar mean = r(mean)
forval i = 1/5 {
        ge adjrnk`i' = (1-rank)^(`i'-1)
        sum adjrnk`i'
        ge lhs`i' = -`i'*r(Var)*neghaz/mean
        reg lhs`i' adjrnk`i'
        sca ci`i' = _b[adjrnk`i']
}
sca li _all
```

The `scalar list` command at the end produces the following:

```
sca    li _all
       ci5 = -.14068989
       ci4 = -.12858764
       ci3 = -.11006521
       ci2 = -.0771886
       ci1 = 0
       mean = 2.0298478
```

which is identical to that produced by the covariance method.

Computing the extended concentration index on grouped data

The grouped-data analogue of equation 9.3 (Wagstaff 2002)[1] is as follows:

$$C(v)=v\sum_{t=1}^{T}f_t\left(1-R_t\right)^{(v-1)}-\frac{v}{\mu}\sum_{t=1}^{T}f_th_t\left(1-R_t\right)^{(v-1)}$$

(9.6)

$$\approx 1-\frac{v}{\mu}\sum_{t=1}^{T}f_th_t\left(1-R_t\right)^{(v-1)}$$

where f_t is the sample proportion in the tth group, h_t is the average level of health or ill health of the tth group, and R_t is its fractional rank, defined as in chapter 8 as follows:

(9.7)
$$R_t=\sum_{\gamma=1}^{t-1}f_\gamma+\tfrac{1}{2}f_t,$$

indicating the cumulative proportion of the population up to the midpoint of each group interval.

This is easily implemented in a spreadsheet, as in table 9.1, taken from Wagstaff (2002). The example involves the distribution of under-five deaths in Bangladesh. The fractional rank variable, R, is derived using the formula above. In this case $v = 4$, and the column headed "(1-R)^(v-1)" gives the adjusted fractional rank for each asset group. The column headed "h" is the under-five mortality rate. The column headed "product" is the product of f, h, and (1-R)^(v-1). The sum of these products (34.67) is then multiplied (in a cell not shown) by v, and divided by μ. The complement of this is the extended concentration index, in this case –0.0847, not dramatically different from $C(2)$, which is equal in this case to –0.0841.

Achievement—trading off inequality and the mean

The measure of "achievement" proposed in Wagstaff (2002) reflects the average level of health and the inequality in health between the poor and the better-off. It is defined as a weighted average of the health levels of the various people in the sample, in which higher weights are attached to poorer people than to better-off people. Thus achievement might be measured by the index:

(9.8)
$$I(v)=\frac{1}{n}\sum_{i=1}^{n}h_iv\left(1-R_i\right)^{(v-1)},$$

---

[1]Note that equation A6 in Wagstaff (2002) contains a typo. Equation 9.6 above is the correct equation.

Table 9.1 *Inequality in Under-Five Deaths in Bangladesh*

Asset group	No. births	f	R	$(1-R)^{\wedge}(v-1)$	h	Product
1	2,950	0.22	0.11	0.71	141.1	21.85
2	3,191	0.24	0.34	0.29	146.9	10.11
3	2,695	0.20	0.56	0.09	135.2	2.36
4	2,581	0.19	0.75	0.02	122.3	0.35
5	2,029	0.15	0.92	0.00	76.0	0.00
	13,446				127.9	34.67

Source: Authors.

which is a weighted average of health levels, in which the weights are as graphed in Figure 9.1 and average to one. This index can be shown to be equal to (Wagstaff 2002) the following:

$$(9.9) \qquad I(v) = \mu(1 - C(v)).$$

When h is a measure of ill health (so high values of $I(v)$ are considered bad) and $C(v) < 0$ (ill health is higher among the poor), inequality serves to raise the value of $I(v)$ above the mean, making achievement worse than it would appear if one were to look just at the mean. If ill-health declines monotonically with income, the greater the degree of inequality aversion, the greater the wedge between the mean, μ, and the value of the index $I(v)$.

Computing the achievement index

Given equation 9.9, there is nothing complicated about this. The Stata code below is the same as the code above for the extended concentration index, except that it adds a line to the loop that computes the achievement index for the current value of v and then adds a second loop that prints out a table, showing for each value of v, the values of $C(v)$ and $I(v)$. This can then be pasted into Excel or Word.

```
sum neghaz
scalar mean = r(mean)
forval i = 1/5 {
        ge adjrnk`i'=(1-rank)^(`i'-1)
        corr neghaz adjrnk`i' , covar
        sca ci`i' = -`i'*r(cov_12)/mean
        sca achiev`i' = mean*(1-ci`i')
}
forval i = 1/5 {
        di `i' _col(5) %5.3f ci`i' _col(20) %5.3f achiev`i'
_col(30)
}
```

For the example of child malnutrition, the last loop produces the following output:

```
1       0.000       2.030
2      -0.077       2.187
3      -0.110       2.253
4      -0.129       2.291
5      -0.141       2.315
```

The first column is the value of v, the second is the value of $C(v)$, and the third is the value of $I(v)$. The latter is equal to μ when there is no aversion to inequality (i.e., $v = 1$). As v increases above 1, measured inequality becomes more and more negative (in this example h is a "bad"), and $I(v)$ rises further and further above μ, meaning that the level of "disachievement" becomes larger and larger.

The spreadsheet computation of the achievement index is similarly straightforward, requiring just an extra cell in the spreadsheet above.

References

Kakwani, N. C., A. Wagstaff, and E. van Doorslaer. 1997. "Socioeconomic Inequalities in Health: Measurement, Computation and Statistical Inference." *Journal of Econometrics* 77(1): 87–104.

Wagstaff, A. 2002. "Inequality Aversion, Health Inequalities and Health Achievement." *Journal of Health Economics* 21(4): 627–41.

Wagstaff, A., E. van Doorslaer, and N. Watanabe. 2003. "On Decomposing the Causes of Health Sector Inequalities, with an Application to Malnutrition Inequalities in Vietnam." *Journal of Econometrics* 112(1): 207–23.

10

Multivariate Analysis of Health Survey Data

The most basic description of health sector inequality is given by the bivariate relationship between a health variable and some indicator of socioeconomic status (SES) captured, for example, by the concentration curve and index. For a finer description, the analyst might want to standardize for demographic factors, such as age and gender (see chapters 5 and 15). Or, the analyst might want to explain the inequality through decomposition into its constituent parts (see chapters 12 and 13). More ambitiously, the analyst might want to test for the existence of a causal relationship between a health variable and SES and to examine the nature of any causality. All of these tasks require moving from bivariate to multivariate analysis. In this chapter, we discuss some issues that generally deserve consideration when undertaking multivariate analysis of survey data for the purpose of learning about health sector inequality or inequity. First, we distinguish between descriptive and causal analysis and identify the statistical issues that are relevant in each case. Second, because health data invariably derive from complex sample surveys, we consider the consequences of sample design for estimation and inference. To illustrate, we use a variety of methods to conduct multivariate analysis of child nutritional status in Vietnam. In the following chapter, we present some of the estimators most commonly used in analysis of health data.

Descriptive versus causal analysis

Descriptive analysis

As always, the appropriate statistical approach depends on the question to be answered. If the analyst is interested in simply describing SES-related inequality in health or health care, then statistical modeling issues are irrelevant. The analyst simply wants to describe how health varies with SES, conditional on other factors such as age, gender, and so on. Ordinary least squares (OLS) can be used to describe how the mean of health varies with SES, conditional on whatever factors the analyst wants to control for. The more variables the analyst controls for, the finer is the description of the relation between health and SES. Issues of omitted variable bias and endogeneity are not relevant. Of course, such simplicity comes at a price. The analyst cannot place any causal interpretation on the estimates. A significant OLS coefficient does not mean that SES has an effect on health, even if the analyst controls for a multitude of observable covariates. It simply means that health is observed to vary as SES varies. There is inequality.

The standardization and the decomposition methods covered in chapters 5 and 15 and in chapters 12 and 13, respectively, are examples of exploratory, or even explanatory, but still descriptive analysis. They are used to describe the distribution, primarily the mean, of health or health care conditional on SES, age, gender, and so forth.

Causal models

If the analyst wants to draw causal inferences, then the approach has to move from a descriptive one to a modeling approach. Causal relationships can arise through a number of pathways. Models and estimators vary in sophistication with the degree of detail of the causal relationship the analyst is aiming to uncover. For example, maternal education can affect child health either directly, through knowledge of healthy behavior, or indirectly, through preferences for child health. If the analyst is interested simply in whether educating women is an effective means of raising child health, irrespective of the mechanism through which it works, then the statistical model, and estimator, can be quite simple. A reduced form approach (see below) is adequate. However, if the analyst wants to establish whether educated mothers are better able to raise healthy children, abstracting from preference effects, then the model, as well as the methods, has to be more sophisticated. A structural model (see below) must be developed and estimated.

The household production model (Becker 1964, 1965) provides a useful framework for causal analysis of health variations (Grossman 1972a, 1972b; Rosenzweig and Schultz 1982, 1983; Schultz 1984; Wagstaff 1986). According to this approach, health, which is of intrinsic value, is "produced" by the household through the input of time and goods, such as food and medical care. The household selects such inputs given its members' physiological predispositions to good/bad health. These health endowments are observable to the household but not to the analyst. As a consequence, regressing outcomes, such as health, on inputs, such as medical care, will not render unbiased estimates of the causal impact of the latter because both the inputs and the outcomes reflect the values of the health endowments.

The most popular empirical strategy is to estimate reduced form demand relations. That is, to regress health outcomes on (exogenous) determinants of health inputs, for example, medical care prices. The resulting coefficients reflect both "technological" relationships between inputs and outcomes, and household preferences for health relative to other "goods." From such a reduced form health function it is not possible to conclude anything about the technological impact of a variable on health. For example, the relationship between female wage rates and child health reflects both the incentive effects of the wage on household time allocation and the effect of time use on child health. Nevertheless, for certain policy questions, reduced form estimation is appropriate. For example, say the analyst wants to know how population health will respond to an increased availability of medical care facilities, taking account both of the technological impact of medical care on health and the behavioral response with respect to utilization. Then, estimation of the reduced form correlation of area variations in medical facilities with individual levels of health is adequate.

If estimates of the health production technology are desired, then the problems of omitted variable bias and unobservable heterogeneity must be confronted. For example, regressing health on health care use, while omitting education, will give a biased estimate of the impact of health care in the likely instance that it is correlated with education. Resolution of the problem demands a sufficiently rich data set. The problem of heterogeneity bias arises from the unobservable health endowment, which induces correlation between the observable and unobservable components of a model of health determination. With cross-section data, correction of the resulting bias requires the availability of instruments, that is, variables that affect the health inputs but, conditional on these, not health itself. Appropriate instruments vary with the specific inputs being considered. At a general level, instruments used in the estimation of health production functions commonly come from geographic variation in market prices, from family endowments, for example, land rights, and from characteristics of public health programs at the regional level (Rosenzweig and Schultz 1983).

Instrumental variable (IV) estimation is fraught with danger. It is easy to claim that an endogenous regressor has been instrumented. It is somewhat more difficult to find a valid instrument. IV estimation should therefore be subjected to stringent testing (Bound, Jaeger, and Baker 1995; Staiger and Stock 1997). The variables proposed as instruments should be significant in a reduced form for the health input. Further, overidentification tests should be used to check whether exclusion of the proposed instruments from the health equation is justified.

Panel data have two important advantages with respect to estimation of health production functions. First, with data on the same individuals at different points in time, it is easier to account for the effect of unobservable health endowments, which generate much of the endogeneity problem. For example, the fixed effects estimator (see below) eliminates the time invariant unobservable effects and is consistent. The second important advantage of panel data is that they allow the time dynamics of health relationships to be investigated. The determination of health is essentially a dynamic process; health today reflects experiences of the past. For causal analysis of the determination of health, panel data are top priority.

Estimation and inference with complex survey data

Most surveys used for analysis of health sector inequalities in developing countries have complex sample designs. Typically, there is random sampling at some level or levels but there might be separate sampling from population subgroups (strata), groups of observations (clusters) may not be sampled independently, and there might be oversampling of certain groups. These three basic features of complex sample design—stratification, cluster sampling, and unequal selection probabilities—were introduced in chapter 2, in which we briefly discussed how the sample design should be taken into account in conducting inference with respect to population means. We now consider whether and how sample design should be taken into account in conducting multivariate analyses. A related issue, which we consider, is that of area effects—controlling for all observable determinants, area of residence exerts an independent effect on health. Such effects are characteristics of the population itself, but their sample importance depends on the sample design.

Stratified sampling

Samples can be stratified in a variety of ways. The design most typically employed in household surveys undertaken in developing countries, for example, the Living Standards Measurement Surveys, is standard stratified sampling. The population is divided into a relatively small number of strata—for example, urban/rural or large geographic regions. A random sample, of predetermined size, is selected independently from each of these strata. The sample proportions accounted for by each strata may or may not correspond to population proportions. In the case that they do not, the overall sample is not representative of the population and the issue of sample weights arises. This is a separate issue from stratification and is considered as such below.

If population means differ across strata, then predetermination of strata sample sizes reduces the sampling variance of estimators of these means. As a result, standard errors on estimates of population means, and other descriptive statistics, should be adjusted downward. In chapter 2, we demonstrated how to do this using the special routines for survey data available in Stata. It turns out that adjustment is not necessary in (nondescriptive) regression analysis and a wide variety of other multivariate modeling approaches, provided stratification is based on variables that are exogenous within the model (Wooldridge 2001, 2002). For example, say a sample stratified by urban/rural is used to estimate the determinants of child nutritional status, measured by height-for-age z-score. Provided, conditional on the regressors, unobservable determinants of height-for-age and of city dwelling are uncorrelated, the OLS estimator, for example, is consistent and efficient, and the usual standard errors are valid. In the likely presence of heteroscedasticity, the analyst would want to make the standard errors robust, but that is another issue. If stratification is based on an endogenous variable, however, then standard errors should be adjusted (Wooldridge 2002).

So, the need to adjust standard errors for stratification is situation specific. In practice, relative to simple standard errors, adjusting for stratification may inflate the standard errors. But with survey data, standard errors robust to heteroscedasticity, and possibly clustering (see below), will be required. Relative to those adjustments, the magnitude of that for stratification is usually modest and normally downward (see box 10.1). So, a conservative strategy is not to make any adjustment. If stratification is exogenous, there is no need for adjustment and, if endogenous, the adjustment will normally increase statistical significance.

It is often sensible to allow for intercept, and possibly slope, differences with respect to factors on which the sample is stratified. But this is in response to differences that exist in the population itself, not to the stratified design of the sample. For example, in many cases it is sensible to include an urban/rural dummy and to interact this with other regressors, to allow for differences in both the mean and responses between urban and rural locations, irrespective of whether the sample is stratified by urban/rural.

COMPUTATION   Stata is the best package available for handling survey design issues. For the example presented in Box 10.1, OLS estimates with stratification adjusted SEs were obtained from the following:

```
svyset , strata(region)
svy, subpop(child): regr depvar varlist
```

where strata(region) instructs that the sample be stratified on the variable region, depvar denotes the dependent variable (height-for-age z-score [*–100] in

Box 10.1 *Standard Error Adjustment for Stratification Regression Analysis of Child Nutritional Status in Vietnam*

In the table below we present OLS coefficients from a regression of height-for-age z-scores (see chapter 4) using a sample of Vietnamese children under 10 years of age. The data are from the 1998 Vietnam Living Standards Survey (VLSS), which was stratified by 10 regions. The specification of the regression is based on that used by Wagstaff, van Doorslaer, and Watanabe (2003) (see also chapter 13). The dependent variable is actually the negative of the z-score (multiplied by 100), such that a positive coefficient indicates a negative correlation with height.

In addition to the OLS point estimates, we present standard errors (SEs) calculated with various degrees of adjustment. Relative to simple OLS SEs (column 2), adjustment for stratification alone (column 3) tends to inflate the SEs appreciably, but not dramatically. In some cases, the adjustment is slightly downward. In no case does the adjustment change the level of significance of the coefficient. In this example, making the SEs robust to heteroscedasticity of general form (column 4) has a very similar effect to that of adjusting for stratification. Besides stratification, the VLSS has a cluster sample design. Adjusting SEs for cluster sampling but not stratification (column 5) has a greater impact than stratification adjustment. In all cases, as expected, the adjustment is upward and in two cases it actually changes the level of significance. Finally, we adjust for both stratification and clustering (column 6). Comparing columns 5 and 6, it is apparent, for this example, that given adjustment for clustering, the marginal impact of stratification adjustment is small. In most cases, but not all, this marginal adjustment is downward. In no case does adjustment for stratification change the level of significance relative to that obtained by adjusting for clustering alone.

For this example, adjusting standard errors for clustering appears to be more important than adjustment for stratification. Although care must be taken not to draw general conclusions from an example, this is consistent with what is generally found in empirical work.

OLS analysis of height-for-age z-scores (*–100), Vietnam 1998 (children <10 years)

	Co-efficient	Standard errors				
		Un-adjusted	Strati-fication adjusted	Hetero. robust	Cluster adjusted	Strat. & cluster adj.
Child's age (months)	3.70***	0.1986	0.2466	0.2470	0.2885	0.2872
Child's age squared (/100)	–2.38***	0.1554	0.1755	0.1758	0.1966	0.1957
Child is male	12.31***	3.2927	3.2708	3.2792	3.3649	3.2844
(log) hhold. consumption per capita	–37.85***	3.9843	4.1046	4.1116	5.4035	5.4582
Safe drinking water	–7.43	4.9533	4.8300	4.8441	9.1538	9.2098
Satisfactory sanitation	–15.53***	5.1009	4.8199	4.8326	**6.1202**	**6.0937**
Years of schooling of household head	–0.87*	0.4804	0.4770	0.4786	**0.7302**	**0.7188**
Mother has primary school diploma	–2.33	4.0598	4.1309	4.1397	6.1913	6.2438
Sample size	5218					

Note: Dependent variable is **negative** of z-score, multiplied by 100. Bold indicates a change in significance level relative to that using unadjusted standard errors. Regression also contains region dummies at the level of stratification. ***, ** and * indicate 1%, 5% and 10% significance according to unadjusted standard errors.
Source: Authors.

the example), `varlist` is a list of regressors, and `subpop(child)` requests that the model be estimated for children (`child=1`) only. Restricting the sample to children and then estimating the model would not give the correct (stratification-adjusted) SEs. Computation for cluster sample adjustment is given below.

Cluster samples

Cluster samples arise from a two-stage (or more) sampling process. In the first stage, groups (clusters) of households are randomly sampled from either the population or the strata. Typically, these clusters are villages or neighborhoods of towns and cities. In the second stage, households are randomly sampled from each of the selected clusters. An important distinction from stratification is that strata are selected deterministically, whereas clusters are selected randomly. A further difference is that typically strata are few in number and contain many observations, whereas clusters are large in number and contain relatively few observations.

As a result of this design, observations are not independent within clusters, although most probably they are across clusters. There is likely to be more homogeneity within clusters than there is across the population as a whole. Within clusters, correlation of both observable and unobservable factors across households can be expected. Although these correlations exist in the population, the sample design increases their sample presence relative to that of a simple random sample. Consequences and remedies depend on the nature of the within-cluster correlation. Much of the analysis is analogous to that of unobservable individual effects in a panel data setting.

CASE 1: EXOGENOUS CLUSTER EFFECTS   Consider the following model:

(10.1) $$y_{ic} = \mathbf{X}_{ic}\boldsymbol{\beta} + \lambda_c + \varepsilon_{ic}, \ E[\varepsilon_{ic} | \mathbf{X}_{ic}, \lambda_c] = E[\varepsilon_{ic}] = 0,$$

where i and c are household (individual) and cluster indicators, respectively; $\mathbf{X}_{ic}$ is a vector of regressors; λ_c are cluster effects; and ε_{ic} idiosyncratic disturbances. If we assume that the cluster effects are independent of the regressors $(E[\lambda_c | \mathbf{X}_{ic}] = E[\lambda_c])$, then so is the composite error $(u_{ic} = \lambda_c + \varepsilon_{ic})$. This is the random effects model.

Conventional point estimators, for example, OLS, probit, and so on, depending on the nature of the dependent variable, are consistent, but inefficiency arises from the cluster-induced correlation in the composite errors which, in addition, requires adjustment of the standard errors. One option is to accept inefficiency and simply adjust the standard errors. In Stata, this is easily implemented through the option `cluster(varname)`, where `varname` defines the clusters. This option, which is available for most estimators, will adjust both for within-cluster correlation and for heteroscedasticity of unknown form.

An alternative strategy is to pursue efficiency by estimating the within-cluster correlation and taking account of this in estimation of the model parameters. In the linear case, for example, the analyst would use generalized least squares (GLS). A Lagrange multiplier test can be used to test the null that the cluster effects are insignificant and OLS is efficient (Wooldridge 2002). In the case of a binary discrete dependent variable, the analyst can estimate the random effects probit.

CASE 2: ENDOGENOUS CLUSTER EFFECTS   The model is equation 10.1, but we relax the assumption of independence between the cluster effects and the regressors. That is, we allow $(E[\lambda_c | \mathbf{X}_{ic}] \neq E[\lambda_c])$. This is the fixed effects model.

For example, in a regression of individual health on health service utilization, we would expect the latter to be correlated with the unobservable cluster-specific quality of those services. In instances in which there is such dependence, regressors are correlated with the composite error and standard estimators are inconsistent. The analyst must purge the cluster effects from the composite error. In a linear context, either include cluster dummies or, equivalently, transform the data by taking differences from within cluster means (i.e., the within-groups estimator). In a binary discrete choice context, the analyst can use the fixed effects logit estimator (Wooldridge 2002) (see chapter 11). Once the cluster effects have been purged from the composite error, there is no need to adjust standard errors for clustering (providing the linear specification of the cluster effects is correct). Adjustment for heteroscedasticity is likely to be a good idea.

The analyst can choose between the random and fixed effects models by reference to a Hausman test of the null of independence between the cluster effects and the regressors (Wooldridge 2002).

Box 10.2 *Taking Cluster Sampling into Account in Regression Analysis of Child Nutritional Status in Vietnam*

We continue with an examination of height-for-age z-scores of Vietnamese children using the 1998 VLSS, which has a cluster sample design. Cluster samples were actually drawn at two levels in this survey. At the first level, within each stratum a random sample of communes was drawn with probability of selection proportional to commune population size. Communes therefore represent the primary sampling units. Within each of the 194 selected communes, two villages/blocks were randomly selected with selection probabilities again proportional to population size. Finally, within each village/block a random sample of 20 households was selected. With this sample design, clusters could be defined at the level of the commune, village/block, or both. For simplicity, we will define clusters at the commune level.

We take three approaches to the cluster sample issue: OLS with standard errors adjusted for within-cluster correlation, random effects, and fixed effects. In each case, standard errors are made robust to heteroscedasticity of general form. The results of the respective z-score regressions are given in the table below.

Comparing the point estimates, it is apparent that the choice of estimator makes little difference for regressors that are clearly individual specific, but there is greater sensitivity in estimates for regressors that can be expected to display stronger within-commune correlation. So, for example, the point estimates for age and gender are near constant across the estimators. The estimate for household consumption is more sensitive, the effect weakening as we move from OLS, which takes no account of commune effects in the point estimates, to fixed effects, which purge the commune effects. This pattern is even more pronounced for indicators of safety of drinking water and sanitation, which can be expected to display fairly limited within-commune variation.

In general, standard errors are smaller for random and fixed effects. This is expected because these methods take into account the cluster effects in the (point) estimation and do not have to inflate the standard errors to allow for these correlated effects. In this example, however, the choice of estimator makes very little difference to levels of significance, reflecting the strength of the effect of some of the regressors.

The Lagrange multiplier test on the random effects model confirms that commune effects are, indeed, important. The Hausman test rejects the assumption of zero correlation between the commune effects and the regressors, indicating the superiority of the fixed effects estimator in this case.

Box 10.2 continued *Regression Analysis of Height-for-Age z-Scores (*-100), Vietnam 1998 (children <10 years)*

	OLS		Random effects		Fixed effects	
	Coeff.	*Cluster adjusted SE*	*Coeff.*	*Robust SE*	*Coeff.*	*Robust SE*
Child's age (months)	3.72***	0.2917	3.74***	0.2451	3.78***	0.2430
Child's age squared (1100)	–2.40***	0.1987	–2.40***	0.1742	–2.44***	0.1732
Child is male	12.26***	3.4527	12.19***	3.2394	12.97***	3.2443
(log) hhold. consumption p.c.	–50.93***	5.1149	–43.17***	4.0778	–30.37***	4.6090
Safe drinking water	–12.55	8.6438	–7.93	4.8984	–2.75	5.4247
Satisfactory sanitation	–22.90***	5.6974	–19.39***	4.8446	–9.77**	4.9364
Years of schooling of HoH	–0.39	0.6628	–0.33	0.4828	–0.55	0.5081
Mother has primary school diploma	2.67	5.3187	1.71	4.1140	1.74	4.3186
Intercept	445.00***	44.5600	377.01***	32.1941	276.19***	35.0991
Sample size	5,218	R^2	0.1527	B-P LM	485.84	(0.000)
				Hausman	50.54	(0.000)

Note: Dependent variable is **negative** of z-score, multiplied by 100.
SE = standard error, Robust SE-robust to general heteroskedasticity.
B-P LM = Breusch-Pagan Lagrange Multiplier test of significance of commune effects (*p*-value).
Hausman = Hausman test of random versus fixed effects (*p*-value).
***, ** & * indicate significance at 1%, 5% & 10%, respectively.
Source: Authors.

COMPUTATION   Results such as those in box 10.2 can be generated in Stata as follows. For OLS with cluster corrected SEs,

```
svyset commune
svy, subpop(child): regr depvar varlist
```

where the svyset command instructs that clusters are defined by the variable commune. If the analysis were not restricted to part of the sample, the appropriate cluster corrected standard errors could be obtained from the following:

```
regr depvar varlist, cluster(commune)
```

To adjust SEs for both clustering and stratification, simply set the survey parameters appropriately,

```
svyset commune, strata(region)
```

and then run the svy: regr command as above. This was used to generate the SEs in the final column of the table in box 10.1. We do not adjust OLS SEs in the table in box 10.2 for stratification because the random and fixed effects estimators do not allow for that. Random effects estimates are obtained most easily from Stata's linear panel data estimator,

```
xtreg depvar varlist, re i(commune)
```

where i(commune) instructs to allow for common effects within each category of the variable commune. The Breusch-Pagan test statistic is obtained by following the command above with xttest0. To obtain (heteroskedasticity) robust SEs, as in the example, the analyst can implement the random effects (GLS) estimator through OLS on transformed data and request robust SEs. First, run the random effects estimator as above, and save the estimates of the variances of the error components,

```
scalar define sigma_e=e(sigma_e)^2
scalar define sigma_u=e(sigma_u)^2
```

Next calculate the variable that will be used to transform the data,

```
sort commune
by commune: gen T=_N
gen theta=1-sqrt(sigma_e/(sigma_e +(T*sigma_u)))
```

where the first two command lines generate a variable indicating the number of observations within each commune, and the third line gives the transformation variable. Now generate the quasi mean deviations (i.e., deviations from the transformed mean) for the dependent variable and each regressor,

```
local vbls "depvar varlist"
foreach var of local vbls {
  by commune: egen m_`var'=mean(`var')
  gen t_`var'=`var'-theta*m_`var'
}
```

Generate the variable from which the intercept will be estimated and run OLS,

```
gen intercept=1-theta
local vars "t_depvar t_var1 t_var2...  ."
regr `vars' intercept, noconstant robust
```

where the local vars contains the names of the transformed dependent variable and the regressors, noconstant requests that the regression be estimated without a constant, and robust requests heteroscedasticity robust SEs.

Fixed effects estimates can be obtained from the panel data command:

```
xtreg depvar varlist, fe i(commune)
```

Or to obtain the same point estimates but robust SEs, use the following:

```
areg depvar varlist, absorb(commune) robust
```

which requests OLS on deviations from commune specific means, that is, the within-groups or fixed-effects estimator.

The Hausman test statistic can be computed by the following:

```
xtreg depvar varlist, fe i(commune)
est store fixed
xtreg depvar varlist, re i(commune)
hausman fixed
```

Explaining community effects

The strategies outlined above for dealing with cluster samples are appropriate when the analyst is interested exclusively in the determinants of health/health care at the individual level. In this case, the cluster sample design is a problem to be overcome. But cluster, or community, effects can be more than nuisance parameters. With respect to health inequality, for example, area variations in health, and their determinants, are of genuine interest. Not least because implementation of public health policies at the community, rather than the individual, level is often more feasible. In this case, a cluster sample design is an advantage rather than a problem. It facilitates examination of cross-community differences in health and their determinants, particularly if the household survey is accompanied by a community-level survey providing information on characteristics of the community.

Options for the analysis of community effects from individual-level data depend on whether the effects are exogenous or endogenous.

CASE 1: EXOGENOUS CLUSTER (COMMUNITY) EFFECTS   In this case, the analyst can explore the determinants of area variation in health outcomes or utilization by including community-level variables, if available, in the model. Define $\lambda_c = \mathbf{Z}_c \gamma + \lambda_c^*$, where $\mathbf{Z}_c$ are observable community-level factors, for example, health care facilities and personnel, quality of water provision and sewage, prices, and so forth and substitute this definition into equation 10.1. The (rewritten) model is as follows:

$$(10.2) \qquad y_{ic} = \mathbf{X}_{ic}\beta + \mathbf{Z}_c\gamma + \lambda_c^* + \varepsilon_{ic}, \ E\left[\varepsilon_{ic} | \mathbf{X}_{ic}, \mathbf{Z}_c, \lambda_c^*\right] = E\left[\varepsilon_{ic}\right] = 0.$$

To maintain the assumption of exogenous community effects, and therefore consistency (but not efficiency) of standard estimators, we now need the unobservable community effects (λ_c^*) to be independent of both the individual- and community-level regressors (i.e., $E\left[\lambda_c^* | X_{ic}, Z_c\right] = E\left[\lambda_c^*\right]$) (Wooldridge 2002). This is likely to be a stronger assumption than that placed on model 10.1 above. Assuming that the observable community factors capture all of the community effect, ($\lambda_c^* = 0, \forall c$) is even stronger. Excepting the latter restrictive case, standard errors still have to be adjusted (upward) for correlation induced by the (unobservable) community effects. However, the efficiency loss from employing OLS, for example, in this setting may not be large (Deaton 1997).

This random effects model is known as the hierarchical model in some fields (see, e.g., Rice and Jones [1997]). Although the models are equivalent, the hierarchical approach places more emphasis on decomposition of the overall variance into that arising at the individual and the community level. This approach is particularly useful in cases in which the analyst wants to focus on such a distinction between individual- and community-level effects.

CASE 2: ENDOGENOUS CLUSTER (COMMUNITY) EFFECTS   In cases in which the (unobservable) community effects are correlated with individual-level regressors, it is not possible to include community-level variables in a model to be estimated from a single cross section. With a dummy variable approach, the community variables would be perfectly correlated with the community dummies. With a fixed-effects approach, community variables would be wiped out of the model along with the unobservable community effects. If one has panel data, then these problems are avoided provided there is sufficient across-time variation in the community-level variables. With a single cross section, a feasible two-stage approach in a linear context is to estimate a fixed-effects model, obtain estimates of the community effects, and then regress these on community-level variables. In the first stage, the bias arising from the community effects is removed from the individual-level analysis of, say, health determination. In the second stage, sources of community variation in health are examined.

In box 10.3 we continue with the example of child nutritional status in Vietnam, examining the sources of community-level variation, assuming in turn exogenous and endogenous community effects.

Box 10.3 *Explaining Community-Level Variation in Child Nutritional Status in Vietnam*

In box 10.2 we saw that commune effects are an important source of variation in height-for-age z-scores of Vietnamese children. The VLSS offers the opportunity to uncover factors underlying these commune effects through the examination of data from commune-level surveys that accompanied, and can be linked to, the household survey data. For demonstration purposes, we limit attention to the characteristics of commune health centers (CHCs). The analysis is necessarily restricted to children living in rural areas and small towns because the commune surveys were conducted in those areas only.

Again we compare OLS, random effects, and fixed effects. In the case of OLS and random effects, the estimates are obtained from entering the CHC characteristics directly into the individual-level regressions. We present, in the table below, the estimates for the CHC regressors only. Estimates for the individual-level regressors are similar to those given in the table in box 10.2. For the fixed-effects model, we take the two-stage approach outlined above. In the table, we present results from the second stage regression of the estimated commune effects on the CHC characteristics. The first stage estimates are similar to those in the table in box 10.2.

The results indicate a lower prevalence of stunting in communes in which the CHC has electricity, a sanitary toilet and, at marginal significance, a child growth chart. The number of inpatient beds available in a CHC and, at lower significance, the employment of a doctor is positively correlated with the prevalence of stunting. These latter results may reflect the targeting on resources in the communes of greatest need.

Analysis of Commune-Level Variation in Height-for-Age z-Scores (*–100), Rural Vietnam 1998 (children <10 years)

Commune health center vbls.	OLS		Random effects		2nd-stage fixed effects	
	Coeff.	Cluster adj. SE	Coeff.	Robust SE	Coeff.	SE
Vitamin A available ≥ 1/2 time	–10.11	6.6530	–6.86143	6.5927	–8.27114	6.7506
Has electricity	–38.79***	11.4558	–50.56***	12.1861	–45.34***	10.7991
Has clean water source	9.57	7.6534	7.2341	8.4061	7.0070	8.7610
Has sanitary toilet	–27.53***	7.0928	–24.50***	7.6694	–24.30***	7.8715
Has child growth chart	–13.85*	7.2046	–10.2623	7.5879	–11.732	7.6292
Number of inpatient beds	1.52*	0.8298	2.12**	0.9242	2.09**	0.9744
Has a doctor	11.39	6.9765	9.6255	7.1834	10.1856	7.5207
Intercept	371.89***	48.8784	344.71***	41.5639	279.13***	41.6264
Sample size	4,099	R^2 0.1313	B-P LM	248.42 (0.0000)		

Note: Dependent variable is **negative** of z-score, multiplied by 100. OLS & random effects = Coefficients on commune-level regressors only are presented. 2nd stage fixed effects = Estimated commune effects from fixed effects regressed on commune vbls.

SE = standard error, robust SE = robust to general heteroskedasticity.

B-P LM = Breusch-Pagan Lagrange Multiplier test of significance of community effects (*p*-value).

***, ** and * indicate significance at 1%, 5% and 10%, respectively.

Source: Authors.

COMPUTATION   OLS and random effects estimates and standard errors can be generated exactly as above, with the inclusion of community-level regressors. The two-stage fixed-effects approach can be implemented in Stata by first running the linear (fixed effects) panel estimator and saving the predicted commune effects:

```
xtreg depvar varlist, fe i(commune)
predict ce, u
```

where ce is the variable name given to the predicted commune effects, u. OLS regression of these commune effects on commune-level variables (*varlist2*) is most easily implemented by using the between-groups panel estimator:

```
xtreg ce varlist2, be i(commune)
```

Sample weights

The probability of observing an individual in a survey may differ from the probability that the individual is randomly selected from the population. There are a number of reasons for this. The survey may be stratified, with strata sample proportions differing from respective population proportions. For example, there may be oversampling of the urban population. Besides sample design, differential nonresponse will lead to a sample that is not representative of the population. For those reasons, survey data typically come with a set of sample weights that, for each observation, indicate the (inverse of the) probability of being a sample member. In a standard stratified sample with differential sampling by strata, weights or expansion factors are given by the ratio of the population size of each stratum to its sample size.

Sample weights must be applied to obtain unbiased estimates of population means, concentration indices, and so forth and correct standard errors for these estimates. Application of the weights allows for the fact that observations with lower sample probabilities represent a greater number of (similar) individuals in the population. With respect to multivariate analysis, the case for applying sample weights is less clear-cut. In part, the appropriateness of weighting depends on the objective of the analysis. As we stressed at the beginning of this chapter, appropriate methods depend on the purpose of the analysis. If regression is being used simply as a descriptive device, and not for estimation of behavioral parameters, then weights should be applied (Deaton 1997). The regression function describes the means of one variable conditional on others. Application of sample weights will ensure that the conditional means estimated are those that would have been estimated from a simple random sample of the population. In this case, weights are applied for the same reason they are used in univariate analysis. For example, in standardization exercises (see chapters 5 and 15), regression is used simply to obtain conditional means, and it would be appropriate to apply sample weights.

If the purpose of the analysis is more ambitious—to uncover causal relationships—then the crucial factor determining whether weights need to be applied in estimating the model parameters is the source of differences between sample and population proportions. If proportions differ because of selection on factors that are exogenous within the model under consideration, then there is no need to apply weights. Unweighted estimators are consistent and more efficient than weighted counterparts (Wooldridge 2002). Usual or, in the presence of heteroscedasticity, robust standard errors are valid. However, if selection is on endogenous factors, then a weighted estimator is required for consistency (Wooldridge 2002). In the case of the linear model, for example, weighted least squares could be used with the data weighted by the inverse of sample probabilities. If the sample weights derive from stratification with differential sampling by strata, then standard errors need to be calculated taking account of both the weights and the stratification. Alternatively, if there are sample weights but not stratification, then (robust) standard errors are calculated by applying the usual formula to the weighted data.

So, as with sample stratification, the need to take account of sample weights in estimation is situation specific. Consider a model of health determination to be estimated from a survey that oversamples the urban population. If, conditional on all regressors, unobservable determinants of health are uncorrelated with city dwelling, then there is no need to apply weights. Conditioning on an urban dummy is sufficient. In this example, the exogeneity assumption might be considered reasonably weak, although its validity would be challenged if migration were strongly influenced by health status. If, however, there were differential sampling by health itself, say the sick were oversampled, then sample weights would need to be applied.

The discussion above assumes parameter homogeneity across the differentially sampled groups. There might be different (conditional) group means, but that is easily dealt with through the inclusion of dummy variables. A more serious problem is differences in slope parameters across groups. Consider the following model:

$$(10.3) \qquad\qquad y_{is} = \mathbf{X}_{is}\beta_s + \varepsilon_{is}$$

where i and s, respectively, indicate individual and group, for example, urban/rural, gender, ethnicity, and so on, and the parameter vector $\boldsymbol{\beta}_s$ is indexed on s, indicating parameter heterogeneity across groups. If differences in parameters across groups are of inherent interest, then the analyst can estimate either a separate model for each group or a single model with dummies for each group and their interactions with other regressors. The former is more general. In both cases, parameter homogeneity can be tested by standard methods.

For various reasons, the analyst might want an estimate of the average effect across the population. Such an average might be defined as follows: $\boldsymbol{\beta} = \dfrac{1}{N}\sum_{s=1}^{S} N_s \boldsymbol{\beta}_s$, that is, the weighted average of the group-specific parameters with weights provided by the population group proportions $\left(\dfrac{N_s}{N}\right)$ (Deaton 1997). If degrees of freedom are not a problem, this parameter can be consistently estimated by applying OLS to each sector to obtain estimates of the sector-specific parameters, $\hat{\boldsymbol{\beta}}_s$, and taking the population-weighted average of these. For degrees of freedom reasons or otherwise, it is often preferred to estimate the average parameter directly from one regression. In the case in which sample group proportions do not correspond to population proportions, it might be anticipated that unweighted OLS on the whole sample will not be consistent for the average parameter defined. That is correct. It is reasonable to ask whether sample weights can solve the problem. The answer is "no." Weighted regression will give an estimate that corresponds to that which would be obtained from a simple random sample, but that is not consistent for the population average parameter, apart from the extreme case in which regressor values are identical across all groups (Deaton 1997).

Box 10.4 *Applying Sample Weights in Regression Analysis*
of Child Nutritional Status in Vietnam

We reproduce the analysis of box 10.2, but with sample weights applied to all estimators. One other difference is that the OLS standard errors are adjusted for stratification because, within a modeling approach, the logic for applying sample weights and for adjusting for stratification is the same. That is, selection on an endogenous variable.

By comparing the estimates presented in the table below with those given in the table in box 10.2, it is apparent that the application of sample weights makes very little difference to the results. A possible explanation is that the application of sample weights is not necessary in this particular example. That is, differential sampling is exogenous, and so the unweighted estimators are consistent.

Weighted Regression Analyses of Height-for-Age z-Scores
Vietnam 1998 (children <10 years)

	OLS		Random effects		Fixed effects	
	Coeff.	Adjusted SE	Coeff.	Robust SE	Coeff.	Robust SE
Child's age (months)	3.90***	0.3218	3.90***	0.2652	3.91***	0.2642
Child's age squared (/100)	−2.51***	0.2206	−2.50***	0.1875	−2.51***	0.1875
Child is male	14.86***	3.5718	14.56***	3.3595	14.89***	3.3731
(log) hhold. consumption p.c.	−50.14***	5.5131	−40.67***	4.3511	−26.05***	5.0196
Safe drinking water	−12.16	10.2770	−6.92	5.1624	−2.07	5.6079
Satifactory sanitation	−22.01***	5.9503	−19.81***	5.3653	−10.48*	5.4439
Years of schooling of HoH	−0.21	0.7355	−0.15	0.5122	−0.42	0.5363
Mother has primary school diploma	3.62	5.6510	3.04	4.2925	2.19	4.4958
Intercept	428.15***	48.9827	347.47***	34.9686	236.12***	38.5646
Sample size 5,218	R^2	0.1496	R^2	0.4320	R^2	0.2457

Note: Dependent variable is **negative** of z-score, multiplied by 100.

Adjusted SE = standard error adjusted for clustering and stratification and robust to heteroskedasticity.

Robust SE = standard error robust to general heteroskedasticity.

***, ** and * indicate significance at 1%, 5% and 10%, respectively.

Source: Authors.

The issue here is parameter heterogeneity, which exists in the population, and is not simply a feature of sample design. Sample weights cannot be used to address an issue that arises from the population itself.

Sensitivity of estimates and their standard errors to the application of weights is examined in box 10.4.

Further reading

Deaton (1997) is a wonderfully useful guide to the analysis of survey data. Wooldridge (2002) and Cameron and Trivedi (2005) are both excellent, comprehensive textbooks covering the relevant econometric theory.

References

Becker, G. 1964. *Human Capital: A Theoretical and Empirical Analysis With Special Reference to Education.* New York: National Bureau of Economic Research.

———. 1965. "A Theory of the Allocation of Time." *Economic Journal* 75: 492–517.

Bound, J., D. Jaeger, and R. Baker. 1995. "Problems with Instrumental Variables Estimation When the Correlation between the Instruments and the Endogenous Explanatory Variables Is Weak." *Journal of American Statistical Association* 90: 443–450.

Cameron, A. C., and P. K. Trivedi. 2005. *Microeconometrics: Methods and Applications.* New York: Cambridge University Press.

Deaton, A. 1997. *The Analysis of Household Surveys: A Microeconometric Approach to Development Policy.* Baltimore, MD: Johns Hopkins University Press.

Grossman, M. 1972a. *The Demand for Health: A Theoretical and Empirical Investigation.* New York: National Bureau of Economic Research.

Grossman, M. 1972b. "On the Concept of Health Capital and the Demand for Health." *Journal of Political Economy* 80: 223–55.

Rice, N., and A. M. Jones. 1997. "Multilevel Models and Health Economics." *Health Economics* 6: 561–75.

Rosenzweig, M. R., and T. P. Schultz. 1982. "Market Opportunities, Genetic Endowments and Infrafamily Resource Allocation: Child Survival in Rural India." *American Economic Review* 72:803–15.

———. 1983. "Estimating a Household Production Function: Heterogeneity, the Demand for Health Inputs, and Their Impact on Birth Weight." *Journal of Political Economy* 91(5): 723–46.

Schultz, T. P. 1984. "Studying the Impact of Household Economic and Community Variables on Child Mortality." *Population and Development Review* 10: 215–35.

Staiger, D., and J. H. Stock. 1997. "Instrumental Variables Regression with Weak Instruments." *Econometrica* 65(3): 557–86.

Wagstaff, A. 1986. "The Demand for Health: Some New Empirical Evidence." *Journal of Health Economics* 5(3): 195–233.

Wagstaff, A., E. van Doorslaer, and N. Watanabe. 2003. "On Decomposing the Causes of Health Sector Inequalities, with an Application to Malnutrition Inequalities in Vietnam." *Journal of Econometrics* 112(1): 219–27.

Wooldridge, J. M. 2001. "Asymptotic Properties of Weighted M-Estimators for Standard Stratified Samples." *Econometric Theory* 17: 451–70.

———. 2002. *Econometric Analysis of Cross Section and Panel Data.* Cambridge, MA: MIT Press.

11

Nonlinear Models for Health and Medical Expenditure Data

Heath sector variables are seldom continuous and fully observed. For example, they can be discrete (e.g., death), censored (e.g., health care expenditure), integer counts (e.g., visits to doctor), or durational (e.g., time to death). Multivariate analysis of such dependent variables requires nonlinear estimation. In this chapter, we consider the main (parametric) nonlinear estimators that are of relevance to the analysis of health sector inequalities. The literature is extensive, and our coverage is necessarily rudimentary, with a focus on practicalities rather than theory.

Binary dependent variables

There are numerous examples of health sector variables that take only two values—dead/alive, ill/not ill, stunted/not stunted, goes to doctor/doesn't go to doctor, and so on. In some cases, there are only two possible values of the underlying characteristic, for example, dead/alive. In other cases, the underlying characteristic is continuous, for example, degrees of illness, but only two categories are observable in the data—ill/not ill.

Let y_i be the characteristic of interest. Conventionally, $y_i = 1$ indicates that observation i possesses the characteristic, for example, illness, and $y_i = 0$ indicates that it does not. In general, a model of binary response can be defined by the following:

$$(11.1) \qquad E[y_i | \mathbf{X}_i] = \Pr(y_i = 1 | \mathbf{X}_i) = F(\mathbf{X}_i \beta)$$

where $E[\ ]$ and $\Pr(\ )$ indicate expected value and probability, respectively. Different functional forms for $F(\ )$ define different specific models. For example, in the linear case, $F(\mathbf{X}_i \beta) = \mathbf{X}_i \beta$, we have the linear probability model (LPM). It is often claimed that the LPM can be consistently estimated by ordinary least squares (OLS). Horrace and Oaxaca (2006) prove that this is true only in the restrictive case that $\mathbf{X}_i \beta$ has a zero probability of lying outside the (0,1) range. A related problem is that the predicted probability given in equation 11.1 is not constrained to the (0,1) range, making results difficult to interpret in such circumstances. A further problem is that the errors are nonnormal and heteroscedastic, and so the estimator is not efficient and conventional standard errors are invalid. That can be (partially) fixed by weighted least squares.

An obvious, and common, response to these problems with OLS is to choose some functional form for $F(\ )$ that constrains estimated probabilities to lie in the (0,1) range. The two most popular choices are the cumulative standard normal distribution, which gives the probit model, and the cumulative standard logistic distribution, which gives the logit model. Thinking about binary responses being driven by some underlying but unobservable (latent) characteristic helps to motivate such models. For example, let y_i^* indicate propensity to contract illness. When this crosses some threshold, say $y_i^* > 0$, the individual is ill. Specifying the latent variable to be a linear function of observable and unobservable factors, $y_i^* = \mathbf{X}_i\beta + \varepsilon_i$, and choosing a distribution for the error term as either standard normal or logistic gives the probit and logit models. Estimation is carried out by maximum likelihood.

Because the normal and logistic distributions are similar, the choice of a probit or logit specification is not important in most cases. Care must be taken not to compare probit and logit coefficients directly, however. In both cases, parameters are estimable only up to a scaling factor, equal to the unknown standard deviation of the error, which is not estimable given the binary nature of the dependent variable. Only the relative, not the absolute, effect of explanatory variables are estimable. Because variances differ between the normal and logistic distributions, logit coefficients must be multiplied by 0.625 to be comparable with probit coefficients (Amemiya 1981). Dividing probit estimates by 2.5 and logit estimates by 4 will make them comparable with those from the LPM (Wooldridge 2002).

Further care must be taken in the interpretation of estimates from latent variable models. The (scaled) parameters β give the (relative) partial effects on the latent index y_i^*, but these effects are usually not of primary interest. The partial effects on the probability of possessing the characteristic are more informative. For example, an estimate of how the probability of being sick changes with income is more easily interpreted than an estimate of how a latent index of sickness propensity varies with income. From equation 11.1, the estimated partial effect of a continuous regressor (X_k) on the (conditional) probability is given by the following:

$$(11.2) \qquad \frac{\partial \Pr\left(\mathbf{X}_i\hat{\beta}\right)}{\partial X_{ki}} = \frac{\partial F\left(\mathbf{X}_i\hat{\beta}\right)}{\partial X_{ki}} = f\left(\mathbf{X}_i\hat{\beta}\right)\hat{\beta}_k,$$

where $f(\ )$ denotes the probability density function and is standard normal and logistic in the probit and logit cases, respectively. For a dummy regressor (X_K), the estimated partial effects can be calculated as follows:

$$(11.3) \qquad F\left(\hat{\beta}_1 X_{i1} + \dots + \hat{\beta}_{K-1} X_{iK-1} + \hat{\beta}_K\right) - F\left(\hat{\beta}_1 X_{i1} + \dots + \hat{\beta}_{K-1} X_{iK-1}\right).$$

It is clear from equations 11.2 and 11.3 that these partial effects are not constants but are observation specific. There are two options, either calculate equations 11.2 and 11.3 at interesting values of all regressors, such as means or medians, or calculate the partial effect for each observation and take the average of these. The latter is preferable, but the former is somewhat more convenient. In large samples, the partial effect at the means should approximate the mean of the partial effects (Greene 2000). Calculating at medians, rather than means, ensures that values of dummy regressors are either 0 or 1 and, for regressors that are nonlinear transformations of variables, for example, quadratics and logs, it avoids the problem that the mean of the transformation is not the transformation of the mean. However, using medians can create problems of interpretation. For example, it may lead to infeasible combinations of the X's, setting all values to zero for a set of mutually exclusive indicators with less than 50 percent of the sample in each category. Such problems are avoided by computing the partial effect for each observation and then taking the mean or median of these.

Box 11.1 *Example of Binary Response Models—Child Malnutrition in Vietnam, 1998*

We compare the linear probability, logit, and probit models in estimating correlates of a discrete state of child malnutrition, defined as height-for-age more than two standard deviations below the average in a well-nourished (U.S.) population (see chapter 4). The data are for children younger than 10 years of age and are taken from the 1998 Vietnam Living Standards Survey (VLSS). This analysis complements that of a continuous measure of nutritional deprivation presented in the previous chapter.

In the following table we present estimates of the parameters of the respective models. Standard errors are adjusted for the clustered nature of the sample and are robust to general heteroscedasticity (see chapter 10). No adjustment is made for stratification, and sample weights are not applied, it being assumed that stratification is on exogenous factors (see chapter 10). There is a great deal of consistency across the estimators in the levels of significance of the coefficients. As suggested above, dividing logit and probit coefficients by 4 and 2.5, respectively, makes them approximately comparable to the LPM coefficients. For the coefficient on the male dummy, that gives 0.0669 (= 0.2675/4) for logit and 0.0646 (= 0.1614/2.5) for probit, which are both larger than the LPM coefficient of 0.0563. More

(continued)

Estimates from Binary Response Models of Stunting, Vietnam 1998 (children <10 years)

Dependent variable = 1 if height-for-age z-score less than –2					
	LPM (OLS)	Logit (MLE)		Probit (MLE)	
	Coeff.	Coeff.	Partial effect	Coeff.	Partial effect
Child's age (months)	0.0079***	0.0403***	0.0100***	0.0245***	0.0097***
	(0.00075)	(0.00394)	(0.00100)	(0.00238)	(0.00100)
Child's age squared (/100)	–0.0053***	–0.0271***	–0.0068***	–0.0165***	–0.0066***
	(0.00058)	(0.00293)	(0.00074)	(0.00177)	(0.00071)
Child is male	0.0563***	0.2675***	0.0661***	0.1614***	0.0639***
	(0.01281)	(0.06072)	(0.01489)	(0.03688)	(0.01451)
(log) hhold. consumption per capita	–0.1849***	–0.9403***	–0.2347***	–0.5639***	–0.2248***
	(0.01726)	(0.09026)	(0.02255)	(0.05301)	(0.02116)
Safe drinking water	–0.0447*	–0.2017*	–0.0504*	–0.1208*	–0.0482*
	(0.02685)	(0.11669)	(0.02906)	(0.07146)	(0.02844)
Satisfactory sanitation	–0.057**	–0.3344***	–0.0822***	–0.1982***	–0.0782***
	(0.02306)	(0.11838)	(0.02860)	(0.06990)	(0.02728)
Years of schooling of head of household	0.0013	0.0047	0.0012	0.0028	0.0011
	(0.00219)	(0.01070)	(0.00267)	(0.00642)	(0.00256)
Mother has primary school diploma	–0.0041	–0.0106	–0.0027	–0.0079	–0.0031
	(0.02008)	(0.09218)	(0.02301)	(0.05571)	(0.02221)
Intercept	1.5681***	5.4812***		3.2734***	
	(0.13511)	(0.69589)		(0.41134)	
Sample size	5,218				

Note: Robust standard errors in parentheses. Adjusted for clustering and heteroskedasticity. Partial effects calculated at medians of regressors.

LPM = linear probability model, OLS = ordinary least squares, MLE = maximum likelihood estimator.

***, **, and * indicate significance at 1%, 5%, and 10%, respectively.

Box 11.1 *continued*

directly, we can compare the partial effects of the regressors on the probability that a child is stunted. For the LPM, these marginal effects are given by the coefficients themselves and so are constants. For the logit and probit models, we have calculated the partial effects at the median values of the regressors. In general, the estimated partial effects from logit and probit are very close and are larger in magnitude than those from the LPM.

In the next table, we summarize the distributions of the partial effects estimated from the probit model. This form of presentation makes it clear that partial effects vary across individuals. For example, the mean effect of satisfactory sanitation is to reduce the probability of stunting by 0.0689, from an estimated population average probability of 0.3737. In absolute terms, the strongest partial effect of satisfactory sanitation is a reduction in the probability by 0.0790, but this is from a predicted baseline probability for that individual of 0.5281. The weakest absolute effect is a reduction in the probability of only 0.0076, but this is large in relation to the respective baseline probability of 0.0118.

Partial effects can be calculated with respect to variables of inherent interest, rather than transformations of these. For example, in the table, we present the partial effect of a currency unit increase in household consumption, as well as the effect of a marginal increase in the log of consumption. Partial effects of variables entered in quadratic form, such as age, can be calculated but are of limited interest. The partial effect of age itself is a function of the partial effects of the first and second powers of age (given in the table). This function can be calculated but, given the quadratic nature of the function, the partial effect changes sign. It is of more interest to examine a picture of the quadratic function and locate its turning point (six years and two months, in this example).

Partial Effects on Probability That Child Is Stunted, Vietnam 1998 (children <10 years)

(derived from probit estimates in table above)

	Mean	Std. dev.	Min	Max
Child's age (months)	0.0086	0.00160	0.0008	0.0098
Child's age squared (/100)	−0.0058	0.00108	−0.0066	−0.0005
Child is male	0.0568	0.01045	0.0046	0.0643
(Log) Household consumption p.c.	−0.1982	0.03675	−0.2250	−0.0174
Household Consumption p.c. (D)	−0.0001	0.00007	−0.0006	−0.0000
Safe drinking water	−0.0430	0.00743	−0.0482	−0.0043
Satisfactory sanitation	−0.0689	0.01240	−0.0790	−0.0076
Years of schooling of head of hhold.	0.0010	0.00018	0.0001	0.0011
Mother has primary school diploma	−0.0028	0.00051	−0.0031	−0.0002

Note: Data are weigted. D = Vietnamese dong.
Source: Authors.

Computation

Stata, like many packages, has preprogrammed routines for probit and logit:

```
probit depvar varlist [pw=weight], robust
logit depvar varlist [pw=weight], robust
```

where `depvar` and *varlist* represent dependent and independent variables, respectively; `[pw=weight]` is optional to give weighted (on `weight`) estimates; and `robust` is optional for heteroscedasticity robust standard errors. If the survey data are from a cluster sample, standard errors can be corrected for within-cluster correlation using the option `cluster(psu)`, where `psu` is a variable identifying the primary sampling units (see chapter 10).[1]

A special routine is available to give probit partial effects at specific regressor values:

```
dprobit depvar varlist [pw=weight], robust
```

By default, this calculates partial effects at the means. To obtain the effects at other values, such as medians, the following can be used:

```
local vars "varlist"
foreach x of local vars {
        qui sum `x' [aw=weight], d
        sca `x'_md=r(p50)
}
matrix define medians=(var1_md, var2_md,....)
dprobit depvar varlist [pw=wt], robust at(medians)
```

where *var1*, *var2* .... are the names of the regressors in `varlist`. There is no such preprogrammed routine for logit partial effects, but Stata's general routine for partial effects, `mfx`, can be used. Simply run a logit and afterward

```
mfx compute, at(median)
```

where `at()` specifies the values at which effects are to be calculated; `mean`, `median`, `zero`, defined values, or a combination of these can be selected. This is much slower than `dprobit`. It can be speeded up by requesting that standard errors not be calculated through the option `nose`.

To calculate partial effects for each observation, run `probit` or `logit`, then obtain predictions of the latent index (xb) and probability of a nonzero dependent variable (p) for each observation by

```
predict xb if e(sample), xb
predict p if e(sample), p
```

where `if e(sample)` is optional and restricts the prediction to observations used in the estimation. Define two locals containing the names of the continuous variables (e.g., `cont1`, `cont2`, etc.) and those of the dummy variables (e.g., `dummy1`, `dummy2`, etc.),

```
local cont "cont1 cont2 ..."
local dummies "dummy1, dummy2, ..."
```

For continuous regressors, define a variable that will be used to transform the coefficients

```
gen t_var=normden(xb)            | for probit
gen t_var=p*(1-p)                | for logit
```

and, using equation 11.2, obtain the partial effects from

```
foreach c of local cont {
        gen pe_`c'=t_var*_b[`c']
}
```

---

[1]If the survey is stratified and the analyst also wishes to take that into account in computation of the standard errors, Stata's survey estimators for probit/logit can be used.

For dummy regressors, use equation 11.3, and obtain the partial effects for pro-bit from the following:

```
foreach d of local dummies {
     gen pe_`d'=p-norm(xb-_b[`d'])
     replace pe_`d'=norm(xb+_b[`d'])-p if `d'==0
}
```

For logit, use

```
foreach d of local dummies {
     gen pe_`d'=p-(exp(xb-_b[`d'])/(1+exp(xb-_b[`d'])))
     replace pe_`d'=(exp(xb+_b[`d'])/(1+exp(xb+_b[`d'])))-p
       if `d'==0
}
```

Finally, obtain summary statistics of the distribution of the following partial effects:

```
summ `cont' `dummies' [fw=weight], detail
```

where [fw=weight] applies weights and should be included where these exist.

This procedure will generate, for example, estimates of the population means of the partial effects. For inference, standard errors of these estimates would have to be generated by the delta method (Wooldridge 2002).

Limited dependent variables

A limited dependent variable is continuous over most of its distribution but has a mass of observations at one or more specific values, such as zero. The most important example in the health sector is medical expenditure, which is zero for many individuals over a survey recall period, such as 12 months. For example, in 1998 the average Vietnamese spent 153,000 Vietnamese dong (D) ($1 = 13,987D) out-of-pocket on medical care during a 12-month period, but 17 percent spent nothing at all.

There are a multitude of statistical approaches to modeling of a limited dependent variable—for example, the two-part model, the Tobit model, the sample selection model, hurdle models, and finite mixture models. For a comprehensive survey, see Wooldridge (2002). Here, we restrict attention to the most popular approaches to modeling medical expenditures. For an excellent survey of this literature, see Jones (2000). Equity analysis of medical expenditures may focus on their income elasticity, on variation in the price elasticity of health care with household income, on the responsiveness of medical expenditure to health shocks, or the extent to which this responsiveness is reduced by unequally distributed insurance coverage.

Two-part model

The most straightforward approach is the two-part model (2PM). In its most popular form, this comprises a probit (or logit) model for the probability that an individual makes any expenditure on health care and OLS, applied only to the subsample with nonzero expenditures, to estimate correlates of the positive level of expenditure. Given that typically the distribution of medical expenditures is right skewed, invariably the log of expenditure is modeled in the second part OLS.

Application of OLS to only part of the sample raises the possibility of sample selection bias. The issue has been the subject of a great deal of discussion (Jones 2000). In summary, consistency of the 2PM for the model parameters rests on strong assumptions. Nonetheless, if the aim is simply to predict conditional means and not to make inferences about individual parameters, then the 2PM may perform reasonably well (Duan et al. 1983). On that basis, the model will often be adequate for analysis of health sector inequalities, where we simply want to *predict*, for example, medical expenditure conditional on income, age, gender, and so on.

Following Jones (2000), let the probability that medical expenditure (y_i) is positive be determined by observable $(\mathbf{X}_{1i})$ and unobservable (ε_{1i}) factors. Let $\ln(y_i)$ be the log of positive medical expenditure, with covariates $\mathbf{X}_{2i}$, and unobservable determinants ε_{2i}. Consistency of the 2PM is predicated on an assumption of conditional mean independence (Jones 2000).

$$(11.4) \qquad E\left[\ln(y_i)|y_i>0,\mathbf{X}_{2i}\beta_2\right]=E\left[\ln(y_i)|\mathbf{X}_{1i}\beta_1+\varepsilon_{1i}>0,\mathbf{X}_{2i}\beta_2\right]=\mathbf{X}_{2i}\beta_2$$

In other words, conditional on expenditure being positive, the unobservable determinants of its log have zero mean. To justify the assumption, either unobservable factors that influence the positive level of expenditures (ε_{2i}) must be independent of those governing the probability of a positive expenditure (ε_{1i}), or the two error terms must have some peculiar joint distribution that gives a conditional distribution centered around zero. The latter would be an extreme and nontestable assumption (Jones 2000). The former assumption can possibly be supported under certain decision-making processes, for example, if the individual decides whether to seek treatment without considering how much to spend during the course of treatment. That rules out the possibility that the individual decides not to seek care because of the anticipated cost of a course of treatment. In support of such a sequential model of decision making, it might be claimed that the patient delegates all treatment decisions to the doctor. Empirically, however, such a defense is weak because typically survey data span a period of calendar time and not the duration of an illness episode (Deb and Trivedi 1997). Even if it is accepted that medical care decisions are made in a sequential manner, correlation between unobservables would still arise in cases in which common variables are omitted from the two stages of the decision-making process (Jones 2000).

The expected level of medical expenditure is given by the following:

$$(11.5) \qquad E\left[y_i|\mathbf{X}_i\right]=\Pr\left(y_i>0|\mathbf{X}_{1i}\right)E\left[y_i|y_i>0,\mathbf{X}_{2i}\right].$$

Unfortunately, this value cannot be estimated directly when the second part of the model is estimated in logs, as is usually the case. This is known as the retransformation problem; we have to get back from logs to levels. Assumption 11.4 is not sufficient to identify 11.5. For possible solutions to the problem, see Jones (2000) and Mullahy (1998). This rather weakens the argument that the 2PM is reasonable when one is interested only in estimating the conditional means.

Tobit model

Whereas the 2PM assumes that two independent decisions lie behind medical expenditures, the Tobit model, at the other extreme, assumes a single decision. The individual chooses the level of medical expenditure that maximizes his or her welfare. Positive expenditures correspond to desired expenditures. Zero expenditure represents a corner solution, in which income and/or preferences for health are so low that spending nothing on health care is best for the individual. The model can be described using the concept of a latent, desired level of expenditure:

$$(11.6) \qquad y_i^* = \mathbf{X}_i \beta + \varepsilon_i, \qquad \varepsilon_i \sim IN(0, \sigma^2).$$

Observed expenditure is assumed to be related to the latent value by the following:

$$(11.7) \qquad y_i = \begin{cases} y_i^* \text{ if } y_i^* > 0 \\ 0 \text{ otherwise.} \end{cases}$$

The assumption of a single decision-making process is most probably strong. It requires that before making contact with the health services, the individual has full information on the costs of alternative courses of treatment. It also rules out the possibility that the initial decision to seek treatment is made solely by the individual, while both the patient and the doctor influence the decision about the amount of treatment.

The Tobit model is estimated by maximum likelihood (ML). As a rule of thumb, Tobit ML estimates may be approximated by the OLS estimates from the 2PM divided by the proportion of nonzero observations in the sample (Greene 2000). Predicted medical expenditure over the whole sample is still based on equation 11.5, but the second term in the product is no longer given by equation 11.4 but by the following:

$$(11.8) \qquad E\left[y_i \mid y_i > 0, \mathbf{X}_i\right] = \mathbf{X}_i \beta + \sigma \lambda_i, \quad \lambda_i = \frac{\phi\left(\mathbf{X}_i\beta / \sigma\right)}{\Phi\left(\mathbf{X}_i\beta / \sigma\right)}$$

where $\phi(\ )$ and $\Phi(\ )$ are the standard normal probability density and cumulative density functions, respectively, and λ_i is known as the inverse Mill's ratio (IMR).

Sample selection model

The sample selection model (SSM), or generalized Tobit, can be considered, somewhat informally, to lie midway between the extremes of the Tobit and the 2PM. Whereas the Tobit assumes a single decision process and the 2PM two independent decisions, the SSM allows for two interdependent decisions. The decision to seek medical care and the choice of how much to spend can be influenced by distinct but correlated observable and unobservable factors. In latent variable form, the model is given by the following:

$$(11.9) \qquad y_{ji}^* = \mathbf{X}_{ji} \beta_j + \varepsilon_{ji}, \qquad j = 1, 2$$

$$(11.10) \qquad y_i = \begin{cases} y_{2i}^* \text{ if } y_{1i}^* > 0 \\ 0 \text{ otherwise.} \end{cases}$$

Assuming the two error terms are jointly normally distributed, the model can be estimated either by the Heckman two-step procedure or by ML. The former involves estimating a probit for the probability of nonzero expenditure, using the results to estimate the IMR and then running OLS on the nonzeros with the estimated IMR included to correct for selection bias. That is, in the second stage, the following is estimated:

$$(11.11) \qquad y_i = \mathbf{X}_{2i}\beta + \rho\sigma_2 \frac{\phi\left(\mathbf{X}_{1i}\hat{\beta}_1\right)}{\Phi\left(\mathbf{X}_{1i}\hat{\beta}_1\right)} + e_{2i,}$$

where ρ is the correlation coefficient between the errors, and σ_2 is the standard deviation of ε_{2i} ($\sigma_1 = 1$). The t-ratio for the IMR provides a test for selection bias. Standard errors must be corrected for the inclusion of the estimated IMR among the regressors. Packages programmed for the Heckman estimator will make the correction automatically. Efficiency gains can be realized through ML estimation.

Although the SSM is, in an informal sense, more general, this comes at the cost of making greater demands on the data with respect to identification. Given the nonlinearity of the IMR, equation 11.11 is identified even if the regressor matrices $\mathbf{X}_1$ and $\mathbf{X}_2$ are identical, but in this case the Mill's ratio will be closely correlated with the other regressors and, consequently, parameters will not be estimated with precision. It is therefore preferable to have a variable that influences the decision of whether to spend anything on health care but, conditional on this, does not influence the positive level of expenditure. Such variables, however, are few and far between.

The Tobit and 2PM avoid this problem but only by assumption. The bottom line is that it is difficult to make an a priori case for any one model of medical expenditures. One should probably be most skeptical of the Tobit model and its assumption of a single decision process driving both zero and positive expenditures. In choosing between the 2PM and the SSM, it is necessary to consider the purpose of the analysis (prediction or parameter estimation), the likely degree of selection bias, and the information available to identify it.

Box 11.2 *Example of Limited Dependent Variable Models—Medical Expenditure in Vietnam, 1998*

We examine correlates of annual out-of-pocket expenditures on health care in Vietnam. We use data from the 1998 VLSS. Almost one-fifth (18%) of the observations made no expenditures on medical care. In addition to this mass at zero expenditure, the distribution has a long right tail. Given such skewness, one would expect a log transformation of the dependent variable to be appropriate, and the results confirm this. We make two comparisons, the 2PM with the SSM taking logs of positive expenditures in each case and the 2PM with the Tobit leaving the dependent variable in levels (see the table below).

Results from the maximum likelihood estimator of the SSM are given. These do not differ substantially from estimates obtained using the Heckman two-step procedure. Estimates of the coefficients of the selection equation display no substantial differences across the estimators. There are no differences in levels of significance. Coefficient estimates for the continuous parts of the models do show some differences, with those from the SSM generally of greater magnitude. There are some differences in levels of significance.

There is a positive and large degree of correlation between the two equation errors (0.847). The null of no correlation, and therefore no selection bias, is firmly rejected. In the absence of any variable that can plausibly be argued to affect the probability of positive expenditure but not its level, the correlation parameter is being identified through functional form alone. Graphical analysis confirms that, in this case, the inverse Mill's ratio is sufficiently nonlinear in its argument to avoid severe collinearity problems.

(continued)

Box 11.2 *continued*

Comparison of Two-Part and Sample Selection Model Estimates of Medical Expenditure, Vietnam 1998

Dependent variables: Participation = 1 if medical expenditure positive; Continuous = log of (positive) expenditure

	Two-part model				Sample selection model			
	Participation (probit)		Continuous (OLS)		Participation (MLE)		Continuous (MLE)	
	Coeff.	*Rob. SE*	*Coeff.*	*Rob. SE*	*Coeff.*	*Rob. SE*	*Coeff.*	*Rob. SE*
body mass index	−0.1382***	0.0332	−0.0800***	0.0254	−0.1117***	0.0297	−0.1430***	0.0283
(body mass index)^2	0.2820***	0.0820	0.1212*	0.0643	0.2265***	0.0728	0.2488***	0.0709
log(rental value of house)	0.3079***	0.0434	0.5065***	0.0264	0.3393***	0.0350	0.6262***	0.0378
satisfactory sanitation	−0.2160***	0.0775	−0.2362***	0.0434	−0.2183***	0.0713	−0.3283***	0.0605
house not of solid materials	0.0900*	0.0528	0.1896***	0.0363	0.0831*	0.0459	0.2279***	0.0428
attended school, no diploma	0.0527	0.1110	−0.2522***	0.0386	0.0173	0.1023	−0.2240***	0.0638
attended school & diploma	0.0985	0.1320	−0.1335***	0.0482	0.0674	0.1221	−0.0839	0.0774
head of hhold has diploma	−0.0563	0.0570	−0.1557***	0.0391	−0.0684	0.0526	0.1761***	0.0462
head of hhold school grade	−0.0025	0.0078	−0.0112**	0.0049	−0.0029	0.0070	−0.0118**	0.0059
					Rho	0.8470	0.0195	
Sample size	27,368		22,645		Wald (Rho=0)	324.6	*p*=0.0000	
Test slope parameters all zero	Wald = 515	*p* = 0.0000	F = 134.2	*p* = 0.0000		Wald = 3448	*p* = 0.0000	

Note: All models also include a 3rd-degree polynomial in age, gender dummy, head of household dummy, quadratic in household size and regional dummies.
MLE = maximum likelihood estimator; Rob. SE = robust to hetero. and clustering standard error;
Rho = coefficient of correlation of errors; Wald (rho = 0) = Wald test of null of rho = 0.
***, **, and * significant at 1%, 5%, and 10%, respectively.

Comparison of the 2PM with the Tobit is a little less comforting (see following table). First, it is apparent that estimation in levels is less appropriate. The coefficient estimates differ substantially between the estimators and the scaling of the OLS coefficients, that is, dividing by the proportion of "positives" does not get us particularly close to the Tobit estimates. Mean predicted expenditure (over the full sample) from the Tobit model, at 374.2, is well above the actual mean of 157.2.

Box 11.2 *continued*

Comparison of Two-Part and Tobit Model Estimates of Medical Expenditures Vietnam 1998

Dependent variable: **Level** *of annual medical expenditure*

	Two-part model (OLS part)			Tobit (MLE)	
	Coeff.	*SE*	*Scaled coeff.*	*Coeff.*	*SE*
Body mass index	–19.21	*15.94*	–23.18	-47.53***	*15.11*
(body mass index)^2	42.11	*41.42*	50.81	100.69***	*37.64*
Log (rental value of house)	211.66***	*24.01*	255.43	249.15***	*8.86*
Satisfactory sanitation	–73.78***	*17.87*	–89.04	–111.55***	*16.05*
House not of solid materials	37.18***	*11.89*	44.87	51.34***	*12.36*
Attended school, no diploma	–54.36**	*22.93*	–65.61	–38.04**	*19.16*
Attended school & diploma	–31.23	*25.35*	–37.69	–6.14	*23.78*
Head of hhold has diploma	–10.14	*27.97*	–12.24	–21.09	*18.30*
Head of hhold school grade	–9.85**	*4.13*	–11.88	–9.03***	*2.13*
Sample size	22,645			27,335	
Test of all slope parameters zero	F = 14.29	*p* = 0.0000		LR = 1887	*p* = 0.0000

Note: All models also include a 3rd degree polynomial in age, gender dummy, head of household dummy, quadratic in household size and regional dummies.

Scaled coeff. = OLS coefficient divided by sample proportion with positive expenditure.

MLE = maximum likelihood estimator; SE = standard error; LR = Likelihood ratio test.

***, **, and * significant at 1%, 5%, and 10%, respectively.

Source: Authors.

Computation

Computation of the 2PM is straightforward. Run a `probit` for the probability of positive expenditure followed by OLS (`regr`) for the log of expenditure on the selected sample. Stata has a preprogrammed routine `heckman` for the SSM. For the (consistent) two-step estimator, use the following:

```
heckman depvar varlist, sel(depvar_s = varlist_s) twostep ///
  mills(imr)
```

where `depvar` is the continuous dependent variable (e.g., expenditures) and `varlist` associated regressors; `depvar_s` is a binary variable identifying the selected sample (those with positive expenditures) and `varlist_s` associated regressors; `mills(imr)` saves the inverse Mill's ratio and calls it `imr`. Omitting the `twostep` option gives the MLE, and with this `robust` and `cluster` adjusted standard errors can be requested.

To examine whether the Mill's ratio is nonlinear over its sample range, the following can be used:

```
predict xbsel if depvar_s==1, xbsel
twoway (scatter xbsel imr if depvar_s==1)
```

To estimate a Tobit model with censoring at zero, as in the example, use the following:

```
tobit depvar varlist, ll(0)
```

Count dependent variables

Many of the variables of interest in the health sector are nonnegative counts of events. For example, visits to the doctor, drugs dispensed, days ill, and so on. A count is a variable that can take only integer-values. Often, as with most health count variables, negative values are not possible. Typically, the distribution of such variables tends to be right skewed, often comprising a large proportion of zeros and a long right-hand tail. The discrete nature of a nonnegative count dependent variable and the shape of its distribution demand the use of particular estimators. For example, least squares would not guarantee that predicted values are nonnegative.

The most basic approach is to assume a Poisson process to describe the probability of observing a specific count of events over a fixed interval. That is, the probability of observing a count of y_i, conditional on a set of explanatory variables, $\mathbf{X}_i$, is assumed to be given by

$$(11.12) \qquad \Pr(y_i|\mathbf{X}_i) = \exp(-\lambda_i)\lambda_i^{y_i}/y_i!$$

where $\exp()$ is the exponential function, $y_i!$ indicates y_i factorial, and λ_i is the conditional mean of the count and is usually specified as

$$(11.13) \qquad \lambda_i = E[y_i|\mathbf{X}_i] = \exp(\mathbf{X}_i\beta).$$

A peculiarity of the Poisson distribution is that its mean and its variance are both equal to its one parameter, λ. This is often restrictive. In health applications, for example, the conditional mean is usually less than the conditional variance. In jargon, there is *overdispersion*. One consequence can be underprediction of the number of observations with zero counts; again, an empirical feature of many health care applications. Overdispersion can be allowed for, or rather imposed, through alternative distributional assumptions. For example, a negative binomial specification maintains the Poisson process (equation 11.12) but extends equation 11.13 to include an error term, for which a (gamma) distribution is assumed. As a result, the (conditional) variance of the count is restricted to be greater than its mean (Cameron and Trivedi 1986). The difference between the variance and mean, that is, the dispersion, can be specified as proportional to the mean (NegBin I) or a quadratic function of the mean (NegBin II) (Cameron and Trivedi 1986). The model can be further generalized by allowing the dispersion to vary across observations with a set of regressors.

Overdispersion is not the only reason a simple Poisson model may underpredict the number of zero counts. There may be a particular process responsible for generating zeros that is distinct from that generating other values of the count variable. One possibility, in the context of health care utilization, is a sequential decision-making process, as discussed in the previous section. This takes us back to the 2PM. In a count framework, the 2PM consists of a probit/logit (or Poisson/ NegBin) to model the probability of a nonzero count followed by a count regression, such as Poisson or NegBin, applied to observations with positive counts only and allowing for the truncation at zero (Pohlmeier and Ulrich 1995). Independence is assumed between the two processes. Other possibilities are "zero-inflated" models and latent class models (Jones 2000, 318–24).

Unobservable heterogeneity, deriving time-invariant individual effects in a panel data context or community effects in a cross section, can be taken into account in estimation of the Poisson model through a random-effects specification. Alternatively, with a fixed-effects specification of the Poisson, individual/community effects are eliminated. These are somewhat analogous to the random- and fixed-effects specification in a linear context discussed in chapter 10. The random effects specification is more efficient but requires an assumption that individual/community effects are independent of the regressors. A fixed-effects specification relaxes the assumption. Apart from taking unobservable heterogeneity into account, these methods have the further important advantage of relaxing the equi-dispersion restriction of the Poisson model (Wooldridge 2002).

Box 11.3 *Example of Count Data Models—Pharmacy Visits in Vietnam, 1998*

Annual visits to a pharmacy or drug peddler in Vietnam provides a good example of a distribution suited to the application of count data models. That is, there are a large number of zeros and a long right tail.

No. of pharmacy visits	*Frequency*
0	20865
1	3980
2	1899
3	846
4	434
5	197
6	79
7	52
8	25
9	5
10+	124

It should be acknowledged that we chose this distribution on the basis of its suitability for count analysis. With many count variables encountered in health applications, the dominance of zero values is much greater than in this example and the best option is simply to dichotomize the variable and use probit or logit to model the probability of a nonzero count.

Estimates and robust standard errors from a NegBin II model of pharmacy visits are given in the first two columns of the following table. NegBin II was chosen over NegBin I by comparison of the log-likelihood values. There is strong evidence of overdispersion as indicated by the magnitude of the dispersion parameter and the LR test, which decisively rejects the Poisson (equi-dispersion) specification.

Moving to a 2PM, there is some loss of significance, with significant effects in the first stage probit only. Restricting the count regression to positive values is not sufficient to remove overdispersion—a Poisson specification is still strongly rejected. Finally, we estimate a fixed-effects Poisson on all observations. The fixed effects are those of 194 communes. Point estimates from the FE Poisson are somewhat similar to those from NegBin II on the full sample, but there are large differences in levels of significance for some interesting variables. In particular, the household consumption effect becomes strongly significant. Apparently, the commune effects had initially confounded this (negative) income effect. *(continued)*

Box 11.3 *continued*

Count Models for Annual Pharmacy Visits, Vietnam 1998

| | NegBin II (all observations) | | Two-part model | | | | Fixed-effects Poisson | |
| | | | Probit | | Truncated NegBin II | | | |
	Coeff.	Rob. SE	Coeff.	Rob. SE	Coeff.	Rob. SE	Coeff.	Rob. SE
Log hhold. consumption per capita	−0.0314	0.0648	−0.0451	0.0432	0.0559	0.1303	−0.0710***	0.0221
Attended school, no diploma	−0.1696**	0.0734	−0.0771	0.0547	−0.1038	0.3238	−0.1422***	0.0263
Attended school & diploma	−0.1486	0.0976	−0.0760	0.0701	−0.0957	0.2928	−0.1171***	0.0327
Body mass index	−0.1640***	0.0401	−0.1006***	0.0242	−0.0818	0.1015	−0.1462***	0.0207
Body mass index^2/100	0.3582***	0.1019	0.2081***	0.0593	0.2117	0.2973	0.3215***	0.0500
Satisfactory sanitation	−0.1792**	0.0748	−0.1065**	0.0443	−0.1445	0.1076	−0.1347***	0.0276
House not built of solid materials	0.1394***	0.0535	0.0399	0.0365	0.1900	0.1807	0.0786***	0.0221
Head of household	0.1187**	0.0485	0.0662***	0.0239	0.0850	0.3022	0.1147***	0.0233
Household size	−0.0401***	0.0119	−0.0352***	0.0080	0.0017	0.0227	−0.0525***	0.0048
Dispersion parameter (alpha)	2.6387	0.1547	n.a.		2.5372		n.a.	
LR test of equidispersion	10,685	$p = 0.0000$	n.a.		41,656	$p = 0.0000$	n.a.	
Sample size	27,365		27,368		7,441		27,176	
Log-likelihood	−25,661.4		−15,287.4		−10,176.5		−28,132.8	

Note: All models also include a 3rd-degree polynomial in age and gender dummy. All models except FE Poisson include region dummies. Rob. SE = robust to hetero. and clustering standard error; Log-L = log likelihood. LR test of equidispersion is NegBin against Poisson (p = p-value). ***, **, and * significant at 1%, 5%, and 10%, respectively.

Source: Authors.

Computation

The Stata programmed routine for the Poisson model is `poisson`. For NegBin models it is

```
nbreg depvar varlist, dispersion(constant) cluster(commune)
```

where `dispersion(constant)` is optional and requests NegBin I; the default is NegBin II . Here the `cluster` option is used to correct standard errors for within-commune correlation. Note that an LR test against Poisson is generated only if the options `robust` or `cluster` are not specified. For the second part of a 2PM, the truncated Poisson or negative binomial can be computed by using the commands `trnpois0` and `trnbin0`, respectively, which can be downloaded from the Stata Web site. In the latter case,

```
trnbin0 depvar varlist if depvar>0, cluster(commune)
```

Random- and fixed-effects Poisson models are obtained from the following:

```
xtpois depvar varlist, fe i(commune)
```

where `i(commune)` specifies common effects for all observations with the same values of the variable `commune`, and the option `fe` requests the fixed-effects model. The default is random effects.

Further reading

For a comprehensive review of econometric analyses of health and health care data, see Jones (2000). A more concise review, along with applications, can be found in Jones and O'Donnell (2002). For a practical guide to health econometrics containing many worked examples and Stata code, see Jones (2007). More generally, Wooldridge (2002) and Cameron and Trivedi (2005) are both excellent microeconometrics textbooks.

References

Amemiya, T. 1981. "Qualitative Response Models: A Survey." *Journal of Economic Literature* 19(4): 481–536.

Cameron, A. C., and P. K. Trivedi. 1986. "Econometric Models Based on Count Data: Comparisons and Applications of Some Estimators and Tests." *Journal of Applied Econometrics* 1: 29–53.

Cameron, A., and R. Trivedi. 2005. *Microeconometrics: Methods and Applications.* New York: Cambridge University Press.

Deb, P., and P. K. Trivedi. 1997. "Demand for Medical Care by the Elderly: A Finite Mixture Approach." *Journal of Applied Econometrics* 12(3): 313–36.

Duan, N., W. G. Manning, C. N. Morris, and J. P. Newhouse. 1983. "A Comparison of Alternative Models of the Demand for Health Care." *Journal of Business and Economic Statistics* 1: 115–26.

Greene, W. 2000. *Econometric Analysis.* Upper Saddle River, NJ: Prentice-Hall Inc.

Horrace, W. C., and R. L. Oaxaca. 2006. "Results on the Bias and Inconsistency of Ordinary Least Squares for the Linear Probability Model." *Economics Letters* 90: 321–27.

Jones, A. M. 2000. Health Econometrics. In *Handbook of Health Economics,* ed. A. J. Culyer and J. P. Newhouse, 265–346. Amsterdam, Netherlands: Elsevier North-Holland.

——— 2007. *Applied Econometrics for Health Economists—A Practical Guide.* Oxford, England: Radcliffe Medical Publishing.

Jones, A. M., and O. O'Donnell. 2002. *Econometric Analysis of Health Data.* Chichester, UK: John Wiley and Sons.

Mullahy, J. 1998. "Much Ado About Two: Reconsidering Retransformation and the Two-Part Model in Health Econometrics." *Journal of Health Economics* 17(3): 247–81.

Pohlmeier, W., and V. Ulrich. 1995. "An Econometric Model of the Two-Part Decision-Making Process in the Demand for Health Care." *Journal of Human Resources* 30(2): 339–61.

Wooldridge, J. M. 2002. *Econometric Analysis of Cross Section and Panel Data.* Cambridge, MA: MIT Press.

12

Explaining Differences between Groups: Oaxaca Decomposition

After inequalities in the health sector are measured, a natural next step is to seek to explain them. Why do inequalities in health exist between the poor and better-off in many countries despite health systems explicitly aimed at eliminating inequalities in access to health care? Why is inequality in the incidence of health sector subsidies greater in one country than in another? Why has the distribution of health or health care changed over time?

In this chapter and the next, we consider methods of decomposing inequality in health or health care into contributing factors. The core idea is to explain the distribution of the outcome variable in question by a set of factors that vary systematically with socioeconomic status. For example, variations in health may be explained by variations in education, income, insurance coverage, distance to health facilities, and quality of care at local facilities. Even if policy makers have managed to eliminate inequalities in some of these dimensions, inequalities between the poor and better-off may remain in others. The decomposition methods reveal how far inequalities in health can be explained by inequalities in, say, insurance coverage rather than inequalities in, say, distance to health facilities. The decompositions in this chapter and the next are based on regression analysis of the relationships between the health variable of interest and its correlates. Such analyses are usually purely descriptive, revealing the associations that characterize the health inequality, but if data are sufficient to allow the estimation of causal effects, then it is possible to identify the factors that generate inequality in the variable of interest. In cases in which causal effects have not been obtained, the decomposition provides an explanation in the statistical sense, and the results will not necessarily be a good guide to policy making. For example, the results will not help us predict how inequalities in Y would change if policy makers were to reduce inequalities in X, or reduce the effect of X and Y (e.g., by expanding facilities serving remote populations if X were distance to provider). By contrast, if causal effects have been obtained, the decomposition results ought to shed light on such issues.

The decomposition method outlined in this chapter, known as the Oaxaca decomposition (Oaxaca 1973), explains the gap in the means of an outcome variable between two groups (e.g., between the poor and the nonpoor). The gap is decomposed into that part that is due to group differences in the magnitudes of the determinants of the outcome in question, on the one hand, and group differences in the effects of these determinants, on the other. For example, poor children may be less healthy not only because they have less access to piped water but also because their parents are less knowledgeable about how to obtain the maximum health benefits from piped water (Jalan and Ravallion 2003; Wagstaff and Nguyen 2003). The decomposition technique considered in the next chapter does not permit such a distinction between the contributions of differences in the magnitudes and the effects of determinants. In its favor, however, it does allow us to decompose inequalities in health or health care across the full distribution of say, income, rather than simply between the poor and the better-off.

Oaxaca-type decompositions

Some preliminaries

Suppose we have a variable, y, which is our outcome variable of interest. We have two groups, which we shall call the poor and the nonpoor. We assume y is explained by a vector of determinants, x, according to a regression model:

$$(12.1) \qquad y_i = \begin{cases} \beta^{poor} x_i + \varepsilon_i^{poor} \text{ if poor} \\ \beta^{nonpoor} x_i + \varepsilon_i^{nonpoor} \text{ if nonpoor} \end{cases}$$

where the vectors of β parameters include intercepts. In the case of a single regressor, drawn in figure 12.1, the nonpoor are assumed to have a more advantageous regression line than the poor. At each value of x, the outcome, y, is better. In addition, the nonpoor are assumed to have a higher mean of x. The result is that the poor have a lower mean value of y than do the nonpoor.[1]

Figure 12.1 *Oaxaca Decomposition*

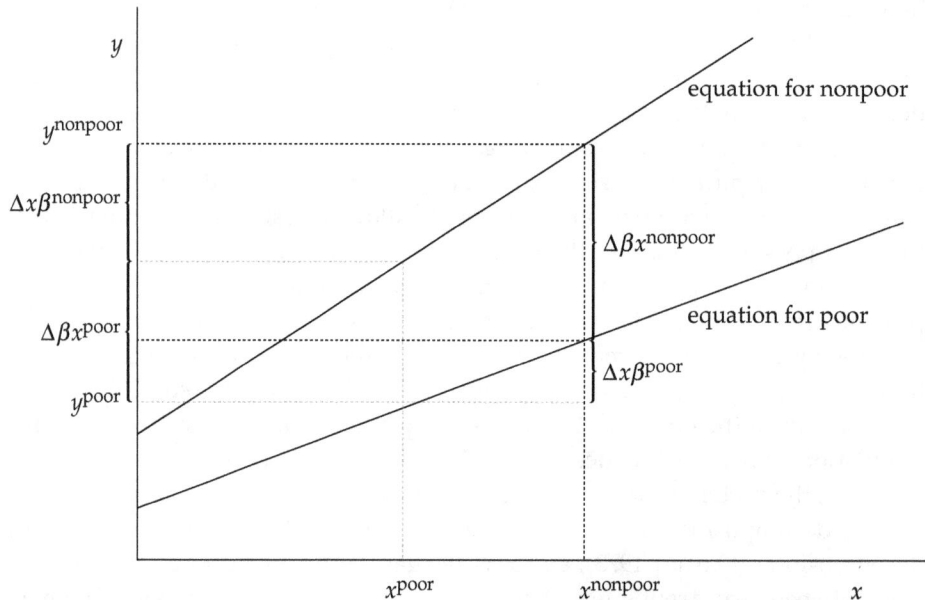

Source: Authors.

---

[1] In the case of the poor, we read off the equation for the poor above x^{poor}, giving a value of y equal to y^{poor}. In the case of the nonpoor, we read off the equation for the nonpoor above $x^{nonpoor}$, giving a value of y equal to $y^{nonpoor}$.

The gap between the mean outcomes, $y^{nonpoor}$ and y^{poor}, is equal to

(12.2)
$$y^{nonpoor} - y^{poor} = \beta^{nonpoor} x^{nonpoor} - \beta^{poor} x^{poor},$$

where $x^{nonpoor}$ and x^{poor} are vectors of explanatory variables evaluated at the means for the nonpoor and the poor, respectively.[2] For example, if we have just two x's, x_1 and x_2, we can write the following:

(12.3)
$$y^{nonpoor} - y^{poor} = \left(\beta_0^{nonpoor} - \beta_0^{poor}\right) + \left(\beta_1^{nonpoor} x_1^{nonpoor} - \beta_1^{poor} x_1^{poor}\right) + \left(\beta_2^{nonpoor} x_2^{nonpoor} - \beta_2^{poor} x_2^{poor}\right)$$
$$= G_0 + G_1 + G_2$$

so that the gap in y between the poor and the nonpoor can be thought of as being due in part to (i) differences in the intercepts (G_0), (ii) differences in x_1 and β_1 (G_1), and (iii) differences in x_2 and β_2 (G_2). For example, G_1 might measure the part of the gap in mean health status (y) due to differences in educational attainment (x_1) and the effects of educational attainment (β_1), and G_2 might measure the part of the gap due to the gap in accessibility to health facilities (x_2) and differences in the effects of accessibility (β_2).

Estimates of the difference in the gap in mean outcomes can be obtained by substituting sample means of the x's and estimates of the parameters β's into equation 12.2. In the rest, we make such a substitution but do not make it explicit in the notation.

Oaxaca's decomposition

We could stop here. But we might want to go further and ask how much of the overall gap or the gap specific to any one of the x's (e.g., G_1 or G_2) is attributable to (i) differences in the x's (sometimes called the explained component) rather than (ii) differences in the β's (sometimes called the unexplained component). The Oaxaca and related decompositions seek to do just that.

From figure 12.1, it is clear that the gap between the two outcomes could be expressed in either of two ways:

(12.4)
$$y^{nonpoor} - y^{poor} = \Delta x \beta^{poor} + \Delta \beta x^{nonpoor}$$

where
$$\Delta x = x^{nonpoor} - x^{poor} \text{ and } \Delta \beta = \beta^{nonpoor} - \beta^{poor}, \text{ or as}$$

(12.5)
$$y^{nonpoor} - y^{poor} = \Delta x \beta^{nonpoor} + \Delta \beta x^{poor}.$$

As the figure makes clear, these decompositions are equally valid. In the first, the differences in the x's are weighted by the coefficients of the poor group and the differences in the coefficients are weighted by the x's of the nonpoor group, whereas in the second, the differences in the x's are weighted by the coefficients of the nonpoor group and the differences in the coefficients are weighted by the x's of the poor group. Either way, we have a way of partitioning the gap in outcomes between

---

[2]Assuming exogeneity, the conditional expectations of the error terms in (12.1) are zero.

the poor and nonpoor into a part attributable to the fact that the poor have worse x's than the nonpoor, and a part attributable to the fact that *ex hypothesi* they have worse β's than the nonpoor.

The decompositions in equations 12.4 and 12.5 can be seen as special cases of a more general decomposition:[3]

$$(12.6) \qquad y^{nonpoor} - y^{poor} = \Delta x \beta^{poor} + \Delta \beta x^{poor} + \Delta x \Delta \beta$$
$$= E + C + CE$$

so that the gap in mean outcomes can be thought of as deriving from a gap in endowments (E), a gap in coefficients (C), and a gap arising from the interaction of endowments and coefficients (CE). Equations 12.4 and 12.5 are special cases in which

$$(12.4) \qquad y^{nonpoor} - y^{poor} = \Delta x \beta^{poor} + \Delta \beta x^{nonpoor} = E + (CE + C)$$

and

$$(12.5) \qquad y^{nonpoor} - y^{poor} = \Delta x \beta^{nonpoor} + \Delta \beta x^{poor} = (E + CE) + C.$$

So, in effect, the first decomposition places the interaction in the unexplained part, whereas the second places it in the explained part.[4]

Related decompositions

We can also write Oaxaca's decomposition as a special case of another decomposition:

$$(12.7) \quad y^{nonpoor} - y^{poor} = \Delta x \left[D\beta^{nonpoor} + (I - D)\beta^{poor} \right] + \Delta \beta \left[x^{nonpoor}(I - D) + x^{poor}D \right],$$

where I is the identity matrix and D a matrix of weights. In the simple case, where x is a scalar rather than a vector, I is equal to one, and D is a weight. In this case, $D = 0$ in the first decomposition, equation 12.4, and $D = 1$ in the second, equation 12.5. In the case in which x is a vector, we have

$$(12.8) \qquad\qquad\qquad D = 0 \text{ (Oaxaca) (equation 12.4')}$$

$$(12.9) \qquad\qquad\qquad D = I \text{ (Oaxaca) (equation 12.5')}$$

Other formulations have been suggested. Cotton (1988) suggested weighting the differences in the x's by the mean of the coefficient vectors, giving us

$$(12.10) \qquad\qquad\qquad \text{diag}(D) = 0.5 \text{ (Cotton)},$$

---

[3]This notation is from Ben Jann's help file for his Stata decompose routine used later in the chapter.

[4]The rationale for this is that the decompositions were devised to look at discrimination in the labor market. The analog of the nonpoor would be whites or males, and the analog of the poor would be blacks or women. In the first decomposition the presumption is that it is blacks and women who are paid according to their characteristics, whereas whites and men receive unduly generous remuneration. In the second decomposition, the presumption is that whites and men are paid according to their characteristics, and it is blacks and women who are discriminated against.

where diag(D) is the diagonal of D. Reimers (1983) suggested weighting the coefficient vectors by the proportions in the two groups, so that if f_{NP} is the sample fraction in the nonpoor group, we have

(12.11)
$$\text{diag}(D) = f_{NP} \text{ (Reimers)}.$$

In addition to Oaxaca's two decompositions and the additional two proposed by Cotton and Reimers, there is a fifth proposed by Neumark (1988), which makes use of the coefficients obtained from the pooled data regression, β^P:

(12.12)
$$y^{nonpoor} - y^{poor} = \Delta x \beta^P + \left[x^{nonpoor} \left(\beta^{nonpoor} - \beta^P \right) + x^{poor} \left(\beta^P - \beta^{poor} \right) \right] \text{ (Neumark)}.$$

Illustration: decomposing poor–nonpoor differences in child malnutrition in Vietnam

We illustrate the decompositions by means of an example. The setting is Vietnam. The aim of the exercise is to explain the difference between the poor and the nonpoor in child malnutrition, measured anthropometrically through height-for-age z-scores (see chapter 4).

We classify (under-10) children as poor if they are below the poverty line of D 1,790,000 (D = Vietnamese dong), which is the classification developed by the World Bank (Glewwe, Gragnolati, and Zaman 2000) and used by the government of Vietnam. On this basis, using sample weights, we have 46 percent of under-10 children being classified as poor. Figure 12.2 shows that poor children (poor = 1) tend to have a height-for-age z-score (HAZ) lower than that of nonpoor children (poor = 0). The mean HAZ values among the nonpoor and poor are –1.44 and –1.86, respectively. A mean of 0.00 would place the group in question at the 50th centile in the U.S. reference sample of well-nourished children (distribution sketched in figures), so even the average nonpoor child in Vietnam is substantially undernourished by U.S. standards. Our focus here is on explaining the gap of 0.42 between the mean HAZ of nonpoor and poor children.

Regression model and its estimation

In our setting, y is the HAZ malnutrition score. As in chapter 13, we use basically the same regression model as Wagstaff, van Doorslaer, and Watanabe (2003) and include the log of the child's age in months (lnage), a dummy indicating whether the child in question is male (sex), dummies indicating whether the child's household has safe drinking water (safewtr) and satisfactory sanitation (oksan), the years of schooling of the child's mother (schmom), and the natural logarithm of household per capita consumption (lnpcexp). Our poverty grouping variable is poor, which takes a value of 1 if the child's household is poor. The first step is to see whether the regression coefficient vector, β, differs systematically between the poor and nonpoor. The relevant Stata commands are as follows:

```
xi: regr haz poor i.poor|lnage i.poor|sex i.poor|safwtr
  i.poor|oksan i.poor|schmom i.poor|lnpcexp [pw=wt]
    testparm poor _I*
```

Figure 12.2 *Malnutrition Gaps between Poor and Nonpoor Children, Vietnam, 1998*

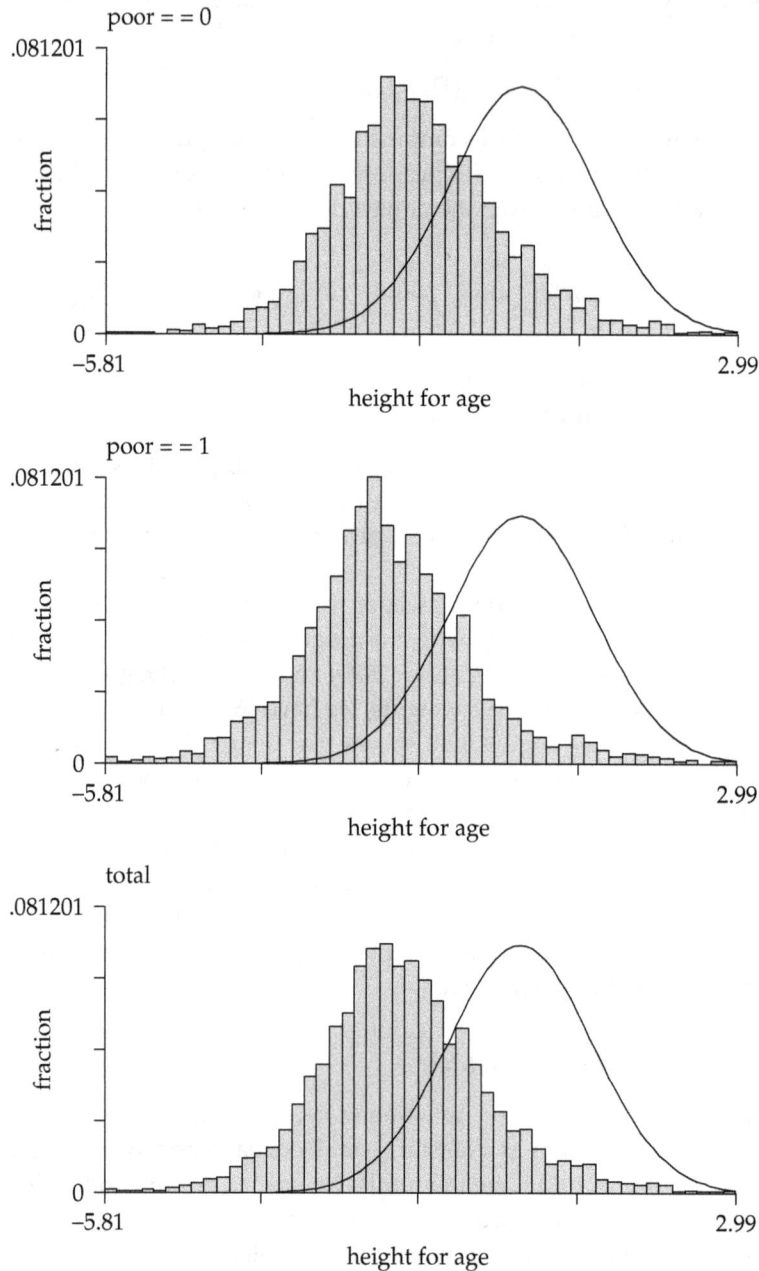

poor == 0

poor == 1

total

Source: Authors.

The first command runs a regression with the poor dummy included alone and interacted with all the x's. The second command tests the hypothesis that the coefficients on the poor dummy and its interactions are simultaneously equal to zero. The F-statistic, with 7 and 5154 degrees of freedom, is 2.03 and has a p-value of 0.0472. Thus the Oaxaca-type approach, which allows for different regression coefficients, makes some sense in this context, although rejection of the null of parameter homogeneity is somewhat marginal.

Decomposition

Ben Jann's Stata routine decompose, which is downloadable from the Stata Web site,[5] allows all the decompositions outlined above to be computed in just one command:

```
decompose haz lnage sex safwtr oksan schmom lnpcexp [pw=wt],
  by(poor) detail estimates
```

The syntax is the same as the regress command, except that after the comma the user has to specify the variable defining the two groups (in our case poor). The first block of output (table 12.1) reports the mean values of y for the two groups, and the difference between them. It then shows the contribution attributable to the gaps in endowments (E), the coefficients (C), and the interaction (CE). In this application, the gap in endowments accounts for the great bulk of the gap in outcomes.

Table 12.1 *First Block of Output from* decompose

Mean prediction high (H):	-1.442
Mean prediction low (L):	-1.861
Raw differential (R) {H-L}:	0.419
- due to endowments (E):	0.406
- due to coefficients (C):	-0.082
- due to interaction (CE):	0.095

Source: Authors.

The second block of output (table 12.2) shows how the explained and unexplained portions of the outcome gap vary depending on the decomposition used. The first and second columns correspond to the Oaxaca decomposition in equations 12.4′ and 12.5′, where $D = 0$ and $D = I$, respectively. The third and fourth columns correspond to Cotton's and Reimers' decompositions, where the diagonal of D equals 0.5 and $f_{NP} = 0.562$ (in our case), respectively. The final column labeled "*" is Neumark's decomposition. Whatever decomposition is used, it is clearly the difference in the mean values of the x's that accounts for the vast majority of the difference in malnutrition between poor and nonpoor children in Vietnam. Differences in the effects of the determinants play a tiny part in explaining malnutrition inequalities.

Table 12.2 *Second Block of Output from* decompose

D:	0	1	0.5	0.562	*
Unexplained (U){C+(1-D)CE}:	0.014	-0.082	-0.034	-0.038	-0.032
Explained (V) {E+D*CE}:	0.406	0.501	0.454	0.458	0.451
% unexplained {U/R}:	3.2	-19.5	-8.1	-9.1	-7.5
% explained (V/R):	96.8	119.5	108.1	109.1	107.5

Source: Authors.

---

[5]From within Stata, give the command findit decompose and follow the links. Another ado file—oaxaca—is available for Stata version 8.2 and later. This has all the functions of decompose with the important addition of providing standard errors for the contributions.

The third block of output (table 12.3) allows the user to see how far gaps in individual x's contribute to the overall explained gap. For example, focusing on the final column corresponding to Neumark's decomposition, we see that the gaps in the two demographic variables actually *favor* the poor, whereas the gaps in the remaining variables all *disfavor* the poor. Of the latter, it is the gap in household consumption that accounts for the bulk of the explained gap. It is not so much the correlates of poverty (poor water and sanitation, low educational levels) that account for malnutrition inequalities between poor and nonpoor children in Vietnam—it is poverty itself, in the form of lack of purchasing power.

Table 12.3 Third Block of Output from decompose

			explained: D =				
Variables	E(D=0)	C	CE	1	0.5	0.543	*
lnage	-0.027	0.282	0.005	-0.022	-0.024	-0.024	-0.024
Sex	-0.004	0.038	0.002	-0.002	-0.003	-0.003	-0.003
safwtr	0.029	0.005	0.004	0.033	0.031	0.031	0.033
oksan	-0.008	0.016	0.056	0.048	0.02	0.022	0.036
schmom	0.029	-0.103	-0.035	-0.006	0.012	0.01	0.009
lnpcexp	0.387	0.551	0.064	0.45	0.419	0.421	0.4
_ cons	0	-0.87	0	0	0	0	0
Total	0.406	-0.082	0.095	0.501	0.454	0.458	0.451

Source: Authors.

The fourth and final block of output (table 12.4) gives the coefficient estimates, means, and predictions for each x for each group, the "high group" in this case being the nonpoor and the "low group" being the poor.

Table 12.4 Fourth Block of Output from decompose

	High model			Low model			Pooled	
Variables	Coef.	Mean	Pred.	Coef.	Mean	Pred.	Coef.	
lnage	-0.321	4.021	-1.291	-0.392	3.952	-1.551	-0.354	
Sex	-0.088	0.513	-0.045	-0.166	0.491	-0.081	-0.122	
Safwtr	0.165	0.421	0.069	0.144	0.221	0.032	0.164	
Oksan	0.195	0.313	0.061	-0.034	0.069	-0.002	0.147	
Schmom	-0.003	7.696	-0.023	0.015	5.739	0.086	0.005	
lnpcexp	0.544	7.99	4.348	0.467	7.162	3.346	0.483	
_ cons	-4.561	1	-4.561	-3.691	1	-3.691	-3.955	
Total			-1.442			-1.861		

Source: Authors.

For the first Oaxaca decomposition (12.4'), columns 2 and 3 of table 12.3 allow us to identify how the gap in each of the β's contributes to the overall unexplained gap. For the other decompositions, the contributions of the individual β's can be found by taking the group difference in the variable specific predictions given in table

Figure 12.3 *Contributions of Differences in Means and in Coefficients to Poor–Nonpoor Difference in Mean Height-for-Age z-Scores, Vietnam, 1998*

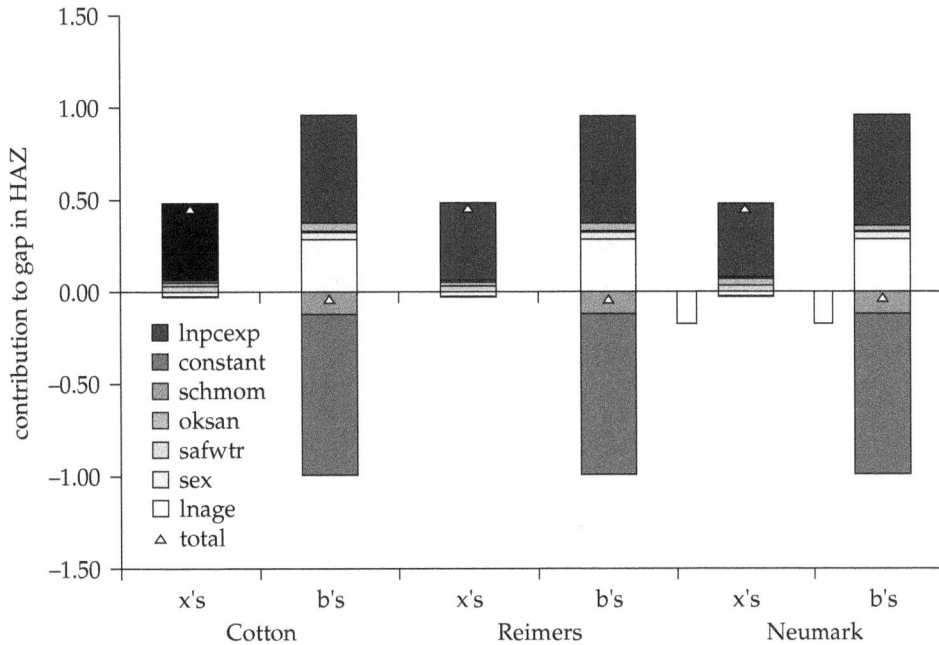

Source: Authors.

12.4 and subtracting the explained part given in table 12.3 from this. A bar chart can then be presented, as in figure 12.3, showing the contribution of the difference in the means of each x and the difference in the coefficients on each x. As far as the means of the x's are concerned, figure 12.3 tells us simply what we already knew from the second block of output: most of the explained part of the malnutrition gap is attributable to the gap in per capita consumption. The triangles in the chart, which indicate the overall contributions of the x's and the β's, also show us something else we already knew: that the bulk of the gap in malnutrition is from gaps in the x's, not gaps in the β's. Figure 12.3 makes clear that the unimportance overall of the unexplained portion is due to offsetting effects from different β's. The poor have a higher intercept in the HAZ equation, but this is largely offset by the fact that the consumption effect is weaker for the poor.

Extensions

The framework above can be extended in a number of ways. One is to explain changes in gaps over time (Makepeace et al. 1999). Wagstaff and Nguyen (2003) use this framework to investigate why child survival continued to improve in Vietnam during the 1990s for the nonpoor but not for the poor.

Another extension would be to take selectivity into account. There are, in fact, two separate selectivity issues that might be explored. The first concerns sample selection. Consider the example of child malnutrition. Because a child's nutritional status influences its survival prospects, it also affects the probability that the child appears in the sample (Lee, Rosenzweig, and Pitt 1997). The resulting selection bias can be dealt with provided data are available to model the selection process. In the example given, this would require fertility history data such that the probability of a child death before the survey date could be modeled as a function of household characteristics. The selection correction term—known as the inverse Mills ratio (IMR) (Wooldridge 2002)—can then be used to adjust the group mean difference in the outcome variable. In the `decompose` routine, this can be done with the option `lambda(varname)`, where *varname* would be that given to the IMR. A second selection problem concerns the selection into the poor and nonpoor groups—group assignment selection. Malnutrition in a child might itself reduce a household's living standards by, for example, keeping the mother at home to look after the child and preventing her from working or by reducing the amount of help the child can provide on the family farm (Ponce, Gertler, and Glewwe 1998). If this is the case, malnutrition may influence the selection of a child into poverty. If the sample selection issue is put aside, the group assignment problem can be dealt with by modeling the probability of being in one group rather than the other, and then using the selection correction terms to adjust the difference in group means. Again, this can be done in the `decompose` routine with the `lambda()` option.

A further extension is the case in which the relationship of interest is nonlinear. Examples include a probit model or a hazard model in the case of modeling child survival. In such cases, one option would be to work with the underlying latent variable that is linear in the covariates. Wagstaff and Nguyen (2003), for example, do their decomposition in terms of the negative of the log of the hazard rate.

The methods described above decompose the difference in the mean of an outcome variable between two groups. Group differences in other parameters of the distribution can also be of interest. For example, with respect to the example of child malnutrition, the difference in mean HAZ scores is arguably less interesting than the difference in the proportion of poor and nonpoor children that are stunted. The general Oaxaca approach can be extended to decompose differences in a full distribution of an outcome into the contribution of differences in the distributions of covariates, on the one hand, and differences in the effects of these covariates, on the other. For example, this can be done using quantile regression (Machado and Mata 2005). Apart from decomposing the full distribution, and not simply the mean, this approach has the advantage of allowing the effect of covariates to differ over the conditional distribution of the outcome. So, for example, one can allow for the possibility that income has a different marginal effect on the nutritional status of malnourished and well-nourished children. The approach has been used to explain the change in the distribution of HAZ scores in Vietnam between 1993 and 1998 (O'Donnell, López-Nicolás, and van Doorslaer 2005; O'Donnell, van Doorlsaer, and Wagstaff 2006).

References

Cotton, J. 1988. "On the Decomposition of Wage Differentials." *Review of Economics and Statistics* 70(2): 236–43.

Glewwe, P., M. Gragnolati, and H. Zaman. 2000. *Who Gained from Vietnam's Boom in the 1990s?* Washington, DC: The World Bank.

Jalan, J., and M. Ravallion. 2003. "Does Piped Water Reduce Diarrhea for Children in Rural India?" *Journal of Econometrics* 112(1): 153–73.

Lee, L.-F., M. Rosenzweig, and M. Pitt. 1997. "The Effects of Improved Nutrition, Sanitation, and Water Quality on Child Health in High-Mortality Populations." *Journal of Econometrics* 77: 209–35.

Machado, J. A. F., and J. Mata. 2005. "Counterfactual Decomposition of Changes in Wage Distributions Using Quantile Regression." *Journal of Applied Econometrics* 20(4): 445–65.

Makepeace, G., P. Paci, P. H. Joshi, and P. Dolton. 1999. "How Unequally Has Equal Pay Progressed Since the 1970s." *Journal of Human Resources* 34(3): 534–56.

Neumark, D. 1988. "Employers' Discriminatory Behavior and the Estimation of Wage Discrimination." *Journal of Human Resources* 23(3): 279–95.

Oaxaca, R. 1973. "Male-Female Wage Differentials in Urban Labor Markets." *International Economic Review* 14: 693–709.

O'Donnell, O., A. López-Nicolás, and E. van Doorlsaer. 2005. "Decomposition of Changes in the Distribution of Child Nutrition Using Quantile Regression: Vietnam 1993–98." Mimeo, University of Macedonia, Thessaloniki, Greece.

O'Donnell, O., E. van Doorlsaer, and A. Wagstaff. 2006. "Decomposition of Inequalities in Health and Health Care." In *Elgar Companion to Health Economics,* ed. A. M. Jones. Chichester, England: Edward Elgar.

Ponce, N., P. Gertler, and P. Glewwe. 1998. "Will Vietnam Grow Out of Malnutrition?" In *Household Welfare and Vietnam's Transition,* ed. D. Dollar, P. Glewwe, and J. Litvack, 257–75. Washington, DC: World Bank.

Reimers, C. W. 1983. "Labor Market Discrimination against Hispanic and Black Men." *Review of Economics and Statistics* 65(4): 570–79.

Wagstaff, A., and N. N. Nguyen. 2003. "Poverty and Survival Prospects of Vietnamese Children under Doi Moi." In *Economic Growth, Poverty and Household Welfare: Policy Lessons from Vietnam,* ed. P. Glewwe, N. Agrawal, and D. Dollar. Washington, DC: World Bank.

Wagstaff, A., E. van Doorslaer, and N. Watanabe. 2003. "On Decomposing the Causes of Health Sector Inequalities, with an Application to Malnutrition Inequalities in Vietnam." *Journal of Econometrics* 112(1): 219–27.

Wooldridge, J. M. 2002. *Econometric Analysis of Cross Section and Panel Data.* Cambridge, MA: MIT Press.

13

Explaining Socioeconomic-Related Health Inequality: Decomposition of the Concentration Index

In the previous chapter we examined methods to explain the difference between two groups in the mean of some outcome variable of interest, which could be health or health care. By defining groups by socioeconomic status and using the method above, we can explain socioeconomic-related inequality in health or health care. But the degree of inequality captured is inevitably limited, given that group differences are examined. Measurement and explanation of inequality in health or health care across the entire distribution of some measure of socioeconomic status would be preferable. In chapter 8 we introduced the concentration index as a measure of socioeconomic-related inequality in health or health care. In this chapter we will explain how such inequality can be explained through decomposition of the concentration index.

Decomposition of the concentration index

For ease of exposition, we will refer to any health sector variable, such as health or health care use or payments, as "health" and to any (continuous) measure of socioeconomic status as "income." Wagstaff, van Doorslaer, and Watanabe (2003) demonstrate that the health concentration index can be decomposed into the contributions of individual factors to income-related health inequality, in which each contribution is the product of the sensitivity of heath with respect to that factor and the degree of income-related inequality in that factor. For any linear additive regression model of health (y), such as

$$(13.1) \qquad y = \alpha + \sum_k \beta_k x_k + \varepsilon ,$$

the concentration index for y, C, can be written as follows:

$$(13.2) \qquad C = \sum_k (\beta_k \bar{x}_k / \mu) C_k + GC_\varepsilon / \mu,$$

where μ is the mean of y, $\bar{x}_k$ is the mean of x_k, C_k is the concentration index for x_k (defined analogously to C), and GC_ε is the generalized concentration index for the error term (ε). Equation 13.2 shows that C is equal to a weighted sum of the concentration indices of the k regressors, where the weight for x_k is the elasticity of y with respect to x_k $\left(\eta_k = \beta_k \dfrac{\bar{x}_k}{\mu} \right)$. The residual component—captured by the last term—reflects the income-related inequality in health that is not explained by systematic variation in the regressors by income, which should approach zero for a well-specified model.

Wagstaff, van Doorslaer, and Watanabe (2003) use equation 13.2 to decompose income-related inequality in child malnutrition in Vietnam in 1993 and 1998. As in chapters 10 and 12, malnutrition is measured by the height-for-age z-scores (HAZ) of children younger than 10 years of age, and the measure of living standards is household consumption per capita. The z-scores are multiplied by –1 such that a greater value indicates more malnourishment. The specification of the regression model (equation 13.1) is very similar to that used in chapters 10 and 12. Here we include commune fixed effects to pick commune-level determinants of nutritional status. A summary of the results is presented in table 13.1. The (negative) concentration indices in the last row show that there was inequality in HAZ to the disadvantage of the poor in each year and that this inequality increased over time. The entries in each column are derived from equation 13.2 and give, for each year, the elasticity of HAZ with respect to each factor, the concentration index for each factor, and the total contribution of each factor to the HAZ concentration index. In each year, most of the consumption-related inequality in HAZ is explained by the direct effect of household consumption and by commune-level correlates of both malnutrition and consumption. The large elasticities of HAZ with respect to these factors are responsible for their large contribution to the HAZ concentration index. In contrast, there is a great deal of consumption-related inequality in access to both safe drinking water and satisfactory sanitation, but there is little sensitivity of HAZ to variation in these factors, and so they make little contribution to the HAZ concentration index.

Table 13.1 *Decomposition of Concentration Index for Height-for-Age z-Scores of Children <10 Years, Vietnam, 1993 and 1998*

	1993			1998		
	Elasticities	*Concentration indices*	*Contri-butions*	*Elasticities*	*Concentration indices*	*Contri-butions*
Child's age (in months)	1.137	0.020	0.023	1.630	0.018	0.030
Child's age squared	−0.634	0.030	−0.019	−0.880	0.028	−0.025
Child = male	0.022	0.003	0.000	0.045	0.014	0.001
(log)household consumption p.c.	−0.936	0.038	−0.035	−1.288	0.040	−0.052
Safe drinking water	−0.003	0.312	−0.001	−0.017	0.256	−0.004
Satisfactory sanitation	−0.009	0.468	−0.004	−0.006	0.508	−0.003
Years schooling household head	−0.017	0.065	−0.001	−0.015	0.094	−0.001
Years schooling mother	−0.037	0.075	−0.003	−0.003	0.108	−0.000
Fixed commune effects	1.477	−0.024	−0.035	1.534	−0.031	−0.047
"Residual"			−0.002			0.002
Total			−0.077			−0.099

Source: Wagstaff, van Doorslaer, Watanabe (2003, table 2).

Computation

The decomposition (equation 13.2) can be computed easily in Stata. First create the weighted fractional rank variable (rank) and estimate concentration index (CI) for the health variable (y) using the code provided in chapter 8. Generate a global X that refers to all the regressors in equation 13.1, estimate this regression, and create a scalar equal to the (weighted) mean of the health variable.

```
global X "varlist"
qui regr y $X [pw=weight]
sum y [aw=weight]
sca m_y=r(mean)
```

Then the factor specific elasticities, concentration indices, and contributions in equation 13.2 can be computed and displayed with the following loop,[1]

```
foreach x of global X {
    qui {
            sca b_`x' = _b[`x']
            corr rank `x' [pw=weight], c
            sca cov_`x' = r(cov_12)
            sum `x' [pw=weight]
            sca elas_`x' = (b_`x'*r(mean))/m_y
            sca CI_`x' = 2*cov_`x'/r(mean)
            sca con_`x' = elas_`x'*CI_`x'
            sca prcnt_`x' = con_`x'/CI
    }
    di "`x' elasticity:", elas_`x'
    di "`x' concentration index:", CI_`x'
    di "`x' contribution:", con_`x'
    di "`x' percentage contribution:", prcnt_`x'
}
```

The final term in equation 13.2 can be obtained as a residual—the difference between the concentration index and the sum of the factor contributions.

Decomposition of change in the concentration index

Wagstaff, van Doorslaer, and Watanabe (2003) also proposed two approaches to explaining changes in income-related inequality over time. A first approach is to apply an Oaxaca-type decomposition (Oaxaca 1973) (see chapter 12). This can also be used to examine differences in inequality across cross-sectional units (van Doorslaer and Koolman 2004). Applying Oaxaca's method to equation 13.2 gives the following:

$$(13.3) \qquad \Delta C = \sum_k \eta_{kt} \left(C_{kt} - C_{kt-1} \right) + \sum_k C_{kt-1} \left(\eta_{kt} - \eta_{kt-1} \right) + \Delta \left(GC_{\varepsilon t} / \mu_t \right),$$

where t indicates time period and Δ denotes first differences. As discussed in chapter 12, the Oaxaca decomposition is not unique and an alternative to equation 13.3 would be to weight the difference in concentration indices by the first period

---

[1]We thank Xander Koolman, who originally wrote this code.

elasticity and weight the difference in elasticities by the second period concentration index.

This approach allows one to decompose change in income-related inequality in health into changes in inequality in the determinants of health, on the one hand, and changes in the elasticities of health with respect to these determinants, on the other. But it does not allow one to disentangle changes going on within the elasticities. To address this limitation, Wagstaff, van Doorslaer, and Watanabe (2003) consider the total differential of equation 13.2, allowing for changes in turn in the regression parameters, the means, and the concentration indices of the regressors. The change in the concentration index can be approximated (for small changes) by the following:

$$(13.4) \quad dC = -\frac{C}{\mu}d\alpha + \sum_k \frac{\bar{x}_k}{\mu}(C_k - C)d\beta_k + \sum_k \frac{\beta_k}{\mu}(C_k - C)d\bar{x}_k + \sum_k \frac{\beta_k \bar{x}_k}{\mu}dC_k + d\frac{GC_\varepsilon}{\mu}.$$

Note that the effect on C of a change in β_k, or in $\bar{x}_k$, depends on whether x_k is more unequally or less unequally distributed than y. This reflects two separate channels of influence—the direct effect of the change in β_k (or $\bar{x}_k$) on C and the indirect effect operating through μ. An increase in inequality in $\bar{x}_k$ (i.e., C_k) will increase the degree of inequality in y. The impact is an increasing function of β_k and $\bar{x}_k$ and a decreasing function of μ.

Wagstaff, van Doorslaer, and Watanabe (2003) use both equation 13.3 and equation 13.4 to decompose the change in income-related inequality in HAZ in Vietnam between 1993 and 1998. The results are summarized in table 13.2. Estimates of the percentage contribution of each determinant to the total change in C (third from last and last columns) are broadly similar across the two methods, with some important discrepancies. The Oaxaca-type method attributes more of the change to

Table 13.2 *Decomposition of Change in Concentration Index for Height-for-Age z-Scores of Children <10 Years, Vietnam, 1993–98*

| | Decomposition of change in concentration index | | | | | | |
| | Total differential approach (13.4) | | | | | Oaxaca-type approach (13.3) | |
	β's	*Means of x's*	*CIs*	*Total*	*Percent*	*Total*	*Percent*
Child's age (in months)	0.003	0.011	−0.002	0.012	−57	0.007	−30
Child's age squared	0.003	−0.010	0.001	−0.006	29	−0.006	26
Child = male	0.001	0.000	0.000	0.001	−5	0.001	−3
Household consumption	−0.005	−0.005	−0.002	−0.011	52	−0.016	74
Safe drinking water	−0.002	0.000	0.000	−0.003	14	−0.003	16
Satisfactory sanitation	0.003	−0.002	0.000	0.001	−5	0.001	−5
Years schooling hhold. head	0.001	0.000	−0.001	0.000	0	0.000	1
Years schooling mother	0.005	0.000	−0.001	0.004	−19	0.003	−11
Fixed commune effects	0.000	−0.014	−0.010	−0.025	119	−0.012	55
"Residual"				0.005	−24	0.005	−24
Total	0.010	−0.021	−0.016	−0.021	100	−0.022	100

Source: Wagstaff, van Doorslaer, and Watanabe (2003, tables 3 and 4).

household consumption, whereas the differential approach gives more weight to changes occurring at the commune level. From the individual components of the total differential method (columns 2–4), we see that whereas changes in the means and concentration indices of the determinants of malnutrition have, on balance, tended to increase income-related inequality in HAZ, the opposite appears to be true of changes in the regression coefficients.

Computation

The components of equation 13.3 could be computed by running the regression and loop given in the previous section for each year of data, labeling the scalars to distinguish between their values in each year and taking the differences between them appropriately weighted, as in equation 13.3. The same general procedure could be used for equation 13.4, but differences between the year-specific regression coefficients and variables means would also have to be computed. That the total differential decomposition holds only for small changes must be kept in mind. Extrapolation to actual changes gives just an approximation to the change in the concentration index.

Extensions

As discussed in chapter 5, one is often interested in income-related inequality in a health sector variable after standardizing for correlates of income, such as age and gender. To assess equity in the distribution of health care (see chapter 15), it is also necessary to standardize for differences in "need." The regression decomposition method is a convenient way of making such a standardization. One simply needs to deduct the contributions of the standardizing variables (included in the regression along with others) from the total concentration index. Van Doorslaer, Koolman, and Jones (2004) have demonstrated that this is equivalent to the two-step approach to indirect standardization discussed in chapter 5. Application of this approach to the measurement of inequity in health care use is discussed in chapter 15. This approach has been used to measure and decompose age-sex standardized income-related inequalities in self-reported health in Canada (van Doorslaer and Jones 2003) and in 13 European countries (van Doorslaer and Koolman 2004); to compare England, Wales, and Scotland during the 1979–1995 period (Gravelle and Sutton 2003); and to investigate the causes of changes in mental health in Great Britain (Wildman 2003).

Standard errors for the various components of the concentration index decomposition may be obtained by bootstrapping (van Doorslaer and Koolman 2004). Jones and Lopez-Nicolas (2004) extend this decomposition to a longitudinal setting, distinguishing between short-term inequality and the covariance between income and health through time.

The decomposition method relies on linearity of the underlying regression model. When the model is inherently nonlinear, it may be possible to base the decomposition on a linear approximation to the model. Van Doorslaer, Koolman, and Jones (2004) have used the "partial effects" representation of nonlinear count models to assess the degree of horizontal inequity in health care use in 12 European countries. This representation has the advantage of being a linear additive model of actual utilization, but it holds only by approximation, and the decomposition is not unique but depends on the values at which partial effects are calculated. The approach is presented and discussed in chapter 15. Alternatively, Wan (2004) generalizes the regression-based decomposition method for application to any inequality measure with few restrictions on the underlying regression model.

References

Gravelle, H., and M. Sutton. 2003. "Income Related Inequalities in Self-Assessed Health in Britain: 1979–1995." *Journal of Epidemiology and Community Health* 57(2): 125–29.

Jones, A.M., and A. Lopez-Nicolas. 2004. "Measurement and Explanation of Socio-Economic Inequality in Health with Longitudinal Data." *Health Economics* 13: 1015–1030.

Oaxaca, R. 1973. "Male-Female Wage Differentials in Urban Labor Markets." *International Economic Review* 14: 693–709.

van Doorslaer, E., and A. M. Jones. 2003. "Inequalities in Self-Reported Health: Validation of a New Approach to Measurement." *Journal of Health Economics* 22.

van Doorslaer, E., and X. Koolman. 2004. "Explaining the Differences in Income-Related Health Inequalities across European Countries." *Health Economics* 13(7): 609–28.

van Doorslaer, E., X. Koolman, and A. M. Jones. 2004. Explaining Income-Related Inequalities in Doctor Utilization in Europe. *Health Economics* 13(7): 629–47.

Wagstaff, A., E. van Doorslaer, and N. Watanabe. 2003. "On Decomposing the Causes of Health Sector Inequalities, with an Application to Malnutrition Inequalities in Vietnam." *Journal of Econometrics* 112(1): 219–27.

Wan, G. 2004. "Accounting for Income Inequality in Rural China: A Regression Based Approach." *Journal of Comparative Economics* 32: 348–63.

Wildman, J. 2003. "Income Related Inequalities in Mental Health in Great Britain: Analysing the Causes of Health Inequality over Time." *Journal of Health Economics* 22(2): 295–312.

14

Who Benefits from Health Sector Subsidies?
Benefit Incidence Analysis

Subsidization of health care from the public purse is commonplace. Ensuring that public spending on health care is pro-poor is a stated goal of international organizations, such as the World Bank, as well as many national governments. This may stem from a desire to ensure the poor have access to health care, considered a basic human right. But pro-poor spending on health care can also be pursued for its instrumental value in raising the health of the population and so the productivity of the labor force and, consequently, economic growth. Public subsidization of health care may also be motivated, or at least justified, by sector-specific equity objectives, such as equal treatment for equal need. Public health care can also be used as an instrument of broader poverty alleviation and redistribution policy when redistribution through cash transfers is severely impeded by information and administrative constraints (Besley and Coate 1991). Whether or not such justifications for public spending on health care are convincing depends on the distribution of the benefits from this spending. Who gains most? Is it the poor? Or does a substantial proportion, even a disproportionate proportion, of the spending go to the economically better-off? These are the questions addressed by benefit incidence analysis (BIA).

BIA describes the distribution of public spending across individuals ranked by their living standards (Aaron and McGuire 1970; Brennan 1976; Meerman 1979; van de Walle and Nead 1995). In its most simplistic form, it is an accounting procedure that seeks to establish who receives how much of the public spending dollars. Recipients are usually distinguished by their relative economic position, but the geographic distribution of spending could also be examined or the distribution across characteristics such as ethnicity or age. A more ambitious form of BIA attempts to estimate the extent to which public spending changes the distribution of final income, that is, income net of taxes and gross of in-kind transfers. As with tax incidence, this requires identification of the behavioral response to public spending (van de Walle 2000). For example, to what extent does public spending on health care crowd out private spending, and how does this vary with income? Or more indirectly, to what extent does public health care change gross incomes by affecting labor supply and saving decisions? Answering such questions requires detailed econometric analysis to identify the counterfactual distribution of income that would exist if there were no public spending on health care. In this chapter, we discuss the more simple form of BIA, which aims to describe the distribution of public health spending across an income distribution that is taken as given. We also confine attention to the distribution of average spending and do not consider the benefit incidence of marginal dollars spent on health care (Lanjouw and Ravallion 1999; Younger 2003).

Living standards need not be measured by income. Any of the measures discussed in chapter 6 could be used. If an ordinal measure, such as a wealth index, is chosen, then it is possible only to determine whether the distribution of public health care is pro-poor or pro-rich and not the extent to which, abstracting from behavioral responses, public spending changes some cardinal measure of inequality in living standards.

Having chosen a measure of living standards, there are three principal steps in a nonbehavioral BIA of public health spending. First, the utilization of public health services in relation to the measure of living standards must be identified. Second, each individual's utilization of a service must be weighted by the unit value of the public subsidy to that service. Finally, the distribution of the subsidy must be evaluated against some target distribution. In this chapter, we discuss each of these three steps in turn.

Distribution of public health care utilization

Microdata from a health or multipurpose household survey are required to estimate the distribution of public health care utilization across individuals in relation to living standards. Three factors deserve particular consideration in relation to the choice of survey. First, it must contain data on both health care use and some measure of living standards. Second, it should distinguish between public and private care. Third, the recall periods for health care utilization should be sufficiently long such that the sample of observed users is not too small but not too long such that recall bias is large. For health services that have a higher frequency of utilization, such as ambulatory care, the optimal recall period is probably in the range of 2 to 4 weeks, and most surveys use a period in this range. For inpatient care, the recall period should be longer. It is typically 12 months.

Only health services that are subsidized from the state-controlled budget should be considered. Public health programs and services financed from Overseas Development Assistance (ODA), user fees, and social insurance are relevant, provided the respective revenues are used at the discretion of the state. Difficulties arise if a survey does not distinguish between public and private care. In that case, private insurance cover, if available, might be used to distinguish between public and private patients. Otherwise, a BIA can be conducted only if the private sector is sufficiently small such that it can be ignored.

Calculation of the public health subsidy

Examination of raw utilization data does not capture variation in the quality of health care received and in payments made. Nor does it facilitate aggregation across services to determine the distribution of the total health sector subsidy. Both extensions require estimates of unit subsidies.

Box 14.1 *Distribution of Public Health Care Utilization in Vietnam, 1998*

Data are from the 1998 Vietnam Living Standards Survey (VLSS). Living standards are approximated by household consumption per equivalent adult. Five categories of health care are examined: inpatient days, hospital outpatient visits, visits to commune health centers, visits to polyclinics, and a residual category (domestic medical visits and visits to "other government facilities"). For all categories, except inpatient care, the survey distinguishes between public and private care. Because there were only 4 private hospitals in Vietnam of a total of more than 800 at the time of the survey (World Bank 2001), we simply assume all inpatient care is public care. Inpatient days are reported for a 12-month reference period, the other categories for the previous 4 weeks.

In the table below, we present, for each category of care, the cumulative percentage of total utilization accounted for by each quintile of household consumption. Figures in bold indicate significant differences from the respective population shares at 5 percent or less. Poorer groups receive less than their population share of hospital care at all quintiles. This is confirmed by tests indicating that the 45-degree line dominates both concentration curves for hospital care. This pro-rich bias is also indicated by the concentration indexes, which are positive and significantly different from zero. In contrast, utilization of commune health centers is pro-poor. There is no significant bias in the utilization of polyclinics and other public health services.

Distribution of Public Health Care Utilization in Vietnam, 1998

| Cumulative shares | Hospital care | | Commune health center visits | Polyclinic visits | Other public health services |
	Outpatient visits	Inpatient days			
Poorest 20%	**8.90%**	**10.29%**	22.65%	22.91%	13.22%
(standard error)	(0.9949)	(1.2141)	(1.8860)	(5.7815)	(2.9644)
Poorest 40%	**23.45%**	**27.74%**	**47.83%**	32.81%	47.09%
	(1.6629)	(2.0465)	(2.4084)	(6.2628)	(6.3806)
Poorest 60%	**43.58%**	**47.66%**	**77.86%**	59.29%	59.00%
	(2.3987)	(2.4772)	(1.9943)	(6.8524)	(6.0599)
Poorest 80%	**66.07%**	**70.36%**	**90.60%**	78.24%	79.63%
	(2.7376)	(2.5702)	(1.4456)	(6.5783)	(4.5689)
Test of dominance against 45° line	–	–	+		
Concentration index (robust standard error)	**0.2436**	**0.1784**	**−0.1567**	0.0401	0.0056
	(0.0368)	(0.0370)	(0.0335)	(0.1042)	(0.0777)

Note: For shares, bold indicates significant difference from population share at 5%. For concentration indexes, bold indicates significant difference from zero at 5%. Standard errors for concentration indexes are robust to heteroskedasticity and within cluster (commune) correlation. Dominance tests: – indicates the 45-degree line dominates the concentration curve (pro-rich)

             + indicates concentration curve dominates 45-degree line (pro-poor)

             Blank indicates nondominance.

Dominance is rejected if there is at least one significant difference in one direction and no significant difference in the other, with comparisons at 19 quantiles and 5% significance level. Quintile shares and their standard errors were computed, along with the dominance tests, using the dominance ado described in chapter 7. Concentration indexes computed as described in chapter 8.

Source: Authors.

Definition of public subsidy

The service-specific public subsidy received by an individual is as follows:

(14.1)
$$s_{ki} = q_{ki}c_{kj} - f_{ki},$$

where q_{ki} indicates the quantity of service k utilized by individual i, c_{kj} represents the unit cost of providing k in the region j where i resides, and f_{ki} represents the amount paid for k by i. The total public subsidy received by an individual is as follows:

(14.2)
$$s_i = \sum_k \alpha_k (q_{ki}c_{kj} - f_{ki}),$$

where α_k are scaling factors that standardize utilization recall periods across services. One might standardize on the recall period that applies for the service accounting for the greatest share of the subsidy. For example, where this is inpatient care, reported over a one-year period, then $\alpha_k = 1$ for inpatient care and, for example, $\alpha_k = 13$ for services reported over a 4-week period.

Unit costs

The starting point for the costing component of a BIA is total public recurrent expenditure on health care. Ideally, this should be disaggregated down to geographic region, then to facility (hospital, health center, etc.) and, finally, to service (inpatient/outpatient, etc.). At this disaggregate level, unit cost is calculated by dividing total recurrent expenditure by total units utilized. If accounts are not sufficiently detailed to allow net public expenditure to be identified by region and facility, then all units of a given service must be weighted by the same unit subsidy estimated. In such circumstances, aggregation across services is the only purpose served by application of unit subsidies. Within a particular service, the distribution of the subsidy and the distribution of raw utilization will differ only in their means. Nevertheless, such aggregation can still be informative, allowing the incidence of the total health sector subsidy to be established and this incidence to be decomposed into that arising from differential use of services and that arising from differential subsidies across services.

Aggregate health accounts data are required to determine total public expenditure on health and its disaggregation to regions and facilities. For accuracy and consistency, the data should come from a unified system of National Health Accounts (NHA). In practice, data limitations mean that this ideal scenario is rarely achieved, although see O'Donnell et al. (2007) for BIA studies based on NHA. Moving from facility-specific to service-specific expenditures can be difficult given the joint use of many health resources across a range of services. The detailed information necessary to distinguish between expenditures on, for example, outpatient and inpatient services might be available only from facility-level cost surveys. Data from such surveys can be used to estimate cost functions from which the unit costs of services can be recovered. Without NHA, disaggregation of public health expenditures down to the service level is likely to prove difficult and require the imposition of various assumptions and approximations. The robustness of results to these approximations should be checked through sensitivity analysis.

Aggregate service utilization figures can either be estimated from survey data or taken from administrative records. The relative accuracy of these two approaches will vary across services and countries. Application of survey utilization rates has the advantage of consistency. Unit cost is calculated by dividing aggregate expenditure by the weighted sum utilization reported in the survey data, where weights are expansion factors indicating how many individuals in the population are represented by each sample observation. Expenditure on each (survey) individual is quantity multiplied by unit cost. Summing these individual expenditures across all observations and applying the population expansion factors, one arrives back at total public expenditure on a service.

User fees

The simplest method of allocating user fees is to divide aggregate user fee revenue reported in official accounts by an estimate of total utilization and to assign the resulting average payment to all users. Equivalently, one can apportion public expenditure net of official user fee revenue in proportion to utilization. If the net public expenditure figures are available at a region-facility-service level, then variation in fee payments across region-facility-service groups is taken into account but not variation across individuals within groups. Individual variation in fees paid can be taken into account if the survey provides reliable data on payments made for public health services. This would be important, for example, if there were fee exemptions for the poor.

Some surveys ask the amount paid for each public health service. In this case, the public subsidy can be calculated as in equations 14.1 and 14.2. Alternatively, if the survey gives only the total amount paid for all public health services, then modify equation 14.2 to

$$(14.2') \qquad\qquad s_i = \sum_k \delta_k q_{ki} c_{kj} - f_i,$$

where f_i is the payment for all public health care and δ_k is a scaling factor that standardizes the recall periods for the utilization variables on the recall period that applies to the total payment variable.

Survey estimates of aggregate user fee revenues may not match the official figures. Apart from sampling and nonsampling error, the discrepancy can be explained by payments that are kept locally and not remitted to the central administration or by unofficial payments that are paid not to the facility but to personnel at the facility. The appropriate treatment of user payments in such cases depends on the objective of the analysis. If it is simply to identify the distribution of net expenditures made by the central government in an accounting fashion, then reported payments in excess of official revenue could be ignored. However, if the aim is to identify the incidence of net benefits from government-supported health services, then one seeks an estimate of the difference between the value of services consumed and the payments made for them by the individual, irrespective of whether all of the payment is remitted to the central government. In the instance that payments, official or unofficial, are made to fill the gap between the cost of the care provided and the available budget, then, in principle, they should be added to both costs and payments and so can be ignored in computation of the subsidy. On the other hand, if the payments are rent extracted by providers, then they reduce the real value of the subsidy to the individual and should be subtracted in calculation of the real subsidy. Most surveys do not distinguish between payments remitted to the center and those kept locally, and it is not possible to discern whether payments are used to raise quality or are rent extraction. The distribution of official user fee revenue remitted to the center could be estimated by scaling all reported payments by the ratio of total official user fee revenue to aggregate payments calculated from survey data. One could test the sensitivity of results to this treatment of payments against subtracting all payments reported in the survey. Waiting and travel time also reduce the net benefit from care received by the individual and should, in principle, be valued and subtracted in computation of the subsidy. Survey data do not, however, usually permit this.

Box 14.2 *Derivation of Unit Subsidies—Vietnam, 1998*

National Health Accounts are not available for Vietnam, and so we estimate unit subsidies from public spending accounts. Total recurrent public expenditure on health was more than 5 trillion Vietnamese dong (D) in 1998 ($1 = D 13,987) (World Bank 2001). That covers all spending on health programs and services provided by public health facilities and financed from the state budget, user charges, social health insurance, and external donors. The public accounts do not disaggregate by facilities within regions. We therefore impose the same unit costs across all users irrespective of their geographic location. Although this is common practice in BIA studies (Castro-Leal et al. 2000), it is regrettable. It means that geographic variations in the quality, as opposed to the quantity, of health care are not taken into account. Such variations can be substantial (Das and Hammer 2005).

At the national level, the public accounts disaggregate central and provincial government recurrent health spending by facility, that is, hospitals, polyclinics, and commune health centers (World Bank 2001). Public spending financed from other sources is not disaggregated by facility. Because health insurance finances hospital care only, total revenue from health insurance is added to the government expenditure on hospitals (World Bank 2001). Officially, user fees are charged for hospital and polyclinic care only. For baseline estimates, we divide total user fee revenue between hospitals and polyclinics in the same proportions as apply for government revenue (World Bank 2001). Finally, total public spending financed from ODA (World Bank 2001) is divided between hospitals, polyclinics, and health centers in the same proportions as apply for central and provincial government expenditures. By that allocation method, we arrive at the facility-specific public expenditures given in the first column of the table below. The total across facilities represents 59 percent of total recurrent public health spending.

Public Health Expenditure, Unit Costs and Subsidies, Vietnam 1998

	Recurrent public exp. D millions	Total utilization '000s	Unit cost D	Total user fees		Mean unit subsidy	
				Official D m.	Reported D m.	Scaled user fees[a] D	Reported user fees[b] D
Hospital care	2,704,424			429,128			
Inpatient		52,779 (days)	49,320		2,464,000	42,988	23,800
Outpatient		35,388 (visits)	2,865		1,154,000	1,990	1,690
Comm. health centers	269,101	43,520 (visits)	6,183		48,762	6,183	5,393
Regional polyclinics	34,062	3,973 (visits)	8,572	7,152	17,039	7,916	6,402
Total allocated	3,007,587			436,280	3,634,960		

Source: Authors' calculations from World Bank, SIDA et al. 2001 and VLSS.
Note: a. Calculated from user fees reported in VLSS scaled to sum to official user fee revenue.
   b. Calculated from actual user fees reported in VLSS (not scaled).

Box 14.2 *(continued)*

As is often the case, the accounts do not distinguish between hospital expenditures on inpatient and outpatient services. Cost function estimates from a survey of 80 percent of public hospitals (Weaver and Deolalikar 2004) give the cost of an inpatient day at more than 17 times that of an outpatient visit. From that estimate of relative cost, plus aggregate public expenditure on hospitals and the total utilization of the respective services, the unit costs of an inpatient day and outpatient visits are derived (see table above, column 3). The unit costs of visits to health centers and to polyclinics are calculated by dividing total public expenditures on these facilities by respective total utilization figures, estimated from the VLSS. The resultant costs seem somewhat high in comparison to the estimated unit cost of a hospital outpatient visit. In a full report, sensitivity of results to these estimates of unit costs would be checked.

There is a tremendous difference between reported payments for public health services and official user fee revenue in Vietnam. The official accounts indicate total user fee revenue of D 436 billion in 1998 (World Bank 2001). This is only one-eighth of the total amount individuals report paying for care in public hospitals, polyclinics, and commune health centers (excluding payments for drugs). In fact, the total amount reported in user payments exceeds total recurrent public expenditure on these services (see table above).

Given the difference between official and reported user payments, we experiment with two methods of calculating the public subsidy. In each case, we apply equations 14.1 and 14.2 above, but use different estimates of individual specific user payments. Under the first method (2nd from final column of the table above), we set user fees in commune health centers to zero (officially they do not exist) and scale reported user fees in hospitals and polyclinics by the ratio of official to reported aggregate user payments for these services. Under the second method (final column), we use the actual user fees reported for all services, not including payments for drugs. Patients are usually responsible for purchasing their own drugs. In both cases, we set negative values of the subsidy to zero.

Each mean unit subsidy given in the table indicates the average, across users, of the subsidy per unit of the respective service. So, for example, when user payments are scaled to sum to official fee revenue, inpatients receive a subsidy, on average, equal to almost D 43,000 per day, or more than 80 percent of the cost. However, the value of this subsidy falls by almost 50 percent if it is calculated on the basis of what patients actually report paying.

Some individuals may report payments in excess of production costs. If one is simply interested in who receives the (positive) subsidies from the health care system, then negative values of the subsidy should be set to zero. However, if one is interested in how the subsidy is financed and, in particular, the extent to which there is cross subsidization, then the distributions of both positive and negative subsidies need to be examined.

Evaluating the distribution of the health subsidy

Once individuals have been categorized by their living standards and the value of the health sector subsidy received by each individual has been calculated, the distribution of the subsidy can be traced in relation to living standards. For example, cumulative shares of the subsidy received by living standard quintiles might be presented (see table in box 14.3). For a more complete picture of the distribution, the health subsidy concentration curve can be graphed as in the figure in Box 14.3.

To evaluate the distribution of the subsidy, the analyst must refer to some target distribution and in doing so impose a distributional objective. One alternative is to compare the distribution of the subsidy with population shares. Do the poorest 20 percent of individuals receive more or less than 20 percent of the subsidy? In the figure in Box 14.3, that amounts to comparing a concentration curve with the 45-degree line. This is appropriate if the goal is to ensure that the subsidy is pro-poor, which requires that the subsidy concentration curve dominate the 45-degree line. If the subsidy were considered part of an individual's final income, then an alternative distributional objective would be for final income to be more evenly distributed than presubsidy income. That is, the subsidy should be inequality-reducing, closing the relative gap in welfare between the rich and the poor. This requires that the subsidy concentration curve dominate the Lorenz curve, which is obviously much less demanding than domination of the 45-degree line. Domination of the Lorenz curve may be referred to as progressivity, or weak progressivity, of the subsidy, as opposed to absolute or strong progressivity in the case that the concentration curve dominates the 45-degree line (Castro-Leal et al. 2000; Sahn and Younger 2000).

The concentration index (see chapter 8) provides a summary measure of absolute progressivity of the subsidy. The Kakwani index, which is defined as twice the area between a concentration curve and the Lorenz curve, can be used as a summary measure of weak progressivity (Kakwani 1977).[1] The index is calculated as $\pi_k = C - G$, where C is the concentration index for the subsidy and G is the Gini coefficient of the living standards measure. The value of π_k ranges from –2 to 1. It is negative (positive) if the concentration curve dominates (is dominated by) the Lorenz curve. In the case in which the concentration lies on top of the Lorenz curve, the Kakwani index is zero.[2]

---

[1] The Kakwani index was originally introduced as a measure of tax progressivity (Kakwani 1977). Its use as a measure of progressivity of health care financing is discussed in chapter 16.

[2] This is a sufficient but not a necessary condition for the Kakwani index to be zero, which could also arise if the concentration and Lorenz curves cross.

Box 14.3 *Distribution of Health Sector Subsidies in Vietnam, 1998*

In the table below, we present cumulative quintile shares of the service-specific subsidies and for the total subsidy across all services. In computing the service-specific quintile shares, we scale all user payments to sum to official user fee revenue (see box 14.2). The subsidy shares are broadly consistent with those for raw service utilization given in the table in box 14.1. Cumulative quintile shares for the total subsidy are given both with and without scaling user payments. Irrespective of the treatment of user payments, the poorest quintile's share of the subsidy is less than 20 percent but greater than its share of total consumption. At higher quintiles, the cumulative subsidy shares deviate from the respective population share only if reported user payments are scaled. However, tests indicate that the subsidy concentration curve is dominated by the 45-degree line under both treatments of user payments and that it always dominates the Lorenz curve. Subsidy concentration curves (with scaled user payments) and the Lorenz curve are graphed in the figure. The concentration curve for the total subsidy follows that of the inpatient subsidy most closely. This reflects the fact that inpatient care receives by far the largest share of public spending in Vietnam (87%—see table below).

Box 14.3 *(continued)*

With one exception (outpatient), the dominance tests and the Kakwani indices services indicate that the subsidies are inequality-reducing or weakly progressive. But only the subsidy to commune health centers is pro-poor or strongly progressive. The subsidy to hospital care and the total subsidy are pro-rich. It may be concluded that public health care subsidies in Vietnam help close the relative gap in welfare between rich and poor but raise the absolute gap.

Distribution of Public Health Care Subsidies in Vietnam, 1998

| Cumulative shares | Equivalent household consumption | Hospital care | | Commune health center | Polyclinic | Other public health services | Total subsidy | |
		Out-patient	Inpatient				Scaled user fees	Reported user fees
Poorest 20%	8.78%	10.21%	10.98%	22.65%*	23.18%*	13.22%	12.29%*	14.81%*
(standard error)	(0.0429)	(1.3456)	(1.3099)	(1.886)	(5.9155)	(2.9644)	(1.1219)	(1.5426)
Poorest 40%	21.38%	24.75%	29.44%*	47.83%*	33.48%	47.09%*	31.87%*	37.70%*
	(0.0880)	(2.1043)	(2.1703)	(2.4084)	(6.3918)	(6.3806)	(1.8559)	(2.4110)
Poorest 60%	37.19%	45.50%*	50.12%*	77.86%*	59.88%*	59.00%*	53.11%*	60.43%*
	(0.1360)	(3.0206)	(2.5461)	(1.9943)	(6.8763)	(6.0599)	(2.1498)	(2.5184)
Poorest 80%	58.17%	67.65%*	73.02%*	90.60%*	78.52%*	79.63%*	74.88%*	81.25%*
	(0.1793)	(3.2196)	(2.5157)	(1.4456)	(6.6011)	(4.5689)	(2.1076)	(2.0504)
Test of dominance								
–against 45° line		–	–	+			–	–
–against Lorenz curve		+	+	+	+	+	+	+
Concentration Index[a] (robust standard error)	0.3229	0.2160	0.1444	–0.1567	0.0298	0.0056	0.1106	0.0115
	(0.0083)	(0.0450)	(0.0378)	(0.0335)	(0.1035)	(0.0777)	(0.0319)	(0.0343)
Kakwani Index (robust standard error)		–0.1069	–0.1785	–0.4797	–0.2932	–0.3174	–0.2124	–0.3115
		(0.0506)	(0.0427)	(0.0376)	(0.1031)	(0.0792)	(0.0365)	(0.0379)
Subsidy shares (scaled user fees)		0.0213	0.8688	0.1010	0.0088		1.0000	

Note: For shares, bold indicates significant difference from population share (5%) and * indicates significant difference from consumption share (5%). For concentration and Kakwani indexes, bold indicates significant difference from zero at 5%. Standard errors for concentration and Kakwani indexes are robust to heteroskedasticity and within cluster (commune) correlation.

Dominance tests: – indicates the 45° line/Lorenz curve dominates the concentration curve
  + indicates concentration curve dominates 45° line/Lorenz curve
  Blank indicates nondominance.

Dominance is rejected if there is at least one significant difference in one direction and no significant difference in the other, with comparisons at 19 quantiles and 5% significance level.

a. Gini index for equivalent household consumption.

(continued)

Box 14.3 (continued)

Concentration Curves for Health Sector Subsidies and Lorenz Curve of Household Consumption, Vietnam 1998

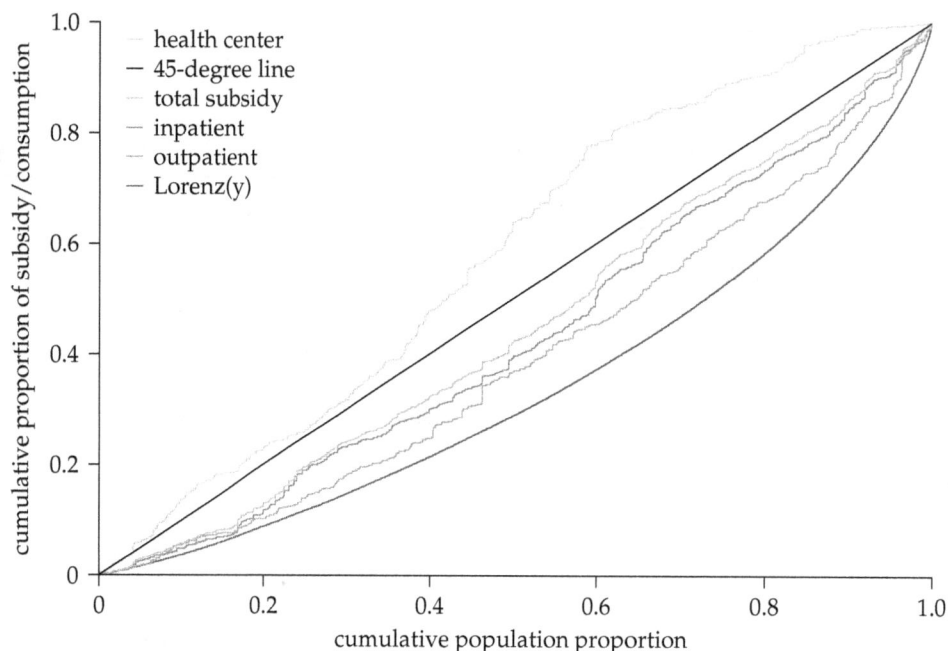

Source: Authors.

Computation

Quintile shares, dominance tests, and concentration indices can be computed as described in chapters 7 and 8. Because a Kakwani index is the difference between a concentration index and a Gini index, both of which can be computed by the convenient regression method (see chapter 8), its value can be computed directly from one convenient regression of the following form:

$$(14.3) \qquad 2\sigma_r^2 \left[\frac{s_i}{\hat{\mu}_s} - \frac{y_i}{\hat{\mu}_y} \right] = \alpha + \beta r_i + u_i,$$

where s_i is the health subsidy to individual i, $\hat{\mu}_s$ is an estimate of its mean, y_i is the living standards measure and $\hat{\mu}_y$ an estimate of its mean, and r_i is the weighted fractional rank in the living standards distribution and σ_R^2 is its variance. The OLS estimate of β is an estimate of the Kakwani index. A standard error for the index can be obtained directly from the convenient regression although in this case, it is not possible to take into account the sampling variability of the estimated means used in the transformation to obtain the left-hand-side variable.

The weighted fractional rank variable (rank) should first be computed as explained in chapter 8. Then, in Stata, the appropriate convenient regression would be estimated as follows:

```
qui sum rank [aw=weight]
sca var_rank=r(Var)
```

```
qui sum subsidy [aw=weight]
sca m_sub=r(mean)
qui sum y [aw=weight]
sca m_y=r(mean)
gen lhs=2*v_rank*(subsidy/m_sub-y/m_y)
regr lhs r [pw=weight], cluster(commune)
```

where y is the (cardinal) living standards measure and, in this case, sample weights and cluster sampling are taken into account.

References

Aaron, H., and M. C. McGuire. 1970. "Public Goods and Income Distribution." *Econometrica* 38: 907–20.

Besley, T., and S. Coate. 1991. "Public Provision of Private Goods and the Redistribution of Income." *American Economic Review* 81(4): 979–84.

Brennan, G. 1976. "The Distributional Implications of Public Goods." *Econometrica* 44: 391–99.

Castro-Leal, F., J. Dayton, L. Demery, and K. Mehra. 2000. "Public Spending on Health Care in Africa: Do the Poor Benefit?" *Bulletin of the World Health Organization* 78(1): 70.

Das, J., and J. Hammer. 2005. "Which Doctor? Combining Vignettes and Item Response to Measure Clinical Competence." *Journal of Development Economics* 78: 348–83.

Kakwani, N. C. 1977. "Measurement of Tax Progressivity: An International Comparison." *Economic Journal* 87(345): 71–80.

Lanjouw, P., and M. Ravallion. 1999. "Benefit Incidence, Public Spending Reforms and the Timing of Program Capture." *World Bank Economic Review* 13(2).

Meerman, J. 1979. *Public Expenditure in Malaysia: Who Benefits and Why?* New York: Oxford University Press.

O'Donnell, O., E. van Doorslaer, R. P. Rannan-Eliya, A. Somanathan, S. R. Adhikari, D. Harbianto, C. G. Garg, P. Hanvoravongchai, M. N. Huq, A. Karan, G. M. Leung, C.-w. Ng, B. R. Pande, K. Tin, L. Trisnantoro, C. Vasavid, Y. Zhang, and Y. Zhao. 2007. "The Incidence of Public Spending on Health Care: Comparative Evidence from Asia." *World Bank Economic Review* 21(1): 93–123.

Sahn, D., and D. Younger. 2000. "Expenditure Incidence in Africa: Microeconomic Evidence." *Fiscal Studies* 21(3): 321–48.

van de Walle, D. 2003. "Behavioral Benefit Incidence Analysis of Public Spending and Social Programs." In *The Impact of Economic Policies on Poverty and Income Distribution: Evaluation Techniques and Tools*, ed. F. Bourguignon and L. A. Pereira da Silva. Washington DC: World Bank and Oxford University Press.

van de Walle, D., and K. Nead, eds. 1995. *Public Spending and the Poor: Theory and Evidence.* Baltimore, MD: Johns Hopkins University Press.

Weaver, M. and A. Deolalikar. 2004. "Economies of Scale and Scope in Vietnamese Hospitals." *Social Science & Medicine* 59(1): 198–208.

World Bank. 2001. *Vietnam Growing Healthy: A Review of Vietnam's Health Sector.* Hanoi: The World Bank.

Younger, S. D. 2003. "Benefits on the Margin: Observations on Marginal Benefit Incidence Analysis." *World Bank Economic Review* 17(1): 89–106.

15

Measuring and Explaining Inequity in Health Service Delivery

Equitable distribution of health care is a principle subscribed to in many countries, often explicitly in legislation or official policy documents (van Doorslaer, Wagstaff, and Rutten 1993). Egalitarian equity goals distinguish between horizontal equity—equal treatment of equals—and vertical equity—appropriate unequal treatment of unequals. In health care, most attention, both in policy and research, has been given to the horizontal equity principle, defined as "equal treatment for equal medical need, irrespective of other characteristics such as income, race, place of residence, etc." (van Doorslaer et al. 2000; Wagstaff and van Doorslaer 2000; Wagstaff, van Doorslaer, and Paci 1991). In this chapter, we discuss measurement and explanation of horizontal inequity in the delivery of health care.

In practice, it is not possible to examine the extent to which the horizontal equity principle is violated without simultaneously specifying a vertical equity norm. Researchers have usually assumed, implicitly or explicitly, that, on average, vertical equity is satisfied. That is, the observed differential utilization of health care resources across individuals in different states of need is appropriate. If that is accepted, then the measurement of horizontal inequity in health care use can proceed in much the same way as the standardization methods covered in chapter 5. For example, one seeks to establish whether there is differential utilization of health care by income after standardizing for differences in the need for health care in relation to income. In empirical analyses, expected utilization, given characteristics such as age, gender, and measures of health status, is used as a proxy for "need." Complications to the regression method of standardization arise because measures of health care utilization typically are nonnegative integer counts (e.g., numbers of visits, hospital days, etc.) with very skewed distributions. As discussed in chapter 11, nonlinear methods of estimation are then appropriate. But the standardization methods presented in chapter 5 do not immediately carry over to nonlinear models. They can be rescued only if relationships can be represented linearly. In this chapter, we therefore concentrate on standardization in nonlinear settings.

Once health care use has been standardized for need, inequity can be measured by the concentration index. Inequity could then be explained by decomposing the concentration index, as explained in chapter 13. In fact, with the decomposition approach, standardization for need and explanation of inequity can be done in one step. We describe this procedure in the final section of the chapter.

Measuring horizontal inequity

There will typically be inequality in the utilization of health care in relation to socioeconomic characteristics, such as income. Typically, in high-income countries poorer individuals consume more health care resources as a result of their lower health status and so greater need for health care. Obviously, such inequality in health care use cannot be interpreted as inequity. In low-income countries, the lack of health insurance and purchasing power among the poor typically mean that their utilization of health care is less than that of the better-off despite their greater need (Gwatkin et al. 2003; O'Donnell et al. forthcoming). In this case, the inequality in health care use does not fully reflect the inequity. To measure inequity, inequality in utilization of health care must be standardized for differences in need. After standardization, any residual inequality in utilization, by income for example, is interpreted as horizontal inequity, which could be pro-rich or pro-poor.

Standardization for differences in need could be done using either the direct or indirect method described in chapter 5. Although with demographic standardization the appropriate standardizing variables are immediately obvious, that is not true for need standardization. Need is a rather elusive concept that has been given a variety of interpretations in relation to the definition of equity in health care delivery (Culyer 1995; Culyer and Wagstaff 1993). By some definitions, measurement of need is not tractable, at least in the context of large-scale household surveys. In practice, researchers have relied on demographics plus health status and morbidity variables (e.g., self-assessed health, presence of chronic conditions, activity limitations, etc.) to proxy need.

Although both direct and indirect methods of standardization could be used, as we argued in chapter 5, when microdata are available there is little to commend the direct approach. Here, we restrict attention to the indirect method, which gives the difference between the actual distribution of use and the distribution that would be expected given the distribution of need. The latter is referred to as the *need-expected* distribution of health care.

When health care use is modelled by linear regression, the standardization procedure is exactly as presented in equations 5.1 through 5.3 of chapter 5. The need variables are included among the x's. The control, or z, variables should include nonneed correlates of health care utilization for which we do *not* want to standardize but which would bias the coefficients on the need variables if omitted from the regression (Gravelle 2003; Schokkaert and van de Voorde 2004). For example, suppose that some groups with poor health (an x variable), for example, people who are disabled or handicapped, receive more generous insurance coverage (a z variable) than the nondisabled. If we were to estimate the standardizing regression excluding a variable capturing the better coverage, then the coefficient on the poor health variable would—to some extent—pick up the effect of more generous cover, over and above the direct effect of greater need. That would overestimate the "appropriate vertical need difference" as embodied in the coefficient of poor health.[1]

Once need-standardized utilization has been estimated, inequity can be tested by determining whether standardized use is unequally distributed by income, for example. Inequity could be measured by estimating the concentration index for need-standardized utilization, which has been referred to as the health inequity

---

[1] The more generous cover to disabled persons may reflect society's concern that these individuals would receive less care than they need in the absence of such a subsidy. We assume here that—holding all other factors such as income and accessibility constant—it is the partial effect of poor health on health care use that, *on average*, reflects the appropriate vertical need difference between those who are in poor health and those who are not.

index (HI_{WV}) (Wagstaff and van Doorslaer 2000). Equivalently, this can be obtained as the difference between the concentration index for actual utilization and that for need-predicted utilization.

This procedure rests on the assumption that once observable need indicators have been controlled for, any residual variation in utilization is attributable to non-need factors. Given that the data available on need indicators typically are limited, that is likely to be a strong assumption. It will result in biased measurement of horizontal inequity in the case that unobservable variation in need is correlated with income. Schokkaert, Dhaene, and Van de Voorde (1998) discuss this issue in the context of the related literature on risk adjustment.

Indirect standardization with nonlinear models

Measures of health care use are typically nonnegative integer counts, for example, number of visits to a doctor or days in a hospital. In a sample, there will typically be a large proportion of observations with no utilization and very few observations, corresponding to individuals falling severely ill, with utilization very much above the mean. Given this, it may be considered appropriate to model the determinants of the use/nonuse probability separately from the number of visits conditional on any use. Although the least squares regression method of indirect standardization could be used with such data, it would not guarantee that the predicted values from the standardizing regression (equation 5.2) lie in the permitted range of (0,1) for binary variables and at or above zero for nonnegative counts (see chapter 11). This can be avoided by using nonlinear estimators.

Let us write a nonlinear model of the relationship between a health care variable, y, which may be binary or a count, and need (x) and control (z) variables in terms of a general functional form G:

$$(15.1) \qquad y_i = G\left(\alpha + \sum_j \beta_j x_{ji} + \sum_k \gamma_k z_{ki}\right) + \varepsilon_i,$$

where G will take particular forms for the probit, logit, Poisson, negative binomial, and so on models. If there were no z variables included in equation 15.1, then predicted values obtained from the model could be interpreted as need-expected utilization. Need-standardized utilization could then be defined as actual use minus need-expected utilization, as in equation 5.3, only in this case the mean of the prediction should be added, rather than the mean of the actual variable, to ensure that the mean of standardized utilization equals that of actual utilization.

However, as argued above, including z variables in the model is probably desired to avoid omitted-variables bias. Doing so in this nonlinear context leads to a problem because the effect of the z variables on need-standardized use can no longer be entirely neutralized by setting them equal to their means or indeed to any other vector of constants. As a result, the variance of the need-standardized use will depend on the values to which the z variables are set in the standardization procedure, and that will affect measures of income-related inequality, such as the concentration index. Accepting this, the analyst could define standardized use as follows:

$$(15.2) \qquad \hat{y}_i^{IS} = y_i - G\left(\hat{\alpha} + \sum_j \hat{\beta}_j x_{ji} + \sum_k \hat{\gamma}_k \bar{z}_k\right) + \frac{1}{n}\sum_{i=1}^{n} G\left(\hat{\alpha} + \sum_j \hat{\beta}_j x_{ji} + \sum_k \hat{\gamma}_k \bar{z}_k\right),$$

where n is the sample size, and we have chosen to set the z variables to their means $(\bar{z}_k)$ in obtaining the predictions. Note that the mean of $\hat{y}_i^{IS}$ is equal to that of y but because G is not linearly additive, its variance would differ if the z variables were set to some other vector of values.

Box 15.1 *Distribution of Preventive Health Care Utilization and Need in Jamaica*

The table below shows the actual need-expected and need-standardized distributions for the probability of reporting at least one preventive visit to a doctor, nurse, or other health practitioner, by quintiles of equivalent expenditure in Jamaica derived from the 1989 Survey of Living Conditions (van Doorslaer and Wagstaff 1998). The indicators used in the prediction of needed health care are demographic variables (7 age-sex dummies), self-assessed health (4 dummies), and functional limitations of activities (7 dummies). It can be seen that the actual distribution observed is clearly pro-rich, and the need-expected distribution is pro-poor. This is a result of the fact that "need," as proxied by demographic and morbidity characteristics, is more concentrated among the lower-income groups. As a result, for the poorest fifth of Jamaicans, the probability of reporting a preventive care contact is 6.5 percent lower than would be expected on average given their need, whereas the richest 20 percent of Jamaicans report a probability of such a contact that is 8.2 percent higher than expected. It is therefore no surprise that the need-standardized distribution shows an even more pro-rich distribution than the actual distribution. After need standardization, the richest quintile's contact probability is twice that of the poorest.

The figures reported in the table for need-predicted use and its difference from actual use are derived from a probit model including control variables, specifically (log) equivalent expenditure and health insurance status, which are set equal to their sample means to obtain the predictions. Need-standardized use is presented both with and without the inclusion of controls in the standardizing model and estimating this by both OLS and probit. In this example, results are not sensitive to either variation. It has been found elsewhere that concentration indices for standardized health care utilization are relatively insensitive to the use of OLS or nonlinear models for standardization (van Doorslaer, Masseria, and OECD Health Equity Research Group 2004; van Doorslaer et al. 2000; Wagstaff and van Doorslaer 2000). That is reassuring given the complications introduced by nonlinear models noted above. Insensitivity to the inclusion of control variables in the standardizing regression may be more specific to this example. Others have found more substantial differences (Gravelle 2003).

Distributions of Actual Need-Predicted and Need-Standardized Preventive Visits to Doctor, Nurse, or Other Health Practitioner, Jamaica 1989

	Probability of using preventive health care in previous 6 months						
	Probit with controls			Need-standardized			
				With controls		Without controls	
Quintile	Actual	Need-predicted	Difference = predicted − actual	Probit	OLS	Probit	OLS
Poorest 20%	0.1717	0.2363	−0.0646	0.1450	0.1457	0.1483	0.1481
2nd poorest 20%	0.2003	0.2158	−0.0155	0.1942	0.1943	0.1952	0.1950
Middle	0.2052	0.2119	−0.0067	0.2029	0.2030	0.2029	0.2029
2nd richest 20%	0.2157	0.1954	0.0203	0.2300	0.2297	0.2282	0.2285
Richest 20%	0.2706	0.1888	0.0817	0.2914	0.2908	0.2889	0.2891
Mean	0.2127	0.2097	0.0030	0.2127	0.2127	0.2127	0.2127
Concentration index/HI_{WV}	0.0928	−0.0452		0.1374	0.1362	0.1318	0.1322
Standard error	0.0122	0.0039		0.0117	0.0117	0.0117	0.0117
t-ratio	7.6249	−11.4721		11.7162	11.6182	11.2663	11.2968

Source: Authors.

Computation

Stata computation for standardization by linear regression is provided in chapter 5. The general procedure is the same in the case of nonlinear models, with the replacement of the OLS command `regr` with the chosen estimator. So, in the case of a probit model, the need-predicted (`yhat`) and need-standardized (`yst`) probability of health care utilization would be generated as follows:

```
qui probit y $X $Z [pw=weight]
foreach z of global Z {
        gen copy_`z'=`z'
        qui sum `z' [aw=weight]
        replace `z' = r(mean)
}
predict yhat
foreach z of global Z {
        replace `z' = copy_`z'
        drop copy_`z'
}
sum m_yhat [aw=weight]
gen yst = y-yhat + r(mean)
```

where X and Z are globals containing lists of need and control variables, respectively. Note that the mean of predicted use and not the mean of actual use is added in generating standardized use. Obviously if control variables were not included, the predictions would be obtained immediately after the model is estimated and neither loop is required.

Quintile means can be estimated using `tabstat` and concentration indices computed as explained in chapter 8.

Explaining horizontal inequity

In chapter 13, we noted that if a health variable is specified as a linear function of determinants, then its concentration index can be decomposed into the contribution of each determinant, computed as the product of the health variable's elasticity with respect to the determinant and the latter's concentration index. This makes it possible to explain socioeconomic-related inequality in health care utilization. In fact, the decomposition method allows horizontal inequity in utilization to be both measured and explained in a very convenient way. The concentration index for need-standardized utilization is exactly equal to that which is obtained by subtracting the contributions of all need variables from the unstandardized concentration index (van Doorslaer, Koolman, and Jones 2004). Besides convenience, the advantage of this approach is that it allows the analyst to duck the potentially contentious division of determinants into need (x) and control (z) variables and so the determination of "justified" and "unjustified," or inequitable, inequality in health care utilization. The full decomposition results can be presented, and the user can choose which factors to treat as x variables and which to treat as z variables.

The decomposition result holds for a linear model of health care. If a nonlinear model is used, then the decomposition is possible only if some linear approximation to the nonlinear model is made. One possibility is to use estimates of the partial effects evaluated at the means (van Doorslaer, Koolman, and Jones 2004). That is, a linear approximation to equation 15.1 is given by

(15.3) $$y_i = \alpha^m + \sum_j \beta_j^m x_{ji} + \sum_k \gamma_k^m z_{ki} + u_i,$$

where the β_j^m and γ_k^m are the partial effects, dy/dx_j and dy/dz_k, of each variable treated as fixed parameters and evaluated at sample means; and u_i is the implied error term, which includes approximation errors. Because equation 15.3 is linearly additive, the decomposition result (Wagstaff, van Doorslaer, and Watanabe 2003) can be applied, such that the concentration index for y can be written as

(15.4) $$C = \sum_j (\beta_j^m \bar{x}_j / \mu) C_j + \sum_k (\gamma_k^m \bar{z}_k / \mu) C_k + GC_u / \mu.$$

Because the partial effects are evaluated at particular values of the variables, for example, the means, this decomposition is not unique. This is the inevitable price to be paid for the linear approximation. Also, unlike the truly linear case, the index of horizontal inequity, HI_{WV}, obtained by subtracting the need contributions in equation 15.4 from the unstandardized concentration index will not equal the concentration index for need-standardized utilization calculated from the estimates of the nonlinear model parameters, as described in the previous section.

Note that equation 15.3 could itself be used to estimate need-standardized utilization and, unlike equation 15.2, its distribution would not depend on the values to which the control variables were set. Need-predicted utilization could be defined as

(15.5) $$\hat{y}_i^X = \hat{\alpha}^m + \sum_j \hat{\beta}_j^m x_{ji} + \sum_k \hat{\gamma}_k^m \bar{z}_k.$$

Then indirectly standardized use would be given by the following:

(15.6) $$\tilde{y}_i^{IS} = y_i - \hat{y}_i^X + \bar{\hat{y}},$$

where $\bar{\hat{y}}$ is the mean of the predictions from equation 15.3 with all variables at actual values. Because equation 15.3 is linearly additive, the z variables cancel in the final two terms of equation 15.6, and the variance of $\tilde{y}_i^{IS}$, unlike that of $\hat{y}_i^{IS}$, does not depend on the values to which those variables are set in the need-prediction equation, 15.5. However, $\tilde{y}_i^{IS}$ will depend on the values of both the x and z variables at which the partial effects are evaluated. There is no escaping the nonuniqueness of the standardization in the context of a nonlinear model including control variables.

Computation

Stata code for the concentration index decomposition based on linear regression is provided in chapter 13. For nonlinear estimators, the partial effects must be calculated from the parameter estimates and then the contributions calculated using these partial effects, as in equation 15.4. For the probit model, Stata has a programmed routine called dprobit that provides partial effects directly (see chapter 11):

```
dprobit y $X $Z [pw=weight]
matrix dfdx=e(dfdx)
```

The matrix command saves the partial effects into a matrix named dfdx. By default, partial effects are calculated at the sample means. They can be computed at another vector of values using the at(*matname*) option (see chapter 11). For other

Box 15.2 *Decomposition of Inequality in Utilization of Preventive Care in Jamaica, 1989*

We decompose the concentration index for any use of preventive health care in Jamaica. The probability of making any use of preventive care is estimated both by least squares, in which the decomposition is exactly as presented in chapter 13, and by probit, in which case we make a linear approximation to the model using the partial effects evaluated at sample means, as in equation 15.3, and then use the decomposition given by equation 15.4. Need and nonneed variables are as described in box 15.1, although, as pointed out above, the decomposition approach allows the user to choose which factors to consider as need proxies. We do not present the full decomposition results but provide, in the table below, the absolute and percentage contributions to the unstandardized concentration index for groups of "need" factors (age-sex dummies, self-assessed health dummies, and functional limitation dummies) and for the two "nonneed" factors. Results are not particularly sensitive to the estimation method. The residual difference between the unstandardized concentration index and the sum of the contributions of all need and nonneed factors is larger for the partial effects probit approach, largely because this gives a slightly larger estimate of the contribution of household expenditure.

The contribution of all need factors is negative, indicating that if utilization were determined by need alone, it would be pro-poor. The aggregate contribution of all need factors is about 47 percent of the unstandardized index. Self-assessed health and functional limitations each contribute roughly twice as much as the age-sex groups. Although the distribution of need pushes utilization in a pro-poor direction, this is more than offset by the direct effect of household expenditure and of insurance coverage. If need were distributed equally, the direct effect of household expenditure on utilization would produce a concentration index 29 to 34 percent greater than that observed. There is also an indirect effect of household expenditure on utilization through health insurance coverage that raises the concentration index by 24 percent of its observed value.

The horizontal inequity index is positive, indicating that for given need, the better-off make greater use of preventive care in Jamaica. The index is not particularly sensitive to the estimation method.

Decomposition of Concentration Index for Access to Preventive Health Care in Jamaica, 1989

| | Contributions to concentration index for any preventive care | | | |
| | OLS | | Probit partial effects | |
	Absolute	Percentage	Absolute	Percentage
Need factors				
Age-sex groups	−0.0083	−8.9	−0.0110	−11.9
Self-assessed health	−0.0169	−18.2	−0.0163	−17.5
Functional limitations	−0.0182	−19.6	−0.0170	−18.3
Subtotal	−0.0434	−46.7	−0.0443	−47.7
Nonneed factors				
Log household expenditure	0.1196	128.8	0.1249	134.5
Health insurance cover	0.0218	23.5	0.0221	23.8
Subtotal	0.1414	152.3	0.1470	158.3
Residual	−0.0052	−5.6	−0.0099	−10.6
Total	0.0928		0.0928	
Horizontal inequity index	0.1362		0.1371	

Source: Authors.

nonlinear models, the partial effects can be calculated using the `mfx` command after running the model (see chapter 11).

The contributions of need factors can then be computed with the following loop:

```
sca need=0
foreach x of global X {
    qui {
        mat b_`x' = dfdx[1,"`x'"]
        sca b_`x' = b_`x'[1,1]
        corr r `x' [aw=weight], c
        sca cov_`x' = r(cov_12)
        sum `x' [aw=weight]
        sca m_`x' = r(mean)
        sca elas_`x' = (b_`x'*m_`x')/m_y
        sca CI_`x' = 2*cov_`x'/m_`x'
        sca con_`x' = elas_`x'*CI_`x'
        sca prcnt_`x' = con_`x'/CI
        sca need=need+con_`x'
    }
    di "`x' elasticity:", elas_`x'
    di "`x' concentration index:", CI_`x'
    di "`x' contribution:", con_`x'
    di "`x' percentage contribution:", prcnt_`x'
}
```

where `CI` is a scalar equal to the unstandardized concentration index computed as in chapter 8. The scalar need will contain the sum of the contributions of all the need factors. The contributions of the nonneed factors can be computed by running the same loop over the global Z containing the nonneed factors and renaming the scalar need to nonneed. The total contributions of all need factors and of nonneed factors and the horizontal inequity index (HI_{WV}) can then be displayed as follows:

```
di "Inequality due to need factors:", need
di "Inequality due to non-need factors:", nonneed
sca HI = CI - need
di "Horizontal Inequity Index:", HI
```

Further reading

Detailed discussion of the issues touched on in this chapter can be found in Wagstaff and van Doorslaer (2000); Gravelle (2003); Schokkaert and van de Voorde (2004); and van Doorslaer, Koolman, and Jones (2004). Standard errors for the contributions to the concentration index decomposition can be obtained by bootstrapping (van Doorslaer, Koolman, and Jones 2004). Gravelle, Morris, and Sutton (2006) make a valuable contribution in placing the empirical study of equity in health care in the context of a social welfare maximization model. That helps to make explicit the links between normative and positive analysis of the distribution of health care, a point that has also been emphasized by Schokkaert and van de Voorde (2004). It also helps clarify the conditions required for the identification of horizontal and vertical equity and to distinguish between the two.

References

Culyer, A. J. 1995. "Need: The Idea Won't Do—But We Still Need It" [editorial]. *Soc Sci Med* 40(6): 727–30.

Culyer, A. J., and A. Wagstaff. 1993. "Equity and Equality in Health and Health Care." *Journal of Health Economics* 12(4): 431–57.

Gravelle, H. 2003. "Measuring Income Related Inequality in Health: Standardisation and the Partial Concentration Index." *Health Economics* 12(10): 803–19.

Gravelle, H., S. Morris, and M. Sutton. 2006. "Economic Studies of Equity in the Consumption of Health Care." In *The Elgar Companion to Health Economics,* ed. A. M. Jones, 193–204. Cheltenham, England: Edward Elgar.

Gwatkin, D. R., S. Rustein, K. Johnson, R. Pande, and A. Wagstaff. 2003. Initial Country-Level Information about Socio-Economic Differentials in Health, Nutrition and Population, Volumes I and II. Washington, DC: World Bank, Health, Population and Nutrition.

O'Donnell, O., E. van Doorslaer, R. P. Rannan-Eliya, A. Somanathan, S. R. Adhikari, D. Harbianto, C. G. Garg, P. Hanvoravongchai, M. N. Huq, A. Karan, G. M. Leung, C-W Ng, B. R. Pande, K. Tin, L. Trisnantoro, C. Vasavid, Y. Zhang, and Y. Zhao. 2007. "The Incidence of Public Spending on Health Care: Comparative Evidence from Asia." *World Bank Economic Review* 21(1): 93–123.

Schokkaert, E., G. Dhaene, and C. Van de Voorde. 1998. "Risk Adjustment and the Trade-off between Efficiency and Risk Selection: An Application of the Theory of Fair Compensation." *Health Economics* 7(5): 465–80.

Schokkaert, E., and C. van de Voorde. 2004. "Risk Selection and the Specification of the Conventional Risk Adjustment Formula." *Journal of Health Economics* 23(6): 1237–59.

van Doorslaer, E., X. Koolman, and A. M. Jones. 2004. "Explaining Income-Related Inequalities in Doctor Utilization in Europe." *Health Economics* 13(7): 629–47.

van Doorslaer, E., C. Masseria, and OECD Health Equity Research Group. 2004. "Income-Related Inequality in the Use of Medical Care in 21 OECD Countries." In *Towards High-Performing Health Systems: Policy Studies,* ed. OECD Health Project, 109–66. Paris: OECD.

van Doorslaer, E., and A. Wagstaff. 1998. "Inequity in the Delivery of Health Care: Methods and Results for Jamaica." Paper prepared for the HDN Network, LAC Region, Equi-LAC—WP#3. World Bank, Washington, DC.

van Doorslaer, E., A. Wagstaff, and F. Rutten. 1993. *Equity in the Finance and Delivery of Health Care: An International Perspective.* Oxford, England: Oxford University Press.

van Doorslaer, E., A. Wagstaff, H. van der Burg, T. Christiansen, D. De Graeve, U.-G. Gerdtham, M. Gerfin, J. Geurts, L. Gross, U. Hakkinen, and J. John. 2000. "Equity in the Delivery of Health Care in Europe and the U.S." *Journal of Health Economics* 19(5): 553–84.

Wagstaff, A., and E. van Doorslaer. 2000. "Measuring and Testing for Inequity in the Delivery of Health Care." *Journal of Human Resources* 35(4): 716–33.

Wagstaff, A., E. van Doorslaer, and P. Paci. 1991. "On the Measurement of Horizontal Inequity in the Delivery of Health Care." *Journal of Health Economics* 10(2): 169–205.

Wagstaff, A., E. van Doorslaer, and N. Watanabe. 2003. "On Decomposing the Causes of Health Sector Inequalities, with an Application to Malnutrition Inequalities in Vietnam." *Journal of Econometrics* 112(1): 219–27.

16

Who Pays for Health Care?
Progressivity of Health Finance

Who pays for health care? To what extent are payments toward health care related to ability to pay? Is the relationship proportional? Or is it progressive—do health care payments account for an increasing proportion of ability to pay (ATP) as the latter rises? Or, is there a regressive relationship, in the sense that payments comprise a decreasing share of ATP? The preferred relationship between health care payments and ATP will vary across individuals with their conceptions of fairness. But identification of the nature of the empirical relationship and quantification of the degree of any progressivity or regressivity is of interest, not only from a wide range of equity perspectives, but also for macroeconomic and political analyses of the health care system.

This chapter provides practical advice on methods for assessing and measuring progressivity in health care finance. Throughout, we measure progressivity through departures from proportionality in the relationship between payments toward the provision of health care and ATP. There are other approaches to the measurement of progressivity (Lambert 1993). The relationship between progressivity and the redistributive impact of health care payments is considered in the next chapter.

Definition and measurement of variables

There are two distinct stages to an analysis of progressivity. First, establish the progressivity of each source of finance. Second, establish the overall progressivity of the system by weighting the progressivity of the separate sources. Two types of data are required: survey data to establish the distribution of payments across households and aggregate data to determine the macroweights to be assigned to each finance source. The most suitable source of survey data is a household income and expenditure survey, which should contain good data on the two central variables: payments toward health care and ability to pay.

Ability to pay

In a developing country context, given the lack of organized labor markets and the high variability of incomes over time, household consumption, or even expenditure, is generally considered to be a better measure of welfare and ATP, than is income (see chapter 6). In principle, ATP should indicate welfare before payments for health care, and so measurement of ATP by consumption requires an assumption, most probably a strong one, that the means of financing health care does not affect saving decisions. Household consumption net of expenditures assumed nondiscretionary, such as those on food, is often used as a measure of welfare (World Health Organization 2000). For the purpose of assessing progressivity, such a measure of ATP can be problematic, depending on the objective, if the nondiscretionary expenditures are, in fact, sensitive to the system of health finance. For example, the relative tax rate imposed on food would be expected to differentially influence household decisions with respect to food spending. Then the distribution of household consumption net of food expenditure is itself a product of the health finance system and does not provide a benchmark against which to assess the distributional impact of that system. But if the objective is simply to assess the degree of proportionality between health payments and some measure of living standards, then household expenditures gross or net of those on food can be used, as preferred.

If one wishes to make an inference about the distributional impact of health finance (World Health Organization 2000), then the measure of ATP should be gross of all health care, tax, and social insurance payments. Out-of-pocket payments for health care should already be included in measures of household consumption/expenditure, but it will be necessary to add direct tax payments, social insurance contributions that contribute to health financing and, possibly, private health insurance premiums. If household income is used to proxy ATP, then it must be gross of tax and social insurance contributions, and one examines the impact of health financing on this benchmark distribution of income.

Adjustment should be made for the size and age structure of the household through application of an equivalence scale (see chapter 6).

Health care payments

Evaluation of progressivity in health care finance requires examination of all sources of health sector funding and not simply those payments that are made exclusively for health care. So, in addition to out-of-pocket (OOP) payments, health insurance contributions, and earmarked health taxes, the distributional burden of all direct and indirect taxes is relevant in cases in which, as is commonly true, some health care is financed from general government revenues. Social insurance contributions should also be considered. One source of revenue, foreign aid, is not relevant because the purpose is to evaluate the distributional impact on the domestic population. Assuming tax parameters have been set for foreign loan repayment, the distributional burden on the current generation of foreign debt financing will be captured through evaluation of the tax distribution.

In summary, there are five main sources of health care finance to be considered: direct taxes, indirect taxes, social insurance, private insurance, and OOP payments.

Progressivity analyses usually seek to determine the distribution of the real economic burden of health finance and not simply the distribution of nominal payments. So, the incidence of payments—who incurs their real cost—must be established, or assumed (Atkinson and Stiglitz 1980). For example, the result of employer contributions to health insurance is most likely lower wages received by employees. The extent to which this is true will depend on labor market conditions, in particular, the elasticities of labor demand and supply. Given that incidence depends on market conditions, it cannot be determined through application of universal rules. However, a fairly conventional set of assumptions follows (Wagstaff et al. 1999):

Payment toward health care	*Incidence*
Personal income and property taxes	legal taxpayer
Corporate taxes	shareholder (or labor)
Sales and excise taxes	consumer
Employer social and private insurance contributions	employee
Employee social insurance contributions	employee
Individual private insurance premiums	consumer

Survey data are unlikely to provide complete information on household tax and insurance payments. For example, income tax payments or social insurance contributions may not be explicitly identified, and payments through sales taxes almost certainly will not be reported. Various approximation strategies are necessary. For example, tax and social insurance schedules can be applied to gross incomes/earnings. The distribution of the sales tax burden can be estimated by applying product-specific tax rates to disaggregated data on the pattern of household expenditure.

Estimates of OOP payments from survey data are potentially subject to both recall bias and small sample bias owing to the infrequency with which some health care payments are made. Survey estimates of aggregate payments tend to show substantial discrepancies from production-side estimates, in cases in which the latter are available. Whether estimates of the distribution, as opposed to the level, of OOP payments are biased depends on whether reporting of OOP payments is related systematically to ATP. Under the possibly strong assumption of no systematic misreporting, survey data can be used to retrieve the distribution of payments, and mismeasurement of the aggregate level can be dealt with through application of a macroweight that gives the best indication of the relative contribution of OOP to total revenues.

Assessing progressivity

The most direct means of assessing progressivity of health payments is to examine their share of ATP as the latter varies. In figure 16.1, for Egypt we show OOP payments for health care as a percentage of total household expenditure by quintile groups of equivalent household expenditure. On average, OOP payments claim about 2 percent of household expenditures, and there is a tendency for this share to rise with total expenditure, indicating some progressivity.

A less direct means of assessing progressivity, defined in relation to departure from proportionality, is to compare shares of health payments contributed by proportions of the population ranked by ATP with their share of ATP. That is, to compare the concentration curve for health payments, $L_H(p)$, with the Lorenz curve for ATP, $L(p)$ (see chapter 7). If payments toward health care always account for the same proportion of ATP, then the share of health payments contributed by any group must correspond to its share of ATP. The concentration curve lies on top of the Lorenz curve. Under a progressive system, the share of health payments contrib-

Figure 16.1 *Out-of-Pocket Payments as a Percentage of Total Household Expenditure—Average by Expenditure Quintile, Egypt, 1997*

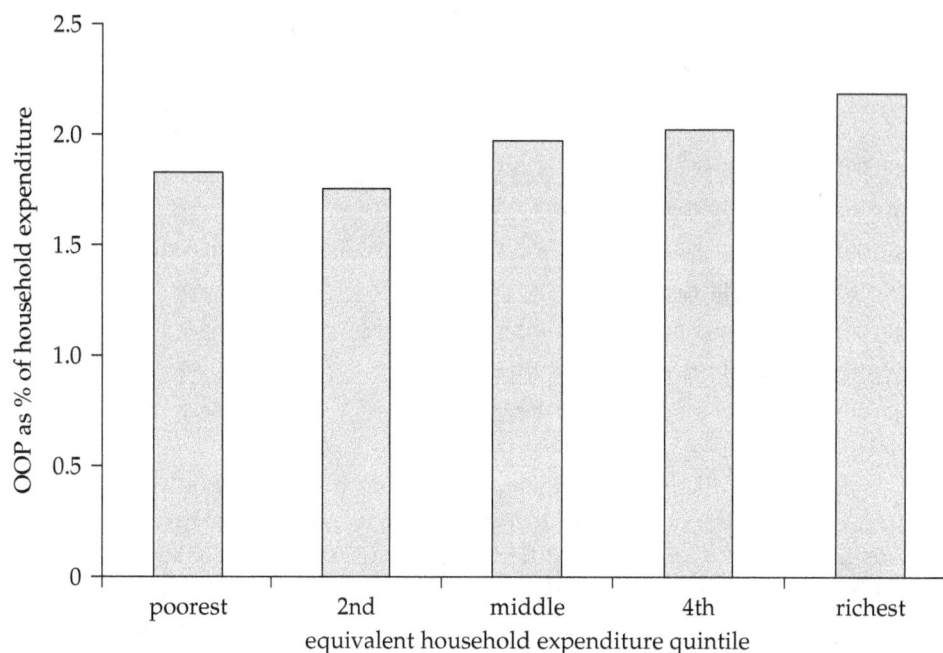

Source: Authors.

Box 16.1 *Progressivity of Health Care Finance in Egypt, 1997*

Health care in Egypt is financed from a number of sources. As is common for developing countries, OOP payments contribute the greatest share of revenue, 52 percent in this case. The next biggest contribution—one-third—is from general government revenues. Social and private health insurance contribute 7 percent and 5.5 percent, respectively, and an earmarked health tax on cigarette sales makes up the remaining 3 percent of revenues going toward the provision of health care.

We assess the progressivity of this system of health finance using data from the 1997 Egypt Integrated Household Survey. In instances in which it is feasible, the incidence assumptions stated above are applied. Payment variables recorded in the survey are as follows: (i) direct personal taxes (income, land, housing, and property taxes), (ii) OOP medical expenses, and (iii) private health insurance premiums. Payment variables estimated from other survey information were (i) sales and cigarette taxes approximated by applying rates to the corresponding expenditures and (ii) social health insurance contributions estimated by applying contribution rates to earnings/incomes of covered workers/pensioners. ATP is approximated by equivalent household expenditure; calculated as total household expenditure, plus direct tax and social insurance contributions, divided by the square root of household size.

In the figures we present the concentration curves for each source of finance, as well as the Lorenz curve for household expenditure. In the first figure (a) the concentration curves for direct and indirect taxes appear to lie outside the Lorenz curve, suggesting that these are progressive sources of finance. The formal tests reported in the table confirm that the Lorenz curve dominates both of these concentration curves. The table also reveals that the cumulative shares of direct and indirect taxes paid at each of the first four quintiles are always significantly less the respective shares of ATP. Again, confirming progressivity. The curve for the earmarked cigarette tax appears to lie inside the Lorenz curve at lower ATP but outside it at higher ATP. The test does not reject the null of nondominance, and therefore proportionality, in this case. Apparently, the difference between the two curves never reaches statistical significance at any point.

Box 16.1 *(continued)*

Concentration Curves for Health Payments and Lorenz Curve for Household Expenditure, Egypt 1997

a. Direct, Indirect, and Cigarette Taxes

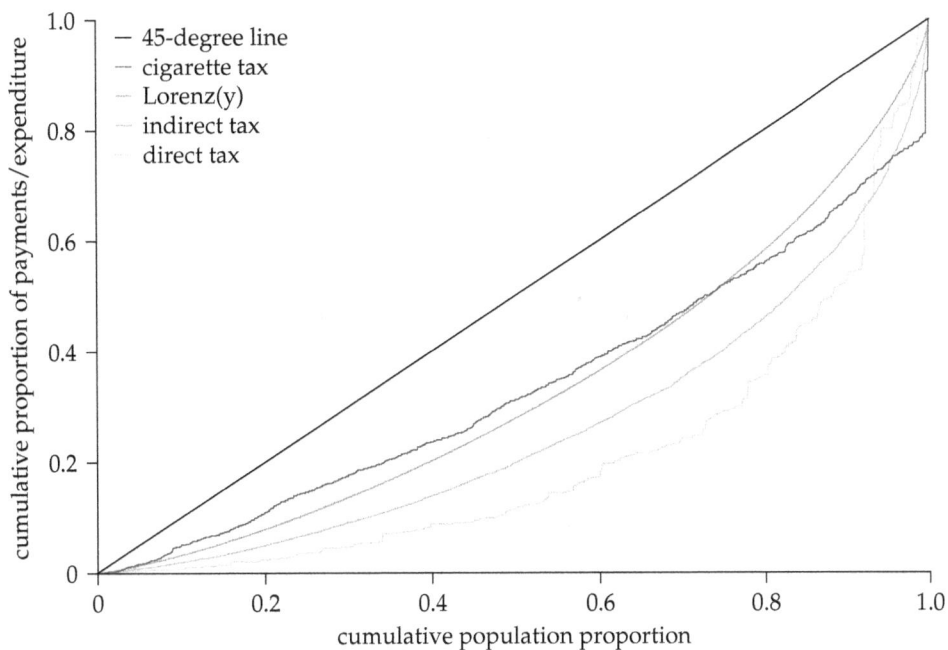

b. Social Insurance Contributions, Private Insurance Premiums, and Out-of-Pocket Payments

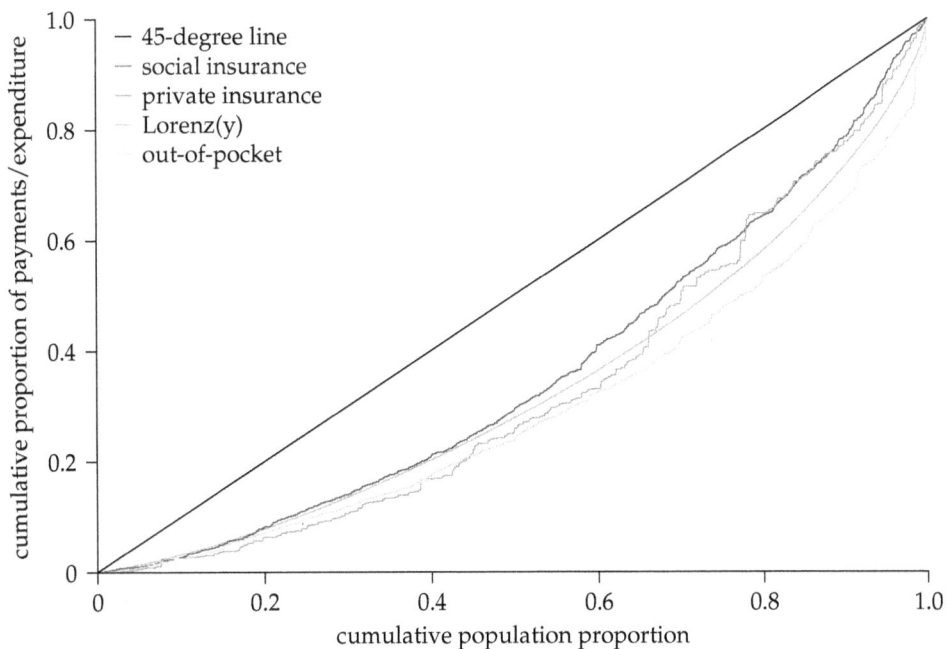

(continued)

In the second figure (b), we present the concentration curves for social insurance contributions, private insurance premiums, and OOP payments. The latter concentration curve appears to lie outside the Lorenz curve, and the test reported in the table confirms that there is dominance. However, unlike for direct and indirect taxes, the cumulative share of OOP payments is not significantly different from the share of ATP at any of the quintiles.[1] Although the concentration curve for private insurance premiums appears to lie below the Lorenz curve at lower ATP, the opposite is true at higher ATP. In fact, the test does not reject nondominance (/proportionality). The concentration curve for social insurance contributions is almost exactly on top of the Lorenz curve (indicating proportionality) up to the middle of the ATP distribution but lies inside the Lorenz curve for the top half of the distribution. This pattern in the top of the distribution leads to the test finding dominance of the concentration curve over the Lorenz curve and so regressivity. The quintile shares confirm that the significant differences are at the higher quintiles.

In summary, there is evidence that direct and indirect taxes plus OOP payments are progressive means of financing health care in Egypt. There is no evidence that the earmarked cigarette tax and private insurance premiums depart significantly from proportionality. Social insurance premiums are regressive but only at the top of the distribution.

---

[1] Despite this, the test finds dominance because we use the multiple comparison approach decision rule, which requires only one significant difference from, in this case, 19 quantile comparison points (see chapter 7).

Distributional Incidence of Sources of Health Finance in Egypt, 1997

Equivalent household expenditure quintile	Equivalent household expenditure	Nonearmarked taxes		Earmarked taxes		Private insurance premiums	OOP payments
		Direct personal taxes	Indirect taxes	Cigarette tax	Social insurance contrbns.		
Poorest 20%	**7.85%**	**2.35%***	**4.96%***	**10.90%***	8.17%	**6.36%**	7.11%
(standard error)	(0.1481)	(0.7609)	(0.2276)	(1.5543)	(0.6241)	(1.4012)	(0.8350)
Poorest 40%	**20.23%**	**8.70%***	**13.86%***	23.54%	21.13%	**16.78%**	17.56%
	(0.3051)	(1.9313)	(0.5304)	(3.1339)	(1.0234)	(2.4107)	(1.6167)
Poorest 60%	**36.46%**	**17.12%***	**27.00%***	38.92%	**40.91%***	33.18%	32.45%
	(0.4761)	(3.0182)	(0.9359)	(5.0465)	(1.5111)	(3.2497)	(2.7124)
Poorest 80%	**58.24%**	**35.60%***	**46.15%***	56.14%	**64.36%***	64.83%	53.44%
	(0.6415)	(5.4012)	(1.4279)	(7.1683)	(1.5481)	(3.6676)	(4.1572)
Test of dominance							
– Against 45° line	–	–	–	–	–	–	–
– Against Lorenz curve		–	–		+		–
Concentration index[a]	0.3345	0.5846	0.4780	0.3283	0.2812	0.3334	0.3988
(robust standard error)	(0.0098)	(0.0395)	(0.0279)	(0.0977)	(0.0202)	(0.0448)	(0.0528)
(*p*-value)	(0.000)	(0.000)	(0.000)	(0.001)	(0.000)	(0.000)	(0.000)
Kakwani index		0.2501	0.1435	−0.0061	−0.0532	−0.0011	0.0644
(robust standard error)		(0.1311)	(0.0460)	(0.1407)	(0.0270)	(0.0748)	(0.0848)
(*p*-value)		(0.059)	(0.002)	(0.965)	(0.051)	(0.988)	(0.449)

Note: For shares: **bold** indicates significant difference from population share (5%)
* indicates significant difference from expenditure share (5%).
Standard errors for concentration and Kakwani indexes are robust to heteroskedasticity and within cluster correlation.
Dominance tests: – indicates the 45-degree line/Lorenz curve dominates the concentration curve
+ indicates concentration curve dominates 45-degree line/Lorenz curve
Blank indicates nondominance.
Dominance is rejected if there is at least one significant difference in one direction and no significant difference in the other, with comparisons at 19 quantiles and 5% significance level.
a. Gini index for equivalent household expenditure.
Source: Authors.

uted by the poor will be less than their share of ATP. The Lorenz curve dominates (lies above) the concentration curve. The opposite is true for a regressive system.

Measuring progressivity

Lorenz dominance analysis is the most general way of detecting departures from proportionality and identifying their location in the ATP distribution. But it does not provide a measure of the magnitude of progressivity, which may be useful when making comparisons across time or countries. Summary indices of progressivity meet this deficiency but require the imposition of value judgments about the weight given to departures from proportionality at different points in the distribution (Lambert 1989). The Kakwani index (Kakwani 1977) is the most widely used summary measure of progressivity in both the tax and the health finance literatures (O'Donnell et al. forthcoming; Wagstaff et al. 1992; Wagstaff et al. 1999).

We gave the definition of the Kakwani index in chapter 14. It is twice the area between a payment concentration curve and the Lorenz curve and is calculated as $\pi_K = C - G$, where C is the concentration index for health payments and G is the Gini coefficient of the ATP variable. The value of π_K ranges from –2 to 1. A negative number indicates regressivity; $L_H(p)$ lies inside $L(p)$. A positive number indicates progressivity; $L_H(p)$ lies outside $L(p)$. In the case of proportionality, the concentration lies on top of the Lorenz curve and the index is zero. But note that the index could also be zero if the curves were to cross and positive and negative differences between them cancel. Given this, it is important to use the Kakwani index, or any summary measure of progressivity, as a supplement to, and not a replacement of, the more general graphical analysis.

In a generalized Kakwani index, the judgment about the weight given to departures from proportionality along the ATP distribution is made explicit through the choice of a parameter (Lambert 1989). An alternative to the simple Kakwani is the Suits index, which gives greater weight to departures from proportionality that occur among households higher up the ATP distribution (Suits 1977).

Progressivity of overall health financing

The progressivity of health financing in total can be measured by a weighted average of the Kakwani indices for the sources of finance, where weights are equal to the proportion of total payments accounted for by each source. Thus, overall progressivity depends both on the progressivity of the different sources of finance and on the proportion of revenue collected from each of these sources.

Ideally, the macroweights should come from National Health Accounts (NHA). It is unlikely, however, that all sources of finance that are identified at the aggregate level can be allocated down to the household level from the survey data. Assumptions must be made about the distribution of sources of finance that cannot be estimated. Their distributional burden may be assumed to resemble that of some other payment source. For example, corporate taxes may be assumed to be distributed as income taxes. In this case, we say that the missing payment distribution has been allocated. Alternatively, we may simply assume that the missing payment is distributed as the weighted average of all the revenues that have been identified. We refer to this as ventilation. Best practice is to make such assumptions explicit and to conduct extensive sensitivity analysis.

Box 16.2 *Measurement of Progressivity of Health Financing in Egypt*

Concentration and Kakwani indices by source of health financing in Egypt are given in the bottom part of the table in box 16.1. All concentration indices are significantly positive confirming, as was clear from the concentration curves and dominance tests, that the better-off contribute absolutely more to the financing of health care than do the poor. The index is largest for direct payments and smallest for social insurance contributions, suggesting that direct taxes are most progressive and social insurance contributions the least so. The Kakwani indices for both direct and indirect tax are statistically significantly positive, marginally so in the case of direct taxes (10 percent), indicating progressivity. For the cigarette tax, private insurance, and OOP payments, the Kakwani indices are not significantly different from zero. In the latter case, this seems inconsistent with the result of the dominance test, which indicates that the OOP concentration curve is dominated by the Lorenz curve. The explanation would appear to be that the curves differ in the top half of the ATP distribution but are near coincident in the bottom half, where the Kakwani index places more weight. The Kakwani index for social insurance contributions is significantly negative at just above the 5 percent significance level. Again, the magnitude of the index is reduced by the near proportionality in the bottom half of the ATP distribution.

We can formally test for the relative progressivity of different sources of finance using dominance methods. The results, which are reported in the table, indicate that the concentration curve for direct taxes is dominated by all the others, and so we can conclude that direct taxes are the most progressive source of finance. Next come indirect taxes, the concentration curve for which is dominated by all the others but for OOP payments. There are no significant differences between the concentration curves for social insurance, private insurance, cigarette taxes, and OOP payments. These sources cannot be ranked in relation to progressivity.

Tests of Dominance between Concentration Curves for Different Sources of Health Finance, Egypt 1997

	Cigarette tax	Private insurance	Out-of-pocket	Indirect taxes	Direct taxes
Social insurance	non-D	non-D	non-D	D	D
Cigarette tax		non-D	non-D	D	D
Private insurance			non-D	D	D
Out-of-pocket				non-D	D
Indirect taxes					D

Note: D indicates that concentration curve of row source dominates (is more progressive than) that of column source. Dominance is rejected if there is at least one significant difference in one direction and no significant difference in the other, with comparisons at 19 quantiles and 5% significance level. Non-D indicates that nondominance between the concentration curves cannot be rejected.
Source: Authors.

Box 16.3 *Derivation of Macroweights and Kakwani Index for Total Health Finance, Egypt, 1997*

The NHA shares of total health revenues in Egypt (1994–5) from various finance sources are given in the table. The table also shows which of the various finance sources can be allocated, either directly or through estimation, from the survey data. In this example, as in most others, the main difficulty concerns the allocation of the 33 percent of all health care finance that flows from general government revenues. Only direct personal and sales taxes, which account for only one-sixth of government revenues, can be allocated down to households. Nonetheless, it is possible to allocate to households, revenues that account for 72 percent of all health care finance.

Box 16.3 *(continued)*

We consider three sets of assumptions about the distribution of unallocated revenues. In case 1, it is assumed that unallocated general government revenues are distributed as the weighted average of those taxes that can be allocated. Essentially, this involves inflating the weight given to the taxes that can be allocated. For example, the weight on domestic sales taxes is inflated from its actual value of 0.0472 of all health finance to a value of 0.2829 (= [4.72/5.5]*0.3298) to reflect the distribution of unallocated revenues. In case 2, we assume that "other income, profits, and capital gains taxes" are distributed as direct personal taxes and that import duties are distributed as sales taxes. It is assumed that the rest of the unallocated revenues are distributed as the weighted average of the allocated taxes. Finally, in case 3, we assume that unallocated revenues are distributed as the weighted average of all allocated payments (and not just allocated taxes). Another interpretation of this case is that the Kakwani index is informative of the overall progressivity of only those health payments that can be allocated to households.

The relative emphasis given to such alternative scenarios should depend on evidence as to the relative validity of the underlying assumptions. In the example, the various assumptions about the distributions of the unallocated revenues makes little difference to the conclusion about the overall progressivity of the health finance system. In every case, the Kakwani index for total payments is only very slightly positive, indicating near proportionality.

Source: Authors.

Health Finance by Source of Progressivity of Overall Health Financing, Egypt 1997

Finance source	Share of total finance	Method of allocation	Kakwani by source	Macroweights		
				Case 1	Case 2	Case 3
General government revenues	32.98%					
Taxes						
a. Income, capital gains, and property	0.78	reported	0.2501	0.0469	0.0552	0.0108
b. Corporate	4.83	ventilated				
		allocated /				
c. Other income, profit, and capital gains	0.62	ventilated				
d. Domestic sales of goods and services	4.72	estimated	0.1435	0.2829	0.2825	0.0649
		allocated /				
e. Import duties	3.64	ventilated				
f. Other	3.22	ventilated				
Nontax revenue	15.16	ventilated				
Earmarked cigarette tax	3.00	estimated	−0.0061	0.0300	0.0300	0.0425
Social insurance	6.67	estimated	−0.0532	0.0667	0.0667	0.0919
Private insurance	5.57	reported	−0.0011	0.0557	0.0557	0.0768
Out-of-pocket payments	51.77	reported	0.0644	0.5177	0.5177	0.7132
Total	100%			1.0000	1.0000	1.0000
% revenues allocated	72.51%					
	Kakwani for total health finance			0.0819	0.0839	0.0527

Derivation of macroweights:

Case 1—Unallocated revenues distributed as the weighted average of allocated taxes.

Case 2—Taxes c. distributed as taxes a. Taxes e. distributed as d. Remainder of unallocated revenues distributed as weighted average of allocated taxes.

Case 3—Unallocated revenues distributed as weighted average of all allocated payments.

Sources: Government of Egypt 1995; Rannan–Eliya 1998.

Computation

Quintile shares, dominance tests, and concentration indices can be computed as described in chapters 7 and 8. Computation for the Kakwani index is provided in chapter 14.

References

Atkinson, A. B., and J. E. Stiglitz. 1980. *Lectures on Public Economics.* New York: McGraw Hill.

Government of Egypt. 1995. *Egypt Government Finance Statistics Yearbook.* Cairo.

Kakwani, N. C. 1977. "Measurement of Tax Progressivity: An International Comparison." *Economic Journal* 87(345): 71–80.

Lambert, P. J. 1989. *The Distribution and Redistribution of Income: A Mathematical Analysis.* Cambridge, MA: Blackwell.

Lambert, P. J. 1993. *The Distribution and Redistribution of Income: A Mathematical Analysis.* Manchester, UK, and New York: Manchester University Press.

O'Donnell, O., E. van Doorslaer, R. Rannan-Eliya, A. Somanathan, S. R. Adhikari, B. Akkazieva, D. Harbianto, C. G. Garg, P. Hanvoravongchai, A. N. Herrin, M. N. Huq, S. Ibragimova, A. Karan, S.-M. Kwon, G. M. Leung, J.-F. R. Lu, Y. Ohkusa, B. R. Pande, R. Racelis, K. Tin, L. Trisnantoro, C. Vasavid, Q. Wan, B.-M. Yang, and Y. Zhao. Forthcoming. "Who Pays for Health Care in Asia?" *Journal of Health Economics.*

Rannan-Eliya, R. 1998. *Egypt National Health Accounts 1994–95,* Special Report No. 3, Partnerships for Health Reform Project. Baltimore, MD: Abt Associates Inc.

Suits, D. 1977. "Measurement of Tax Progressivity." *American Economic Review* 67: 747–52.

Wagstaff, A., E. van Doorslaer, S. Calonge, T. Christiansen, M. Gerfin, P. Gottschalk, R. Janssen, C. Lachaud, R. Leu, and B. Nolan. 1992. "Equity in the Finance of Health Care: Some International Comparisons." *Journal of Health Economics* 11(4): 361–88.

Wagstaff, A., E. van Doorslaer, H. van der Burg, S. Calonge, T. Christiansen, G. Citoni, U. G. Gerdtham, M. Gerfin, L. Gross, U. Hakinnen, P. Johnson, J. John, J. Klavus, C. Lachaud, J. Lauritsen, R. Leu, B. Nolan, E. Peran, J. Pereira, C. Propper, F. Puffer, L. Rochaix, M. Rodriguez, M. Schellhorn, G. Sundberg, and O. Winkelhake. 1999. "Equity in the Finance of Health Care: Some Further International Comparisons." *Journal of Health Economics* 18(3): 263–90.

World Health Organization. 2000. *World Health Report 2000.* Geneva, Switzerland: World Health Organization.

17

Redistributive Effect of Health Finance

Contributions toward the finance of health care may redistribute disposable income. This redistribution may be intended or unintended. Even in the latter case, policy makers may be interested in the degree to which it occurs because of consequences for the distribution of goods and services other than health care and, ultimately, for welfare. Redistribution can occur when payments toward the financing of health care are compulsory and independent of utilization, most obviously when health care is partly financed from government tax revenues. If tax liabilities rise disproportionately with gross incomes, then the posttax distribution of income will be more equal than the pretax distribution. When health care payments are made voluntarily, they do not have a redistributive effect on economic welfare. Payments are made directly in return for a product—health care. It would not make sense to consider the welfare-reducing effect of the payments made while ignoring the welfare-increasing effect of the health care consumption deriving from those payments. This begs the question of the extent to which out-of-pocket payments for health care should be considered voluntary. It might be argued that the moral compulsion to purchase vital health care for a relative is no less strong than the legal compulsion to pay taxes. But in most instances, there is discretion in the purchase of health care in response to health problems.

Redistribution can be vertical and horizontal. The former occurs when payments are disproportionately related to ability to pay. The extent of vertical redistribution can be inferred from measures of progressivity discussed in the previous chapter. Horizontal redistribution occurs when persons with equal ability to pay contribute unequally to health care payments. In this chapter, we describe how the total redistributive effect of compulsory health payments can be measured and how this redistribution can be decomposed into its vertical and horizontal components.

Decomposing the redistributive effect

One way of measuring the redistributive effect of any compulsory payment on the distribution of incomes is to compare inequality in prepayment incomes—as measured by, for instance, the Gini coefficient—with inequality in postpayment incomes (Lambert 1989). The redistributive impact can be defined as the reduction in the Gini coefficient caused by the payment. Thus,

$$(17.1) \qquad\qquad RE = G^X - G^{X-P},$$

where G^X and G^{X-P} are the prepayment and postpayment Gini coefficients, respectively, where X denotes prepayment income, or more generally some measure of ability to pay, and P denotes the payment. Aronson, Johnson, and Lambert (1994) have shown that this difference can be written as

$$(17.2) \qquad\qquad RE = V - H - R \,,$$

where V is vertical redistribution, H is horizontal inequity, and R is the degree of reranking. Because there are few households in any sample with exactly the same prepayment income, one needs to artificially create groups of prepayment equals, within intervals of prepayment income, to distinguish and compute the components of equation 17.2. The vertical redistribution component, which represents the redistribution that would arise if there were horizontal equity in payments, can then by defined as

$$(17.3) \qquad\qquad V = G^X - G^0 \,,$$

where G^0 is the between-groups Gini coefficient for postpayment income. This can be computed by replacing all postpayment incomes with their group means. V itself can be decomposed into a payment rate effect and a progressivity effect,

$$(17.4) \qquad\qquad V = \left(\frac{g}{1-g}\right) K_E \,,$$

where g is the sample average payment rate (as a proportion of income) and K_E is the Kakwani index of payments that would arise if there were horizontal equity in health care payments. It is computed as the difference between the between-groups concentration index for payments and G^X. In effect, the vertical redistribution generated by a given level of progressivity is "scaled" by the average rate g.

Horizontal inequity H is measured by the weighted sum of the group (j) specific postpayment Gini coefficients, G_j^{X-P}, where weights are given by the product of the group's population share and its postpayment income share, α_j.

$$(17.5) \qquad\qquad H = \sum_j \alpha_j G_j^{X-P}.$$

Note that because the Gini coefficient for each group of prepayment equals is nonnegative, H is also nonnegative. Because it is subtracted in equation 17.2, horizontal inequity H can only reduce redistribution, not increase it. This simply implies that any horizontal inequity will always make a postpayment distribution of incomes more unequal than it would have been in its absence.

Finally, R captures the extent of reranking of households that occurs in the move from the prepayment to the postpayment distribution of income. It is measured by

$$(17.6) \qquad\qquad R = G^{X-P} - C^{X-P} \,,$$

where C^{X-P} is a postpayment income concentration index that is obtained by first ranking households by their prepayment incomes and then, within each group of prepayment "equals," by their postpayment income. Note again that R cannot be negative, because the concentration curve of postpayment income cannot lie below the Lorenz curve of postpayment income. The two curves coincide (and the two indices are equal) if no reranking occurs.

All in all, the total redistributive effect can be decomposed into four components: an average rate effect (g), the departure-from-proportionality or progressivity effect (K_E), a horizontal inequity effect H, and a reranking effect R. Practical execution of this decomposition requires an arbitrary choice of income intervals to define "equals." Although this choice will not affect the total $H+R$, it will affect the relative magnitudes of H and R. In general, the larger are the income intervals, the greater will be the estimate of horizontal inequity and the smaller will be the estimate of reranking (Aronson, Johnson, and Lambert 1994). That makes the distinction between H and R rather uninteresting in applications.[1] More interesting is the quantification of the vertical redistribution V, both in absolute magnitude and relative to the total redistributive effect, and its separation into the average rate and progressivity effects. Van Doorslaer et al. (1999) make this decomposition of the redistributive effect of health finance for 12 OECD countries.

Box 17.1 *Redistributive Effect of Public Finance of Health Care in the Netherlands, the United Kingdom, and the United States*

To illustrate the redistributive effect of health finance and its decomposition, we present results for three countries—the Netherlands, the United Kingdom, and the United States—taken from van Doorslaer et al. (1999). For each country, we show the redistributive effect of compulsory payments toward publicly financed health care. Public finance predominates in the finance of health care in both the Netherlands and the United Kingdom, but the source differs. The Netherlands relies mainly on social insurance, whereas most finance in the United Kingdom comes from general taxation. Although the majority of health care finance is private in the United States, there is a substantial contribution from public funds, with two-thirds of this from general taxation.

The figures in the first row of the table indicate that public finance of health care brings about redistribution from rich to poor in the United Kingdom and the United States but from poor to rich in the Netherlands. In both the United Kingdom and the United States, vertical redistribution is very large in comparison with the total redistribution. If there were no horizontal inequity, redistribution from rich to poor would be only 2.4 percent and 5 percent greater than its actual magnitude in the United Kingdom and United States, respectively. In the Netherlands, vertical redistribution is from poor to rich, and horizontal inequity and reranking adds a further 6.6 percent of the redistribution in that direction. In absolute value, the redistribution is largest in the Netherlands because public payments for health care are larger relative to income—8.2 percent of income, compared with only 3.6 percent in the United Kingdom and 6 percent in the United States. It is interesting that the United States spends relatively more public dollars on health care than does the United Kingdom, despite the United Kingdom being a predominantly publicly funded system. This difference in the scale of public spending is responsible for the greater redistributive effect in the United States. Public finance is more progressive in the United Kingdom, indicated by the Kakwani index, but there is less of it.

Source: Authors.

Decomposition of Redistributive Effect of Public Finance of Health Care in the Netherlands, the United Kingdom, and the United States

		Netherlands (1992)	United Kingdom (1992)	United States (1987)
Redistributive effect	RE = GX – GX–P	–0.0096	0.0044	0.0063
Vertical redistribution effect	V = [g/(1–g)]*KE	–0.0089	0.0045	0.0066
Vertical redistribution as % of RE	(V/RE)*100	93.40	102.40	105.00
Total payment as fraction of income	g	0.0821	0.0361	0.0604
Kakwani index assuming horizontal equity	KE	–0.0999	0.1221	0.0979

Source: van Doorslaer et al. 1999.

---

[1] See Duclos, Jalbert, and Araar (2003) for an alternative approach that avoids this limitation.

Computation

Let y be prepayment income and wt be the sample weight variable. Create the weighted fractional rank (r), and estimate the Gini coefficient (gini) for prepayment income using, for example, the covariance approach (see chapter 8),

```
egen   rank1 = rank(y), unique
sort rank1
qui sum wt
gen wi=wt/r(sum)
gen cusum=sum(wi)
gen wj=cusum[_n-1]
replace wj=0 if wj==.
gen r=wj+0.5*wi

qui sum y [aw=wt]
sca m_y=r(mean)
qui cor r y [aw=wt], c
sca gini=2*r(cov_12)/m_y
```

Let X be a global containing all the compulsory health payments variables for which the decomposition is to be undertaken. For taxes, we wish to identify the redistributive effect only of that part of taxation that is used to fund health care. So, all tax payments must be scaled by tax-funded expenditure on health care as a proportion of aggregate general government expenditure on all goods and services. Generate a variable representing postpayment income for each payment, and estimate the Gini coefficient for that variable. Finally, compute the redistributive effect for each payment as the difference between the pre- and postpayment Gini indices. This can all be done in the following loop:

```
foreach x of global X {
    qui {
            gen ypost_`x'=y-`x'
            sum ypost_`x' [aw=wt]
            sca my_`x'=r(mean)
            egen   rank_`x' = rank(ypost_`x'), unique
            sort rank_`x'
            gen cusum_`x'=sum(wi)
            gen wj_`x'=cusum_`x'[_n-1]
            replace wj_`x'=0 if wj_`x'==.
            gen r_`x'=wj_`x'+0.5*wi
            corr r_`x' ypost_`x' [aw=wt], c
            sca gini_`x'=2*r(cov_12)/my_`x'
            sca re_`x'=gini-gini_`x'
    }
}
```

For the decomposition of the redistributive effect, households must be grouped into prepayment "equals." To do this, create a variable that categorizes households according to prepayment income intervals of fixed width. For example, to break the sample into 100 groups, each spanning an interval of income of fixed width, the following may be used:

```
qui sum y
local max=r(max)
kdensity y [aw=wt], n(100) nograph
local width=r(scale)
egen ygroup=cut(y), at(0(`width')`max') icodes
recode ygroup .=99
```

where the kdensity command is used simply to create the width of the income intervals and the egen command creates the categorical variable, ygroup.

To compute the concentration index of postpayment income, which is subtracted from the Gini coefficient for prepayment income in calculation of the reranking term (equation 17.6), we need to rank the groups by prepayment income and then rank households within the groups by postpayment income. With households ranked in this way, the appropriate weighted fractional rank must be computed. The concentration index can then be estimated by the covariance method and the reranking term computed. This is all done in the following loop:

```
foreach x of global X {
    qui {
            drop cusum_`x' wj_`x' r_`x'
            sort ygroup rank_`x'
            gen cusum_`x'=sum(wi)
            gen wj_`x'=cusum_`x'[_n-1]
            replace wj_`x'=0 if wj_`x'==.
            gen r_`x'=wj_`x'+0.5*wi
            corr r_`x' ypost_`x' [aw=wt], c
            sca ci_`x'=2*r(cov_12)/my_`x'
            sca rr_`x'=gini_`x' - ci_`x'
    }
}
```

To compute the Kakwani index in equation 17.4, the data can be collapsed to (weighted) group means and the between-groups concentration index for payments estimated at that level. First, create a constant (grpsize) that will indicate the group sizes when the data are collapsed, and preserve before collapsing the data so that they can be restored later to the household level.

```
gen grpsize=1
preserve
collapse (mean) y $X (sum) grpsize [aw=wt], by(ygroup)
```

At this level, the group sizes are the appropriate weights for computations at the level of group means. For these weights, create the weighted fractional rank to be used in estimation of the concentration index.

```
egen rank1 = rank(y), unique
sort rank1
qui sum grpsize
gen wi=grpsize/r(sum)
gen cusum=sum(wi)
gen wj=cusum[_n-1]
replace wj=0 if wj==.
gen r=wj+0.5*wi
```

Now the between-groups concentration index can be estimated and the Kakwani index computed as the difference between this and the Gini coefficient for prepayment income.

```
foreach x of global X {
    qui {
        sum `x' [aw=grpsize]
        sca m_`x'=r(mean)
        corr r `x' [aw=grpsize], c
        sca ci2_`x'=2*r(cov_12)/m_`x'
        sca k_`x'=ci2_`x' - gini
    }
}
```

The household-level data can then be restored with the `restore` command. The vertical redistribution effect (equation 17.4) can now be computed and this expressed as a percentage of the total redistribution effect.

```
foreach x of global X {
    qui sum `x' [aw=wt]
    sca g_`x'=r(mean)/m_y
    sca v_`x'=(g_`x'/(1-g_`x'))*k_`x'
    sca v100_`x'=(v_`x'/re_`x')*100
}
```

The results of the decomposition can then be displayed.

```
foreach x of global X {
    di "Decomposition of redistributive effect of `x'
payments"
    di "Redistributive effect:", re_`x'
    di "Vertical redistribution:", v_`x'
    di "Vertical redistribution as % total redist. effect",
v100_`x'
    di "Payments as a fraction of total income, g", g_`x'
    di "Horizontal inequity", v_`x'-rr_`x'-re_`x'
    di "Reranking", rr_`x'
}
```

References

Aronson, J. R., P. Johnson, and P. J. Lambert. 1994. "Redistributive Effect and Unequal Tax Treatment." *Economic Journal* 104: 262–70.

Duclos, J.-Y., V. Jalbert, and A. Araar. 2003. "Classical Horizontal Inequity and Reranking: An Integrated Approach." In *Research on Economic Inequality: Fiscal Policy, Inequality and Welfare*, ed. J. A. Bishop and Y. Amiel, 65–100. Amsterdam, Netherlands: Elsevier.

Lambert, P. J. 1989. *The Distribution and Redistribution of Income: A Mathematical Analysis.* Cambridge, MA: Blackwell.

van Doorslaer, E., A. Wagstaff, H. van der Burg, T. Christiansen, G. Citoni, R. Di Biase, U. G. Gerdtham, M. Gerfin, L. Gross, U. Hakinnen, J. John, P. Johnson, J. Klavus, C. Lachaud, J. Lauritsen, R. Leu, B. Nolan, J. Pereira, C. Propper, F. Puffer, L. Rochaix, M. Schellhorn, G. Sundberg, and O. Winkelhake. 1999. "The Redistributive Effect of Health Care Finance in Twelve OECD Countries." *Journal of Health Economics* 18(3): 291–313.

18

Catastrophic Payments for Health Care

Health care finance in low-income countries is still characterized by the dominance of out-of-pocket payments and the relative lack of prepayment mechanisms, such as tax and health insurance. Households without full health insurance coverage face a risk of incurring large medical care expenditures should they fall ill. This uninsured risk reduces welfare. Further, should a household member fall ill, the out-of-pocket purchase of medical care would disrupt the material living standards of the household. If the health care expenses are large relative to the resources available to the household, this disruption to living standards may be considered catastrophic. One conception of fairness in health finance is that households should be protected against such catastrophic medical expenses (World Health Organization 2000).

Ideally, longitudinal data would be used to estimate the extent to which living standards are seriously disrupted by the purchase of medical care in response to illness shocks. That would allow one to identify how spending on nonmedical goods and services changes following some health shock (Gertler and Gruber 2002; Wagstaff 2006). But often only cross-section data are available. Some approximation to the disruptive effect of health expenditures on material living standards must then be made. A popular approach has been to define medical spending as "catastrophic" if it exceeds some fraction of household income or total expenditure in a given period, usually one year (Berki 1986; Russell 2004; Wagstaff and van Doorslaer 2003; Wyszewianski 1986; Xu et al. 2003). The idea is that spending a large fraction of the household budget on health care must be at the expense of the consumption of other goods and services. This opportunity cost may be incurred in the short term if health care is financed by cutting back on current consumption or in the long term if it is financed through savings, the sale of assets, or credit. With cross-section data, it is difficult to distinguish between the two. Besides this, there are other limitations of the approach. First, it identifies only the households that incur catastrophic medical expenditures and ignores those that cannot meet these expenses and so forgo treatment. Through the subsequent deterioration of health, such households probably suffer a greater welfare loss than those incurring catastrophic payments. Recognizing this, Pradhan and Prescott (2002) estimate exposure to, rather than incurrence of, catastrophic payments. Second, in addition to medical spending, illness shocks have catastrophic economic consequences through lost earnings. Gertler and Gruber (2002) find that in Indonesia earnings losses are more important than medical spending in disrupting household living standards following a health shock. Notwithstanding these limitations, medical spending in excess of a substantial fraction of the household budget is informative of at least part of the catastrophic economic consequences of illness, without fully identifying the welfare loss from lack of financing protection against health shocks. In this chapter, we describe measures of catastrophic health payments based on this approach.

Catastrophic payments—a definition

The two key variables underlying the approach are total household out-of-pocket (OOP) payments for health care and a measure of household resources. Income, expenditure, or consumption could be used for the latter. Of these, only income is not directly responsive to medical spending. That may be considered an advantage. However, the health payments-to-income ratio is not responsive to the means of financing health care, and that may be considered a disadvantage. Consider two households with the same income and health payments. Say one household has savings and finances health care from their savings, whereas the other has no savings and must cut back on current consumption to pay for health care. This difference is not reflected in the ratio of health payments to income, which is the same for both households. But the ratio of health payments to total household expenditure will be larger for the household without savings. Assuming that the opportunity cost of current consumption is greater, the "catastrophic impact" is greater for the household without savings and, to an extent, this will be reflected if expenditure, but not if income, is used as the denominator in the definition of catastrophic payments.

If total household expenditure is used as the denominator, the catastrophic payments are defined in relation to the health payments budget share. A potential problem is that this budget share may be low for poor households in low-income countries. The severity of the budget constraint means that most resources are absorbed by items essential to sustenance, such as food, leaving little to spend on health care. This derives from the first limitation of the catastrophic payments approach identified above. Households that cannot afford to meet catastrophic payments are ignored. A partial solution is to define catastrophic payments not with respect to the health payments budget share but with respect to health payments as a share of expenditure net of spending on basic necessities. The latter has been referred to as "nondiscretionary expenditure" (Wagstaff and van Doorslaer 2003) or "capacity to pay" (Xu et al. 2003). The difficulty lies in the definition of expenditure that is nondiscretionary. A common approach is to use household expenditure net of food spending as an indicator of living standards. Of course, not all food purchases are nondiscretionary. But nonfood expenditure may better distinguish between the rich and the poor than does total expenditure.

Let T be OOP payments for health care, x be total household expenditure, and $f(x)$ be food expenditure, or nondiscretionary expenditure more generally. Then, a household is said to have incurred catastrophic payments if T/x, or $T/[x-f(x)]$, exceeds a specified threshold, z. The value of z represents the point at which the absorption of household resources by spending on health care is considered to impose a severe disruption to living standards. That is obviously a matter of judgment. Researchers should not impose their own judgment but rather should present results for a range of values of z and let the reader choose where to give more weight. The value of z will depend on whether the denominator is total expenditure or nondiscretionary expenditure. Spending 10 percent of total expenditure on health care might be considered catastrophic, but 10 percent of nondiscretionary expenditure probably would not. In the literature, when total expenditure is used as the denominator, the most common threshold that has been used is 10 percent (Pradhan and Prescott 2002; Ranson 2002; Wagstaff and van Doorslaer 2003), with the rationale that this represents an approximate threshold at which the household is forced to sacrifice other basic needs, sell productive assets, incur debt, or become impoverished (Russell 2004). World Health Organization researchers have used 40 percent (Xu et al. 2003) when "capacity to pay" (roughly, nonfood expenditure) is used as the denominator.

Measuring incidence and intensity of catastrophic payments

Measures of the incidence and intensity of catastrophic payments can be defined analogous to those for poverty. The incidence of catastrophic payments can be estimated from the fraction of a sample with health care costs as a share of total (or nonfood) expenditure exceeding the chosen threshold. The horizontal axis in figure 18.1 shows the cumulative fraction of households ordered by the ratio T/x from largest to smallest.[1] Reading off this graph at the threshold z, one obtains the fraction H of households with health care budget shares that exceed the threshold z. This is the catastrophic payment head count. Define an indicator, E, which equals 1 if $T_i/x_i > z$ and zero otherwise. Then an estimate of the head count is given by

(18.1)
$$H = \frac{1}{N} \sum_{i=1}^{N} E_i \, ,$$

where N is the sample size.

This measure does not reflect the amount by which households exceed the threshold. Another measure, the catastrophic payment overshoot, captures the average degree by which payments (as a proportion of total expenditure) exceed the threshold z. Define the household overshoot as $O_i = E_i((T_i / x_i) - z)$. Then the overshoot is simply the average:

(18.2)
$$O = \frac{1}{N} \sum_{i=1}^{N} O_i \, .$$

In figure 18.1, O is indicated by the area under the payment share curve but above the threshold level. It is clear that although H captures only the incidence of any catastrophes occurring, O captures the intensity of the occurrence as well. They are related through the mean positive overshoot, which is defined as follows:

(18.3)
$$MPO = \frac{O}{H} \, .$$

Because this implies that $O = H \times$ MPO, it means that the catastrophic overshoot equals the fraction with catastrophic payments times the mean positive overshoot—the incidence times the intensity. Obviously, all of the measures above can also be defined with x-$f(x)$ as denominator.

---

[1]The figure is basically the cumulative density function for the reciprocal of the health payments budget share with the axes reversed.

Figure 18.1 *Health Payments Budget Share against Cumulative Percent of Households Ranked by Decreasing Budget Share*

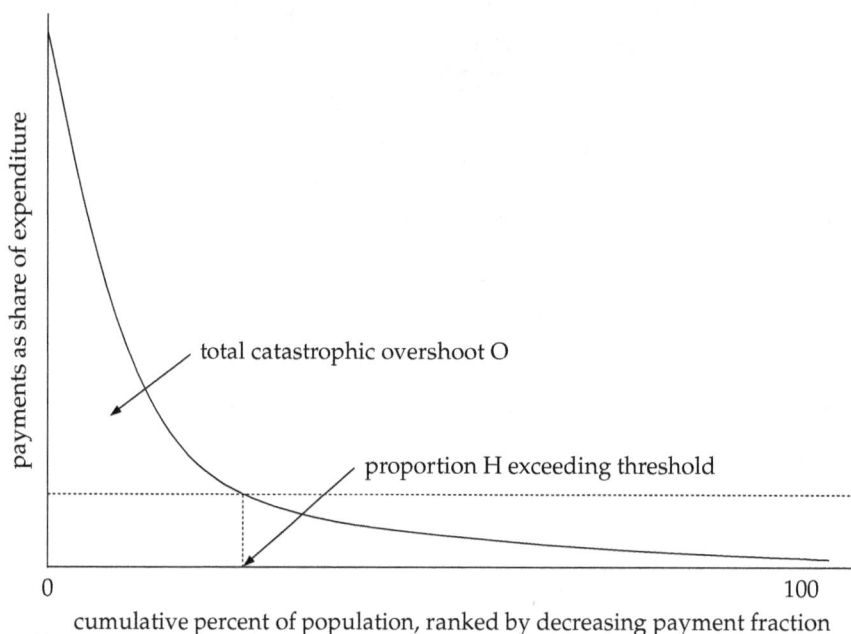

Source: Authors.

Box 18.1 *Catastrophic Health Care Payments in Vietnam, 1993*

The table below presents measures of the incidence and intensity of catastrophic payments for health care in Vietnam estimated from the 1998 Vietnam Living Standards Survey. Catastrophic payments are defined for health payments as a share of both total household expenditure and nonfood expenditure, using various threshold budget shares. As the threshold is raised from 5 percent to 25 percent of total expenditure, the estimate of the incidence of catastrophic payments (*H*) falls from 33.8 percent to 2.9 percent, and the mean overshoot drops from 2.5 percent of expenditure to only 0.3 percent. Standard errors are small relative to the point estimates, which is to be expected for a reasonable sample size (5,999 in this case). Unlike the head count and the overshoot, the mean overshoot among those exceeding the threshold (MPO) need not decline as the threshold is raised. Those spending more than 5 percent of total expenditure on health care, on average spent 12.5 percent (5% + 7.48%). Those spending more than 25 percent of the household budget on health care, on average spent 35.5 percent.

For a given threshold, both the head count and the overshoot are higher, as they must be, when catastrophic payments are defined with respect to health payment relative to nonfood expenditure. This is also illustrated graphically in the figure, which shows the health budget share curves for both definitions. For any budget share, the OOP/[nonfood exp.] curve is always to the right of the OOP/[total exp.] curve. For instance, for more than 15 percent of households, health spending was at least a quarter of nonfood expenditure, but health spending was a quarter of total expenditure for only 3 percent of households.

Estimates of the incidence and intensity of catastrophic payments in 14 Asian counties are given by van Doorslaer et al. (forthcoming).

Box 18.1 (continued)

Incidence and Intensity of Catastrophic Health Payments, Vietnam 1998
Defined with Respect to Total and Nonfood Expenditure, Various Thresholds

Catastrophic payments measures	Threshold budget share, z				
Out-of-pocket health spending as share of total expenditure	*5%*	*10%*	*15%*	*25%*	*40%*
Head count (*H*)	33.77%	15.11%	8.47%	2.89%	—
standard error	0.61%	0.46%	0.36%	0.22%	
Overshoot (*O*)	2.53%	1.39%	0.81%	0.30%	—
standard error	0.08%	0.06%	0.05%	0.03%	
Mean positive overshoot (MPO)	7.48%	9.18%	9.58%	10.46%	—
As share of nonfood expenditure					
Head count (*H*)	—	—	29.37%	15.10%	5.97%
standard error			0.59%	0.46%	0.31%
Overshoot (*O*)	—	—	4.35%	2.24%	0.76%
standard error			0.13%	0.09%	0.05%
Mean positive overshoot (MPO)	—	—	14.81%	14.83%	12.66%

Health Payments Total and Nonfood Budget Share against Cumulative Percentage
of Households Ranked by Decreasing Budget Share, Vietnam 1998

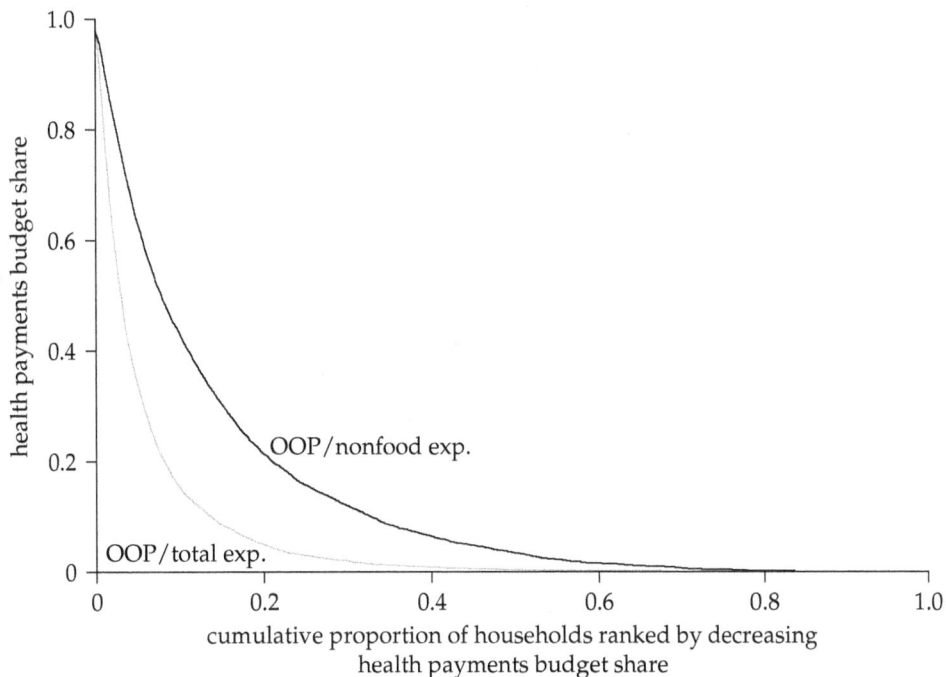

Source: Authors.

Distribution-sensitive measures of catastrophic payments

As noted above, if health spending is income elastic, nonfood expenditure may be preferred for the denominator of the budget share to better detect catastrophic payments among the poor. But the measures introduced in the previous section are insensitive to the distribution of catastrophic payments. In the head count, all households exceeding the threshold are counted equally. The overshoot counts all dollars spent on health care in excess of the threshold equally, irrespective of whether they are made by the poor or by the rich. If there is diminishing marginal utility of income, the opportunity cost of health spending by the poor will be greater than that by the rich. If one wishes to place a social welfare interpretation on measures of catastrophic payments, then it might be argued that they should be weighted to reflect this differential opportunity cost.

The distribution of catastrophic payments in relation to income could be measured by concentration indices for E_i and O_i. Label these indices C_E and C_O. A positive value of C_E indicates a greater tendency for the better-off to exceed the payment threshold; a negative value indicates that the worse-off are more likely to exceed the threshold. Similarly, a positive value of C_O indicates that the overshoot tends to be greater among the better-off. One way of adjusting the head count and overshoot measures of catastrophic payments to take into account the distribution of the payments is to multiply each measure by the complement of the respective concentration index (Wagstaff and van Doorslaer 2003). That is, the following weighted head count and overshoot measures are computed:

(18.4) $$H^W = H \cdot \left(1 - C_E\right) \text{ and}$$

(18.5) $$O^W = O \cdot \left(1 - C_O\right).$$

The measures imply value judgments about how catastrophic payments incurred by the poor are weighted relative to those incurred by the better-off. The imposition of value judgments is unavoidable in producing any distribution-sensitive measure. In fact, it could be argued that a distribution-insensitive measure itself imposes a value judgment—catastrophic payments are weighed equally irrespective of who incurs them. The particular weighting scheme imposed by equation 18.4 is that the household with the lowest income receives a weight of two, and the weight declines linearly with rank in the income distributions so that the richest household receives a weight of zero. So, if the poorest household incurs catastrophic payments, it is counted twice in the construction of H^W; whereas if the richest household incurs catastrophic payments, it is not counted at all. A similar interpretation holds for equation 18.5. Obviously, different weighting schemes could be proposed to construct alternatives to these rank-dependent weighted head count and overshoot indices.

If those who exceed the catastrophic payments threshold tend to be poorer, the concentration index C_E will be negative, and this will make H^W greater than H. From a social welfare perspective and given the distributional judgments imposed, the catastrophic payment problem is worse than it appears simply by looking at the fraction of the population exceeding the threshold because it overlooks the fact that it tends to be the poor who exceed the threshold. However, if it is the better-off individuals who tend to exceed the threshold, C_E will be positive, and H will overstate

Box 18.2 *Distribution-Sensitive Measures of Catastrophic Payments in Vietnam, 1998*

In the table below we present the concentration indices and the rank-weighted head count and overshoot measures for the same example of Vietnam. The distribution of catastrophic payments clearly depends on whether health payments are expressed as a share of total expenditure or of nonfood expenditure. In the former case, catastrophic payments rise with total expenditure, with the exception only of the head count at the 5 percent threshold. This reflects the fact that the OOP health payments budget share tends to rise with total household resources in low-income countries (van Doorslaer et al. 2007). As a result, the rank-weighted head count and overshoot are smaller than the unweighted indices given in the table in box 18.1. But when health payments are assessed relative to nonfood expenditure, the concentration indices are negative, with one exception, indicating that the households with low nonfood expenditures are more likely to incur catastrophic payments defined in this way. As a consequence, the weighted indices are larger than the unweighted indices in the table in box 18.1. The difference between the total and nonfood expenditure results is due to the income inelasticity of food expenditures.

Distribution-Sensitive Catastrophic Payments Measures, Vietnam 1998

Out-of-pocket health spending as share of total expenditure	Threshold budget share, z				
	5%	10%	15%	25%	40%
Concentration index, C^E	−0.0315	0.0270	0.0971	0.2955	—
Rank-weighted head count, H^W	34.84%	14.70%	7.65%	2.03%	—
Concentration index, C^O	0.0960	0.1845	0.2821	0.4594	—
Rank-weighted overshoot, O^W	2.28%	1.13%	0.58%	0.16%	—
As share of nonfood expenditure					
Concentration index, C^E	—	—	−0.1299	−0.1020	−0.0116
Rank-weighted head count, H^W	—	—	33.19%	16.64%	6.04%
Concentration index, C^O	—	—	−0.0681	−0.0197	0.0809
Rank-weighted overshoot, O^W	—	—	4.65%	2.28%	0.69%

Source: Authors.

the problem of the catastrophic payments as measured by H^W. A similar interpretation holds for comparisons between O and O^W.

Computation

Computation of the catastrophic payments measures introduced above is straightforward with standard statistical packages such as Stata or SPSS. Here we present the appropriate Stata code. Let oop be the household OOP health payments variable. The total household expenditure variable is x and nonfood expenditure, or some other definition of nondiscretionary expenditure, xnf. Besides variables indicating the sample design parameters where they exist, these are the only variables required for the analysis.

Create a variable for the health payments budget share (oopshare) and subsequently the indicator of catastrophic payments, E_i (count#), and the overshoot, O_i (over#), for each of the desired threshold values, z,

```
gen oopshare=oop/x
forvalues i = 5 10 to 25 {
      gen count`i'=(oopshare>(`i'/100))
      gen over`i'=count`i'*(oopshare-(`i'/100))
}
```

The head count, H, and the mean overshoot, O, are simply the means of count# and over#. In the case that the sample has a complex design, the appropriate estimates of the population means and their standard errors would be obtained from the following:

```
svyset psu [pw=wt], strata(strata)
svy: mean count* over*
```

where psu is the variable indicating the primary sampling unit, wt is the sample weight, and strata is the variable indicating the characteristic on which the sample is stratified (see chapter 2). The mean positive overshoot (MPO) is obtained from the following:

```
forvalues i = 5 10 to 25 {
            svy, subpop(count`i'): mean over`i'
}
```

Measures of catastrophic payments defined with respect to nonfood expenditure can easily be obtained by simply replacing x with xnf in the denominator of the OOP budget share. One may also want to change the threshold values in this case.

Concentration indices for the variables count# and over# can be computed by the convenient regression or covariance methods presented in chapter 8. To facilitate computation of the rank-weighted head count, H^W, and mean overshoot, O^W, one may store the concentration indices for the various threshold values in matrices. For example, a matrix of concentration indices (ci) for the count variables could be produced as follows:

```
sum r [aw=wt]
sca v_rank=r(Var)

foreach var of varlist count* {
      sum `var' [aw=wt]
      sca m_`var'=r(mean)
      gen d_`var'=(2*v_rank)*(`var'/m_`var')
      quietly {
            regr d_`var' rank
            matrix coefs=get(_b)
            gen ci_`var'=coefs[1,1]
            if "`var'"=="count5" {
                  matrix ci=coefs[1,1]
            }
            if "`var'"~="count5" {
                  matrix ci=(ci, coefs[1,1])
            }
      }
}
```

where the variable r is the weighted fractional rank computed as in chapter 8. A matrix of concentration indices for the overshoot variable at various thresholds could be produced by repeating the loop with count* replaced by over* following varlist and count5 replaced by over5.

A matrix containing the weighted head counts (wh) could then be created with the following:

```
qui svy: mean count*
matrix h=e(b)
matrix wh=(h[1,1]*(1-ci[1,1]),h[1,2]*(1-ci[1,2]), h[1,3]*
   (1-ci[1,3]),h[1,4]*(1-ci[1,4]),h[1,5]*(1-ci[1,5]))
```

The unweighted head counts, concentration indices, and weighted head counts can then be displayed.

```
matrix list h
matrix colnames ci = ci5 ci10 ci15 ci20 ci25
matrix list ci
matrix colnames wh = wh5 wh10 wh15 wh20 wh25
matrix list wh
```

To produce a graph such as that in box 18.1, create the complement of the OOP budget share (compshare), then use this as the sortvar() in a glcurve command to generate the weighted fractional rank (p) for households sorted in decreasing order of the OOP budget share. Then do a connected scatter plot of the budget share against this rank. This can be done for both the share of total and nonfood expenditure as follows:

```
gen compshare = 1-oopshare
glcurve oopshare [aw=wt], pvar(p) sortvar(compshare) nograph
label variable p "OOP/total exp."
gen compshare1 = 1-oopshare1
glcurve oopshare1 [aw=wt], pvar(p1) sortvar(compshare1)
nograph
label variable p1 "OOP/non-food exp."
#delimit ;
twoway (connected p oopshare, sort msize(tiny)) (connected p1
   oopshare1, sort msize(tiny)),
  ytitle(health payments budget share)
  xtitle(cumulative proportion of population ranked by
  decreasing health payments budget share) ;
```

Further reading

Going beyond measurement, one would want to know what characteristics make a household vulnerable to incurring catastrophic payments. An analysis of the correlates of catastrophic payments in six Asian countries is presented in O'Donnell (2005).

References

Berki, S. E. 1986. "A Look at Catastrophic Medical Expenses and the Poor." *Health Affairs* 138–45.

Gertler, P., and J. Gruber. 2002. "Insuring Consumption against Illness." *American Economic Review* 92(1): 51–70.

O'Donnell, O., E. van Doorslaer, R. P. Rannan-Eliya, A. Somanathan, C. G. Garg, P. Hanvora-vongchai, M. N. Huq, A. Karan, G. M. Leung, K. Tin, and C. Vasavid. 2005. "Explaining the Incidence of Catastrophic Payments for Health Care: Comparative Evidence from Asia." EQUITAP Working Paper #5. Erasmus University, Rotterdam, Netherlands, and Institute of Policy Studies, Colombo, Sri Lanka.

Pradhan, M., and N. Prescott. 2002. "Social Risk Management Options for Medical Care in Indonesia." *Health Economics* 11: 431–46.

Ranson, M. K. 2002. "Reduction of Catastrophic Health Care Expenditures by a Community-Based Health Insurance Scheme in Gujarat, India: Current Experiences and Challenges." *Bulletin of the World Health Organization* 80(8): 613–21.

Russell, S. 2004. "The Economic Burden of Illness for Households in Developing Countries: A Review of Studies Focusing on Malaria, Tuberculosis, and Human Immunodeficiency Virus/Acquired Immunodeficiency Syndrome." *American Journal of Tropical Medicine and Hygiene* 71(Supp. 2): 147–55.

van Doorslaer, E., O. O'Donnell, R. P. Rannan-Eliya, A. Somanathan, S. R. Adhikari, B. Akkazieva, D. Harbianto, C. G. Garg, P. Hanvoravongchai, A. N. Herrin, M. N. Huq, S. Ibragimova, A. Karan, T.-j. Lee, G. M. Leung, J.-f.R. Lu, C.-w. Ng, B. R. Pande, R. Racelis, S. Tao, K. Tin, L. Trisnantoro, C. Vasavid, B.-m. Yang, and Y. Zhao. Forthcoming. "Catastrophic Payments for Health Care in Asia." *Health Economics.*

Wagstaff, A. 2006. "The Economic Consequences of Health Shocks: Evidence from Vietnam." *Journal of Health Economics* 26(1): 82–100.

Wagstaff, A., and E. van Doorslaer. 2003. "Catastrophe and Impoverishment in Paying for Health Care: with Applications to Vietnam 1993–98." *Health Economics* 12: 921–34.

World Health Organization 2000. *World Health Report 2000.* Geneva, Switzerland: World Health Organization.

Wyszewianski, L. 1986. "Financially Catastrophic and High Cost Cases: Definitions, Distinctions and Their Implications for Policy Formulation." *Inquiry* 23(4): 382–94.

Xu, K., D. E. Evans, K. Kawabate, R. Zeramdini, J. Klavus, and C. J. L. Murray. 2003. "Household Catastrophic Health Expenditure: A Multicountry Analysis." *Lancet* 362: 111–17.

19

Health Care Payments and Poverty

In the previous chapter we examined the issue of catastrophic payments for health care—the disruption to material living standards due to large out-of-pocket (OOP) payments for health care in the absence of adequate health insurance coverage. In the extreme, OOP payments could lead to poverty. This is not reflected in standard methods of measuring poverty, which compare total household expenditure with a poverty line that is not sensitive to highly variable health care needs. A household that at times of illness diverts expenditure to health care to an extent that its spending on basic necessities falls below the poverty threshold will not be counted as poor. Nor will a household that lives below the poverty threshold but borrows to cover health care expenses such that its total expenditure is raised above the poverty threshold. It has been estimated that 78 million people in Asia are not currently counted as poor despite the fact that their per capita household expenditure net of spending on health care expenditure falls below the extreme poverty threshold of $1 per day (van Doorslaer et al. 2006).

In this chapter we describe and illustrate methods to adjust measures of poverty to take into account spending on health care. In essence, this involves the measurement of poverty on the basis of household expenditure net of OOP spending on health care. The justification of this approach is that spending on health care is a response to a basic need that is not adequately reflected in the poverty line. The stochastic nature of health care needs means that they cannot be captured by a constant poverty line. Admittedly, not all spending on health care is for essential treatment. To the extent that it is not, the subtraction of all health spending from household resources before assessing poverty will result in an overestimate of poverty. But ignoring all health spending will result in an underestimate. Some households are classified as nonpoor simply because high expenses of vital health care raise total spending above the poverty line, while spending on food, clothing, and shelter is below the subsistence level.

Under two conditions, the difference between poverty estimates derived from household resources gross and net of OOP payments for health care may be interpreted as a rough approximation of the impoverishing effect of such payments (Wagstaff and Van Doorslaer 2003). These conditions are (i) OOP payments are completely nondiscretionary and (ii) total household resources are fixed. Under these conditions, the difference between the two estimates would correspond to poverty due to health payments. Neither of the two conditions holds perfectly. A household that chooses to spend excessively on health care is not pushed into poverty by OOP payments. A household may borrow, sell assets, or receive transfers from friends or relatives to cover health care expenses. Then, household expenditure gross of OOP payments does not correspond to the consumption that would be realized in the absence of those payments. For those and other reasons, a simple comparison between poverty estimates that do and do not take into account OOP health payments cannot be interpreted as the change in poverty that would arise from some policy reform that eliminated those payments. Nonetheless, such a comparison is indicative of the scale of the impoverishing effect of health payments.

Health payments–adjusted poverty measures

Let T be per capita household OOP spending on health care, and let x be the per capita living standards proxy that is used in the standard assessment of poverty—household expenditure, consumption, or income. For convenience, we will refer to the latter as household expenditure. Figure 19.1 provides a simple framework for examining the impact of OOP payments on the two basic measures of poverty—the head count and the poverty gap. The figure is a variant on Jan Pen's "parade of dwarfs and a few giants" (see, e.g., Cowell 1995). The two parades plot household expenditure gross and net of OOP payments on the y-axis against the cumulative proportion of individuals ranked by expenditure on the x-axis. For this stylized version of the graph, we assume that households keep the same rank in the gross and net of OOP expenditure distribution. Obviously, in reality rerankings will occur (see below). The point on the x-axis at which a curve crosses the poverty line (PL) gives the fraction of people living in poverty. This is the poverty head count ratio (H). This measure does not capture the "depth" of poverty, that is, the amount by which the poor households fall short of reaching the poverty line. A measure that does take that into account is the poverty gap (G), defined as the area below the poverty line but above the parade.

Figure 19.1 *Pen's Parade for Household Expenditure Gross and Net of OOP Health Payments*

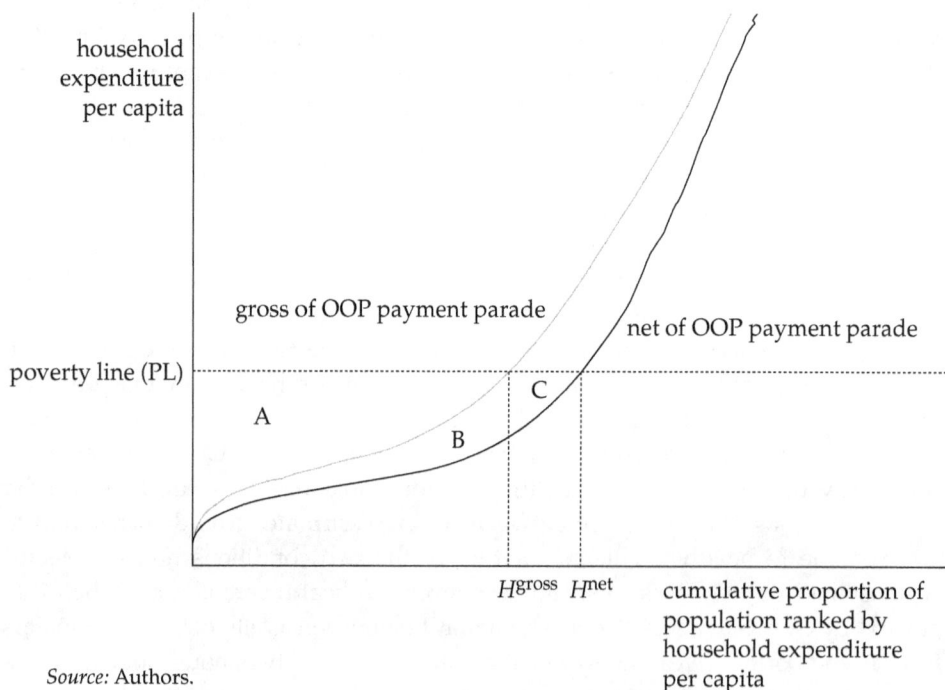

Using household expenditure gross of OOP payments for health care, the poverty head count is H^{gross} and the poverty gap is equal to the area A. If OOP payments are subtracted from household expenditure before poverty is assessed, then the head count and gap must both rise—to H^{net} and $A+B+C$, respectively. So $H^{net} - H^{gross}$ is the fraction of individuals that are not counted as poor despite their household resources net of spending on health care lying below the poverty line. The respective underestimate of the poverty gap is $B+C$. The poverty gap increases both because those already counted as poor appear even poorer once health payments are netted out of household resources (area B) and because some who were not counted as poor on the basis of gross expenditures are assessed as poor after OOP payments (area C) are taken into account.

Let x_i be the per capita total expenditure of household i. An estimate of the gross of health payments poverty head count ratio is

$$(19.1) \qquad H^{gross} = \frac{\sum_{i=1}^{N} s_i p_i^{gross}}{\sum_{i=1}^{N} s_i},$$

where $p_i^{gross} = 1$ if $x_i < PL$ and is 0 otherwise, s_i is the size of the household, and N is the number of households in the sample. Define the gross of health payments individual-level poverty gap by $g_i^{gross} = p_i^{gross}(PL - x_i)$, then the mean of this gap in currency units is

$$(19.2) \qquad G^{gross} = \frac{\sum_{i=1}^{N} s_i g_i^{gross}}{\sum_{i=1}^{N} s_i}.$$

The net of health payments head count is given by replacing p_i^{gross} with $p_i^{net} = 1$ if $(x_i - T_i) < PL$ (and 0 otherwise) in equation 19.1. In the next section, we discuss whether the poverty line should be adjusted downward when assessing poverty on the basis of expenditure net of health payments. The net of health payments poverty gap is given by replacing g_i^{gross} in equation 19.2 with $g_i^{net} = p_i^{net}(PL - (x_i - T_i))$.

When making comparisons across countries with different poverty lines and currency units, it is convenient to normalize the poverty gap on the poverty line as follows:

$$(19.3) \qquad NG^{gross} = \frac{G^{gross}}{PL}.$$

The net of payments normalized gap is defined analogously. The intensity of poverty alone is measured by the mean positive poverty gap,

$$(19.4) \qquad MPG^{gross} = G^{gross} / H^{gross}.$$

In other words, the poverty gap (G) is equal to the fraction of the population who are poor (H) multiplied by the average deficit of the poor from the poverty line (MPG). The mean positive poverty gap can also be normalized on the poverty line.

Defining the poverty line

To compute poverty counts and gaps, a poverty line needs to be established. Poverty lines are either absolute or relative (Ravallion 1998). An absolute poverty line defines poverty in relation to an absolute amount of household expenditure per capita. An extreme absolute poverty line indicates the cost of reaching subsistence nutritional requirements (e.g., 2,100 calories a day) only. More generous poverty lines make some allowance for nonfood needs. A relative poverty line is defined as some fraction of mean or median household expenditure. If such a poverty line were used in the present context, basically the analysis would amount to consideration of how health payments affect the distribution of expenditure. This may be of some interest, but it is likely that primary interest lies in how taking health payments into account affects poverty assessed against an absolute standard.

It might be argued that if poverty is to be assessed on the basis of household expenditure net of OOP payments for health care, then the poverty line should also be adjusted downward. This would be correct if the poverty line allowed for resources required to cover health care needs. Poverty lines that indicate resources required to cover only subsistence food needs clearly do not. Higher poverty lines may make some indirect allowance for expected health care needs, but they can never fully reflect these needs, which are inherently highly variable, both across individuals and across time. A common procedure for constructing a poverty line involves calculating expenditure required to meet subsistence nutrition requirements and the addition of an allowance for nonfood needs (Deaton 1997). More directly, the mean total expenditure of households just satisfying their nutritional requirements may be used as the poverty line. Implicitly, this takes into account the expected spending on health care of those in the region of food poverty. But there will be tremendous variation across households in health status and therefore in their health care needs, which will not be reflected in the poverty line. This may be less of a problem in high-income countries, in which explicit income transfers exist to cover the living costs of disability. But such transfers seldom exist in low-income countries. Further, the health care needs of a given household are stochastic over time. A person falling seriously ill faces health care expenses well above the average. Meeting these expenses can easily force spending on other goods and services below the poverty threshold level.

So, there is no reason to adjust a subsistence food poverty line, but higher poverty lines may make some implicit allowance for expected health care needs and, in this case, it would make sense to adjust the poverty line downward when assessing poverty on expenditure net of health payments. One option is to adjust the poverty line downward by the mean health spending of households with total expenditure in the region of the poverty line (Wagstaff and van Doorslaer 2003). If that practice

---

Box 19.1 *Health Payments–Adjusted Poverty Measures in Vietnam, 1998*

A demonstration of the sensitivity of poverty measures in Vietnam to the treatment of health payments is presented in the table below. The estimates are derived from the 1998 Vietnam Living Standards Survey and are taken from a study of the effect of health payments on the measurement of poverty in 11 Asian countries (van Doorslaer et al. 2006). Estimates are presented for the $1.08 and $2.15 per person per day poverty lines used by the World Bank for international poverty comparisons. The first of these is the poverty threshold used in the definition of the Millennium Development Goal with respect to extreme poverty. At the 1993 purchasing power parity exchange rate, the thresholds convert to 941,772 and 1,883,546 Vietnamese dong per year in 1998 prices. The living standards measure used is per capita household consumption. We do not adjust either poverty line when assessing poverty on the basis of household consumption net of health payments. The lower poverty line is sufficiently strict such that it would not cover even expected health care costs. The higher poverty line is not adjusted

Box 19.1 *(continued)*

because the analysis was part of an international comparison and, as explained above, adjustment would have created perverse results across countries.

When assessed on the basis of total household consumption, 3.6 percent of the population of Vietnam is estimated to be in extreme poverty (<$1.08). If OOP payments for health care are netted out of household consumption, this percentage rises to 4.68 percent. So about 1 percent of the Vietnamese population is not counted as living in extreme poverty but would be considered poor if spending on health care is discounted from household resources. This represents a substantial rise of 30 percent in the estimate of extreme poverty. The estimate of the poverty gap also rises by almost 30 percent, from 5,549 dong to 7,159 dong. Expressed as a percentage of the poverty line, the poverty gap increases from 0.59 percent of the $1.08 line to 0.76 percent when health payments are netted out of household consumption. The mean positive poverty does not increase. It falls slightly. This suggests that the rise in the poverty gap is due to more households being brought into poverty (area C in figure 19.1) and not because of a deepening of the poverty of the already poor (area B in figure 19.1).

At the $2.15 per day poverty line, the pattern of results is the same, but the relative difference in poverty is less and the intensity of poverty, as measured by MPG, no longer falls when poverty is assessed on consumption net of health care costs.

Standard errors are small relative to the point estimates, and for all measures the difference in the estimate of poverty based on household consumption gross and net of health payments is statistically significantly different from zero at 5 percent or less.

Measures of Poverty Based on Consumption Gross and Net of Spending on Health Care, Vietnam 1998

	Gross of health payments (1)	Net of health payments (2)	Difference Absolute (3)=(2)−(1)	Difference Relative [(3)/(1)]*100
$1.08 per day poverty line				
Poverty head count	3.60%	4.68%	1.08%	30.06%
standard error	0.58	0.69	0.23	
Poverty gap ('000 dong)	5.549	7.159	1.610	29.02%
standard error	1.258	1.374	0.260	
Normalized poverty gap	0.59%	0.76%	0.17%	29.99%
standard error	0.13	0.15	0.03	
Normalized mean positive gap	16.38%	16.25%	−0.13%	-0.80%
standard error	1.80	1.49		
$2.15 per day poverty line				
Poverty head count	36.91%	41.35%	4.45%	12.05%
standard error	1.65	1.62	0.33	
Poverty gap ('000 dong)	174.646	206.934	32.288	18.49%
standard error	12.806	13.634	1.827	
Normalized poverty gap	9.27%	10.99%	1.71%	18.28%
standard error	0.68	0.72	0.10	
Normalized mean positive gap	25.12%	26.57%	1.44%	5.74%
standard error	0.92	0.91		

Source: Authors.

is adopted, then obviously some households who spend less on health care than this average can be drawn out of poverty when it is assessed on expenditure net of health care payments. That practice is not advisable if comparisons are being made across countries or time and the standard poverty line has not been adjusted to reflect differences in mean health payments in the region of food poverty. For example, the World Bank poverty lines of $1 or $2 per day clearly do not reflect differences across countries in poor households' exposure to health payments. Subtracting country-specific means of health spending from these amounts would result

---

Box 19.2 *Illustration of the Effect of Health Payments on Pen's Parade, Vietnam, 1998*

Figure 19.1 is a stylized version of the Pen Parade representation of the income distribution. When health payments produce reranking in the income distribution, it is still possible to visualize the effect of health care payments on the parade using what we refer to as a "paint drop" chart (Wagstaff and Van Doorslaer 2003). An example is given in the figure below for Vietnam in 1998. The graph shows the Pen Parade for household consumption gross of health payments. Household consumption is expressed here as multiples of a national extreme poverty line (PL) based on minimum food requirements, which is above the $1.08 threshold. For each household, the vertical bar, or "paint drip," shows the extent to which the subtraction of health payments reduces consumption. If a bar crosses the poverty line, then a household is not counted as poor on the basis of gross consumption but is poor on the basis of net consumption.

The graph shows that health payments are largest at higher values of total consumption, but it is households in the middle and lower half of the distribution that are brought below the poverty line by health payments.

Effect of Health Payments on Pen's Parade of the Household Consumption Distribution, Vietnam 1998

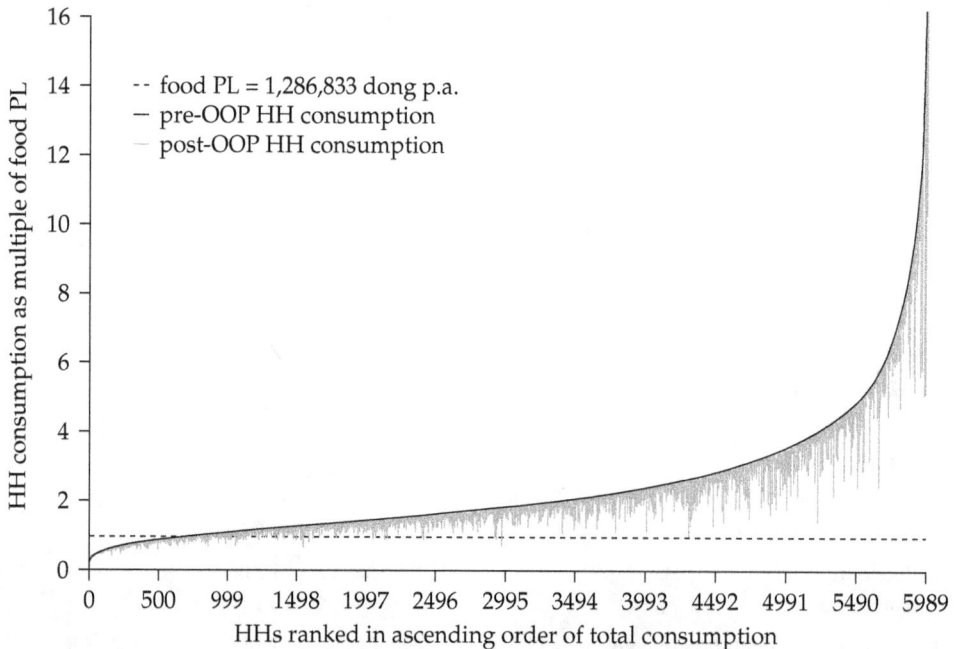

Source: Authors.

in lower poverty lines, and so less poverty, in countries that protect low-income households the least from the cost of health care.

Computation

Computation of the poverty head count and gap measures is straightforward and very similar to that of the corresponding catastrophic payments measures presented in the previous chapter. We describe computation in Stata, but it could easily be done in any statistical package. Assume that the data set is at the household level. Poverty is assessed on household resources on a per capita or per equivalent adult basis if an equivalence scale is applied. Let x be total household consumption (/expenditure/income) per capita, and pcoop be household OOP payments for health care per capita. Define a scalar for the poverty line value (PL) and generate household-level variables indicating gross of health payments poverty status (gross _ h), poverty gap (gross _ g), and normalized gap (gross _ ng):

```
sca PL = ###
gen gross_h = (x < PL)
gen gross_g = gross_h*(PL - x)
gen gross_ng = gross_g/PL
```

If the goal is to estimate poverty at more than one poverty line, another scalar can simply be created for the poverty line value and respective poverty indicator and gap variables. Now a variable can be created equal to per capita household consumption less OOP payments for health care, and the poverty indicator and gap variables can be generated on the basis of this variable:

```
gen net_x = x - pcoop
gen net_h = (net_x < PL)
gen net_g = net_h*(PL - net_x)
gen net_ng = net_g/PL
```

Differences between the two sets of poverty variables can then be computed:

```
gen diff_h = net_h - gross_h
gen diff_g = net_g - gross_g
gen diff_ng = net_ng - gross_ng
```

Sample means of the generated variables give estimates of the poverty head count and gap before and after taking into account health payments and the difference between the two. Stata's survey estimator can be used to obtain the standard errors of these point estimates.

```
svyset psu [pw=wt], strata(strata) || _n
svy: mean gross_h net_h diff_h gross_g net_g diff_g gross_ng
  net_ng diff_ng1
```

where psu is the variable indicating the primary sampling unit (if cluster sampling is used) and, in the case that the sample is stratified, strata identifies stratifying characteristic. By convention, poverty estimates are made for numbers of individuals and not for households. If the data set is at the household level, the sample weight variable should be multiplied by the household size. Application of this weight (wt) will then give estimates for numbers of individuals. If the sample is self-weighting, then the household size should be used as the weight in computation.

The mean positive gap can be estimated by taking the mean gap over all households below the poverty line:

```
svy, subpop(gross_h): mean gross_g gross_ng
svy, subpop(net_h): mean net_g net_ng
```

There exists an ado file, sepov, which can be downloaded from the Stata Web site, that estimates the poverty head count and gap with standard errors without having to generate indicator and gap variables as was done above. The syntax is

```
sepov x [pw=wt], p(PL1) strata(strata) psu(psu)
sepov net_x [pw=wt], p(PL1) strata(strata) psu(psu)
```

This will not, however, provide a standard error for the difference in the estimates.

A figure such as that in box 19.2 can be generated most conveniently in a spreadsheet program such as Excel. It requires first sorting all households in the sample by gross of health payment total expenditure and copying both the gross and net of health payment household expenditure variables into an Excel worksheet. This is easily done simply by cutting and pasting. A cumulative distribution variable (weighted, if necessary) and the poverty line(s) can easily be generated in Excel. A line chart showing the distributions of the gross and net of payment expenditures by the cumulative proportion of households can then be generated.

References

Cowell, F. A. 1995. *Measuring Inequality*. London and New York: Prentice Hall/Harvester Wheatsheaf.

Deaton, A. 1997. *The Analysis of Household Surveys: A Microeconometric Approach to Development Policy*. Baltimore, MD: Johns Hopkins University Press.

Ravallion, M. 1998. "Poverty Lines in Theory and Practice." LSMS Working Paper No. 133, World Bank, Washington, DC.

van Doorslaer, E., O. O'Donnell, R. P. Rannan-Eliya, A. Somanathan, S. R. Adhikari, D. Harbianto, C. G. Garg, A. N. Herrin, M. N. Huq, S. Ibragimova, A. Karan, C.-w. Ng, B. R. Pande, R. Racelis, S. Tao, K. Tin, L. Trisnantoro, C. Vasasvid, and Y. Zhao. 2006. "Effect of Health Payments on Poverty Estimates in 11 Countries in Asia: An Analysis of Household Survey Data." *The Lancet* 368(14): 1357–64.

Wagstaff, A., and E. van Doorslaer. 2003. "Catastrophe and Impoverishment in Paying for Health Care: with Applications to Vietnam 1993–98." *Health Economics* 12: 921–34.